Clinical Manual for Management of Bipolar Disorder in Children and Adolescents

Clinical Manual for Management of Bipolar Disorder in Children and Adolescents

Edited by

Robert A. Kowatch, M.D., Ph.D.

Mary A. Fristad, Ph.D., A.B.P.P.

Robert L. Findling, M.D.

Robert M. Post, M.D.

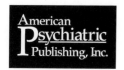

American Psychiatric Publishing, Inc.

Washington, DC
London, England

Note: The authors have worked to ensure that all information in this book is accurate at the time of publication and consistent with general psychiatric and medical standards, and that information concerning drug dosages, schedules, and routes of administration is accurate at the time of publication and consistent with standards set by the U.S. Food and Drug Administration and the general medical community. As medical research and practice continue to advance, however, therapeutic standards may change. Moreover, specific situations may require a specific therapeutic response not included in this book. For these reasons and because human and mechanical errors sometimes occur, we recommend that readers follow the advice of physicians directly involved in their care or the care of a member of their family.

Books published by American Psychiatric Publishing, Inc., represent the views and opinions of the individual authors and do not necessarily represent the policies and opinions of APPI or the American Psychiatric Association.

If you would like to buy between 25 and 99 copies of this or any other APPI title, you are eligible for a 20% discount; please contact APPI Customer Service at appi@psych.org or 800-368-5777. If you wish to buy 100 or more copies of the same title, please e-mail us at bulksales@psych.org for a price quote.

Copyright © 2009 American Psychiatric Publishing, Inc.
ALL RIGHTS RESERVED

Manufactured in the United States of America on acid-free paper
12   11   10   09   08   5   4   3   2   1
First Edition

Typeset in Adobe's AGaramond and Formata.

American Psychiatric Publishing, Inc., 1000 Wilson Boulevard,
Arlington, VA 22209-3901; www.appi.org

Library of Congress Cataloging-in-Publication Data
Clinical manual for management of bipolar disorder in children and adolescents / edited by Robert A. Kowatch…[et al.]. — 1st ed.
      p. ; cm.
   Includes bibliographical references and index.
   ISBN 978-1-58562-291-7 (alk. paper)
   1. Manic-depressive illness in children—Treatment. 2. Manic-depressive illness in adolescence—Treatment. I. Kowatch, Robert A.
[DNLM: 1. Bipolar Disorder—diagnosis. 2. Bipolar Disorder—therapy. 3. Adolescent. 4. Child. WM 207 C641 2009]
   RJ506.D4C593 2009
   618.92′89506—dc22

                                                                    2008042043

British Library Cataloguing in Publication Data
A CIP record is available from the British Library.

Contents

List of Tables and Figures

Contributors

Stephanie Danner, Ph.D.
Postdoctoral Researcher, Department of Psychiatry, The Ohio State University, Columbus, Ohio

Benjamin W. Fields, M.A., M.Ed.
Graduate Research Associate and Doctoral Candidate in Clinical Psychology, The Ohio State University, Columbus, Ohio

Robert L. Findling, M.D.
Professor of Psychiatry and Pediatrics and Director, Division of Child and Adolescent Psychiatry, University Hospitals Case Medical Center, Discovery and Wellness Center for Children, Case Western Reserve University, Cleveland, Ohio

Elisabeth A. Frazier, B.S.
The Ohio State University, Columbus, Ohio

Mary A. Fristad, Ph.D., A.B.P.P.
Professor, Departments of Psychiatry and Psychology; Director, Research and Psychological Services, Division of Child and Adolescent Psychiatry, The Ohio State University, Columbus, Ohio

Robert A. Kowatch, M.D., Ph.D.
Professor of Psychiatry and Pediatrics; Director, Psychiatry Research, Division of Child and Adolescent Psychiatry, Cincinnati Children's Hospital Medical Center, Cincinnati, Ohio

Robert M. Post, M.D.
Adjunct Clinical Professor of Psychiatry, George Washington University and Penn State Schools of Medicine

Matthew E. Young, M.A.
Graduate Research Associate, Departments of Psychology and Psychiatry, The Ohio State University, Columbus, Ohio

Disclosure of Competing Interests

The following contributors to this book have indicated a financial interest in or other affiliation with a commercial supporter, a manufacturer of a commercial product, a provider of a commercial service, a nongovernmental organization, and/or a government agency, as listed below:

Robert L. Findling, M.D.—*Research support, consultant, and speaker's bureau:* Abbott, AstraZeneca, Bristol-Myers Squibb, Celltech-Medeva, Cypress Biosciences, Forest, GlaxoSmithKline, Johnson & Johnson, Lilly, New River, Novartis, Organon, Otsuka, Pfizer, Sanofi-Aventis, Sepracore, Shire, Solvay, Supernus Pharmaceuticals, Wyeth.

Mary A. Fristad, Ph.D., A.B.P.P.—The author receives royalties from a book: *Children's Interview for Psychiatric Syndromes (CHIPS).*

Robert A. Kowatch, M.D., Ph.D.—*Research support:* Stanley Research Foundation, National Institute of Mental Health; National Institute of Child Health and Human Development; *Consultant/Advisory board:* Child Adolescent Bipolar Foundation, Kappa, Medscape, Physicians Postgraduate Press; *Editor: Current Psychiatry; Speaker's bureau:* Astra-Zeneca.

Robert M. Post, M.D.—*Consultant:* Abbott, AstraZeneca, Bristol-Myers Squibb, Glaxo; *Speaker's bureau:* Abbott, AstraZeneca, Bristol-Myers Squibb, Glaxo.

The following contributors have no competing interests to report:
Stephanie Danner, Ph.D.
Benjamin W. Fields, M.A., M.Ed.
Elisabeth A. Frazier, B.S.
Matthew E. Young, M.A.

Preface

There are in fact two things, science and opinion; the former begets knowledge, the latter ignorance.

Hippocrates (ca. 460–377 B.C.E.)

This book was written to provide clinically useful information about the diagnosis and management of bipolar disorder in children and adolescents. Increasing numbers of evidence-based reports about pediatric bipolar disorder have been published; a recent PubMed search found more than 4,000 articles about this disorder, a ninefold increase over the last five decades, with the largest increase occurring in the last decade (see Figure 1).

Pediatric bipolar disorder is a serious medical illness, similar to diabetes, that has an underlying biological diathesis and responds to environmental influences such as family stressors and sleep deprivation. In type 1 diabetes mellitus, a patient's blood sugar levels may change in response to psychosocial stressors, whereas in pediatric bipolar disorder, frank manic or depressive episodes may occur in response to psychosocial stressors. The past dualism of "nature versus nurture" must be replaced with the more accurate "nurture enhancing or igniting nature" in patients burdened with this disorder.

This book evolved out of our first text, *Pediatric Bipolar Disorder: A Handbook for Clinicians,* published in 2003. This new book has been extensively revised and expanded. We have the good fortune to include several excellent new chapters by Dr. Mary Fristad of Ohio State University. Dr. Fristad is an expert in the family and psychosocial aspects of pediatric bipolar disorder, and her and her team's contributions to this manual have been enormous and helped complete the inclusion of the important psychosocial aspects of this disorder.

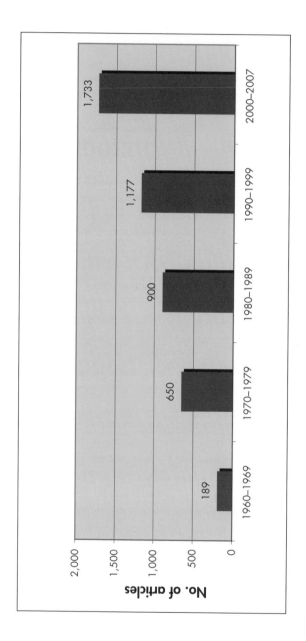

Figure 1.   PubMed articles: bipolar disorder in children and adolescents ages 0–18 years.

1

Introduction

Robert A. Kowatch, M.D., Ph.D.

Bipolar disorders in children and adolescents are serious psychiatric disorders that often disrupt the lives of the affected children and adolescents and their families. Children and adolescents with bipolar disorder have significantly higher rates of morbidity and mortality than do those without bipolar disorder, including psychosocial morbidity with impaired family and peer relationships (Geller and Luby 1997; Geller et al. 2000; Lewinsohn et al. 1995), impaired academic performance with increased rates of school failure and school dropout (Weinberg and Brumback 1976), increased levels of substance abuse (Wilens et al. 2004), increased rates of suicide attempts and completions (Goldstein et al. 2005; Lewinsohn et al. 2000), legal difficulties, and multiple hospitalizations (Akiskal et al. 1985; Geller and Luby 1997). It is extremely important that this disorder is recognized and diagnosed so that these patients and their families can receive appropriate psychiatric care.

Prevalence of Pediatric Bipolar Disorders

The lifetime prevalence of bipolar disorder in adolescents in the United States, based on a recent review of published and unpublished studies from community-based epidemiological studies (Goodwin and Jamison 2007), is between 1.0% and 1.4%. This rate is very similar to the 1.1% rate for bipolar I disorder found among adults in the National Comorbidity Survey Replication (Merikangas et al. 2007). No similar large epidemiological studies have examined the lifetime prevalence of bipolar disorder in children younger than 12 years.

In more specialized psychiatric settings, such as a pediatric psychopharmacology clinic, the occurrence, or "base rate," of pediatric bipolar disorder, ranging from 10% to 30% of patients, is orders of magnitude greater than that found in the general population (Youngstrom and Duax 2005). Wozniak et al. (1995) reported that of 262 children consecutively referred to a specialty pediatric psychopharmacology clinic, 16% met DSM-III-R (American Psychiatric Association 1987) criteria for mania. Isaac (1992) reported that 8 of 12 students in a special education class met DSM-III-R criteria for a bipolar disorder. On child or adolescent inpatient units, it is often found that 30%–40% of the patients have bipolar disorder (Youngstrom and Duax 2005). How often one sees bipolar disorder in children and adolescents largely depends on the type of practice that a clinician has.

Recently, there has been increased recognition of the bipolar spectrum disorders in adults, which include mania, hypomania, recurrent brief hypomania, sporadic brief hypomania, and cyclothymia (Judd et al. 2003). The lifetime prevalence of bipolar spectrum disorders in adults ranged from 2.6% to 6.5% across 12 international studies (Goodwin and Jamison 2007; Merikangas et al. 2007). Several groups have validated similar bipolar spectrum disorders in children and adolescents (Axelson et al. 2006; Quinn and Fristad 2004), and bipolar spectrum disorders likely occur at the same rate as in adults, with a prevalence of approximately 4%.

Age at Onset

Perlis and colleagues (2004) assessed the age at onset of mood symptoms in 1,000 well-characterized adult bipolar patients enrolled in the National Institute of Mental Health's Systematic Treatment Enhancement Program for Bipolar Disorder (STEP-BD). Clinical course, comorbidity, functional status, and quality of life were compared for groups with very early (younger than 13 years), early (ages 13–18 years), and adult (older than 18 years) onset of mood symptoms. Perlis et al. reported that 28% of these patients experienced very early onset, and 38% experienced early onset. Earlier onset was associated with greater rates of comorbid anxiety disorders and substance abuse, more recurrences, shorter periods of euthymia, greater likelihood of suicide attempts and violence, and greater likelihood of being in a mood episode at study entry. Very early or early onset of bipolar disorder might herald a more severe disease course in terms of chronicity and comorbidity.

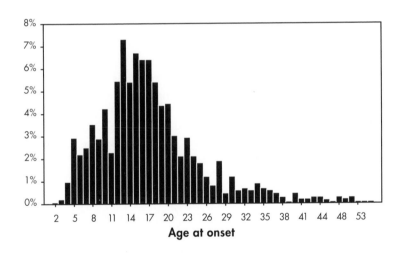

Figure 1–1. Age at onset of bipolar disorder (National Institute of Mental Health Systematic Treatment Enhancement Program for Bipolar Disorder; STEP-BD).

Note. Mean age at onset = 17.37 ± 8.67.
Source. Reprinted from Perlis RH, Miyahara S, Marangell LB, et al.: "Long-Term Implications of Early Onset in Bipolar Disorder: Data From the First 1000 Participants in the Systematic Treatment Enhancement Program for Bipolar Disorder (STEP-BD)." *Biological Psychiatry* 55:875–881, 2004. Copyright 2004, with permission from Society of Biological Psychiatry and Elsevier.

In several large, well-characterized samples of younger children with bipolar disorder (Axelson et al. 2006; Birmaher et al. 2006; Findling et al. 2001; Geller et al. 2004; Wozniak et al. 2005), the mean reported age at onset for bipolar disorder was 7.3±3 years, further validating the STEP-BD findings that bipolar disorder does occur in young children and adolescents.

What emerges from these studies is that pediatric bipolar disorder is a psychiatric disorder that can occur in younger children and that an earlier age at onset indicates a more serious form of this disorder ("the younger the age at onset, the worse the disorder").

References

Akiskal HS, Downs J, Jordan P, et al: Affective disorders in referred children and younger siblings of manic-depressives: mode of onset and prospective course. Arch Gen Psychiatry 42:996–1003, 1985

American Psychiatric Association: Diagnostic and Statistical Manual of Mental Disorders, 3rd Edition, Revised. Washington, DC, American Psychiatric Association, 1987

Axelson D, Birmaher B, Strober M, et al: Phenomenology of children and adolescents with bipolar spectrum disorders. Arch Gen Psychiatry 63:1139–1148, 2006

Findling RL, Gracious BL, McNamara NK, et al: Rapid, continuous cycling and psychiatric comorbidity in pediatric bipolar I disorder. Bipolar Disord 3(Aug):202–210, 2001

Geller B, Luby J: Child and adolescent bipolar disorder: a review of the past 10 years. J Am Acad Child Adolesc Psychiatry 36:1168–1176, 1997

Geller B, Bolhofner K, Craney JL, et al: Psychosocial functioning in a prepubertal and early adolescent bipolar disorder phenotype. J Am Acad Child Adolesc Psychiatry 39:1543–1548, 2000

Geller B, Tillman R, Craney JL, et al: Four-year prospective outcome and natural history of mania in children with a prepubertal and early adolescent bipolar disorder phenotype. Arch Gen Psychiatry 61:459–467, 2004

Goldstein TR, Birmaher B, Axelson D, et al: History of suicide attempts in pediatric bipolar disorder: factors associated with increased risk. Bipolar Disord 7:525–535, 2005

Goodwin FK, Jamison KR: Manic-Depressive Illness: Bipolar Disorders and Recurrent Depression, 2nd Edition. Oxford, UK, Oxford University Press, 2007

Isaac G: Misdiagnosed bipolar disorder in adolescents in a special educational school and treatment program. J Clin Psychiatry 53:133–136, 1992

Judd LL, Akiskal HS, Schettler PJ, et al: The comparative clinical phenotype and long term longitudinal episode course of bipolar I and II: a clinical spectrum or distinct disorders? J Affect Disord 73:19–32, 2003

Lewinsohn PM, Klein DN, Seeley JR: Bipolar disorders in a community sample of older adolescents: prevalence, phenomenology, comorbidity, and course. J Am Acad Child Adolesc Psychiatry 34:454–463, 1995

Lewinsohn PM, Klein DN, Seeley JR: Bipolar disorder during adolescence and young adulthood in a community sample. Bipolar Disord 2:281–293, 2000

Merikangas KR, Akiskal HS, Angst J, et al: Lifetime and 12-month prevalence of bipolar spectrum disorder in the National Comorbidity Survey Replication [published erratum appears in Arch Gen Psychiatry 64:1039, 2007]. Arch Gen Psychiatry 64:543–552, 2007

Perlis RH, Miyahara S, Marangell LB, et al: Long-term implications of early onset in bipolar disorder: data from the first 1000 participants in the Systematic Treatment Enhancement Program for Bipolar Disorder (STEP-BD). Biol Psychiatry 55:875–881, 2004

Quinn CA, Fristad MA: Defining and identifying early onset bipolar spectrum disorder. Curr Psychiatry Rep 6:101–107, 2004

Weinberg WA, Brumback RA: Mania in childhood: case studies and literature review. Am J Dis Child 130:380–385, 1976

Wilens TE, Biederman J, Kwon A, et al: Risk of substance use disorders in adolescents with bipolar disorder. J Am Acad Child Adolesc Psychiatry 43:1380–1386, 2004

Wozniak J, Biederman J, Kiely K, et al: Mania-like symptoms suggestive of childhood-onset bipolar disorder in clinically referred children. J Am Acad Child Adolesc Psychiatry 34:867–876, 1995

Wozniak J, Biederman J, Kwon A, et al: How cardinal are cardinal symptoms in pediatric bipolar disorder? An examination of clinical correlates. Biol Psychiatry 58:583–588, 2005

Youngstrom EA, Duax J: Evidence-based assessment of pediatric bipolar disorder, part I: base rate and family history. J Am Acad Child Adolesc Psychiatry 44:712–717, 2005

2

Definitions

Robert A. Kowatch, M.D., Ph.D.

Pediatric Bipolar Disorder in the Context of DSM-IV-TR

The current criteria for mania—those from DSM-IV-TR (American Psychiatric Association 2000)—were developed for adult patients with bipolar disorders, and none of these criteria take into account developmental differences between adults and children/adolescents with this disorder. The DSM-IV-TR diagnostic classification system for bipolar disorders is fairly complex and involves five types of episodes (manic, hypomanic, mixed, depressed, unspecified), four severity levels (mild, moderate, severe without psychosis, severe with psychosis), and three course specifiers (with or without interepisode recovery, seasonal pattern, rapid cycling). Many children and adolescents are labeled "bipolar" without careful consideration of the diagnostic complexities and subtypes of this disorder. The symptoms of bipolarity in children and adolescents can be difficult to establish because symptom expression varies depending on the context and phase of the illness, development affects symptom expression, and the various psychotropic medications that the patient is taking cause mood and behavioral effects.

Bipolar disorder is defined in DSM-IV-TR by the history of a manic episode or a hypomanic episode (American Psychiatric Association 2000). According to DSM-IV-TR, a manic episode is a period of an abnormally and persistently elevated, expansive, or irritable mood that lasts at least 1 week. The duration of the episode can be shorter and still meet the criterion if hospitalization is necessary for the manic symptoms. During the episode of mania, the patient also must have marked impairment in occupational or school functioning, in social activities, or in relationships with others, or require hospitalization to prevent the patient from harming himself or herself or others. The diagnosis of a manic episode in a child or an adolescent requires both a significant change in mood and the presence of manic symptoms that impair the patient's functioning. A single manic episode will result in a DSM-IV-TR diagnosis of bipolar I disorder, single manic episode (Figure 2–1).

Many adolescents with bipolar disorder may present first with an episode of major depression and then develop manic episodes subsequently (see Figure 2–2).

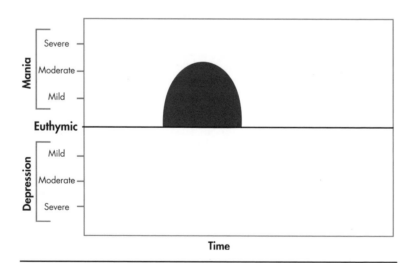

Figure 2–1.   Bipolar I disorder: single manic episode.

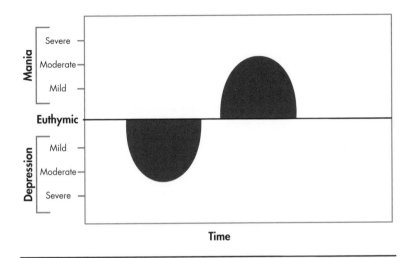

Figure 2–2.   Bipolar I disorder: depression followed by mania.

Several research studies have found that children and adolescents with bipolar disorder often present with a mixed or "dysphoric" picture characterized by frequent short periods of intense mood lability and irritability rather than classic euphoric mania (Geller et al. 1995; Wozniak et al. 1995). A mixed episode is characterized by both manic and depressive symptoms for at least 1 week. A child or an adolescent who is experiencing a mixed episode and who has had an episode of mania or major depression in the past is classified as having bipolar I disorder, most recent episode mixed.

Clinicians often describe pediatric bipolar disorders as the "rapid-cycling" subtype. Several research groups have reported that bipolar children cycle far more frequently than four episodes per year (Findling et al. 2001; Masi et al. 2007; Wozniak et al. 1995). In 81% of a well-defined group of patients, Geller and colleagues (2000) reported continuous daily cycling from mania or hypomania to euthymia or depression. Findling et al. (2001) reported that in a sample of 90 children with bipolar I disorder (mean age = 10.8 years), the mean age at first manic episode was 6.7 years, and a high rate of rapid cycling also was present. The picture that emerges from several independent research groups is that prepubertal children with bipolar disorder typically have multiple daily mood swings and that irritability is much more common than euphoria (Geller et al. 2000; Wozniak and Biederman 1997). In a similar sample of adolescents with bipolar disorder, Dilsaver and colleagues (2005) found that mixed states are extremely common in adolescents with bipolar disorder as well. The pattern of mood cycling across their lifetimes may include periods of mania, hypomania, depression, and euthymia. An example of mood cycling across a lifetime is illustrated in Figure 2–3.

A child or an adolescent who has had one or more major depressive episodes, no episodes of mania, and at least one episode of hypomania is classified in DSM-IV-TR as having bipolar II disorder. Bipolar II disorder, during which an episode of hypomania occurs, is more common in children and adolescents than is bipolar I disorder. A hypomanic episode is characterized in DSM-IV-TR as an abnormally and persistently elevated, expansive, or irritable mood that lasts at least 4 days. An example of bipolar II disorder is presented in Figure 2–4.

In contrast to bipolar I disorder, the illness caused by bipolar II disorder is not severe enough to cause *marked impairment* in occupational functioning (school functioning in children and adolescents), to interfere with social activities or relationships with others, or to necessitate hospitalization, and no psychotic features are present. The features of manic and hypomanic episodes are compared in Table 2–1.

Cyclothymia is a disorder in which hypomanic episodes occur without a history of major depressive episodes. In cyclothymia, the child or adolescent is not without symptoms for more than 2 months at a time. An example of cyclothymia is presented in Figure 2–5.

Retrospective studies of adults with cyclothymia have shown that adolescence is the most common age at onset for cyclothymia. A significant proportion of adolescents with cyclothymia also are at risk to progress to bipolar disorder. In a study by Akiskal et al. (1985) of the offspring of adults with bipolar disorder, 7 of 10 adolescents with cyclothymia progressed to mania or hypomania within 3 years of diagnosis.

Phenomenology and Course

Whenever controversies arise in a scientific field, it is always helpful to examine the data. Four well-described, independently obtained data sets in younger

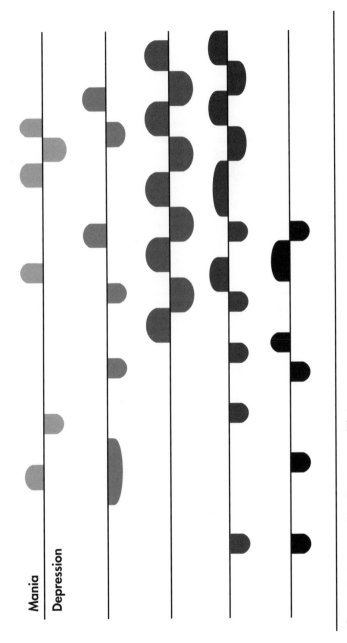

Figure 2–3. Mood cycling across a lifetime.

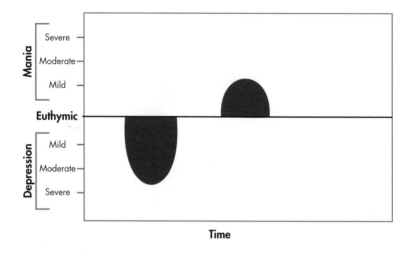

Figure 2–4.   Bipolar II disorder: depression followed by hypomania.

Table 2–1.   Mania versus hypomania

Criterion	Manic episode	Hypomanic episode
Mood symptoms	Abnormally and persistently elevated, expansive, or irritable mood	Abnormally and persistently elevated, expansive, or irritable mood
Duration	At least 7 days	At least 4 days
Number of symptoms	3 or more (4 if mood only irritable)	Same as for manic episode
Impairment	Marked	Does *not* cause marked impairment; unequivocal change in functioning; observable by others

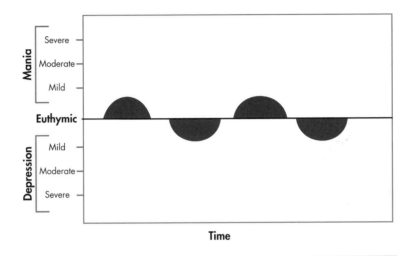

Figure 2–5. Cyclothymia.

patients with bipolar disorder—from Case Western Reserve University, Washington University, Massachusetts General Hospital/Harvard University, and Western Psychiatric Institute and Clinic—illustrate the phenomenology and course of bipolar disorder in youths. The subjects were all assessed by expert raters with a well-validated version of the Schedule for Affective Disorders and Schizophrenia for School-Aged Children (K-SADS) and DSM-IV-TR criteria.

In the Case Western Reserve University data set, Findling and colleagues (2001) studied 90 outpatients with a mean age of 10 years who met the full DSM-IV-TR diagnostic symptom criteria for bipolar I disorder. This study was significant for its thorough diagnostic evaluation and careful clinical characterization of these subjects. The diagnosis of bipolar I disorder was established in these patients by 1) an interview based on the Present and Lifetime Version (K-SADS-PL) or Epidemiologic Version (K-SADS-E) of the K-SADS administered by a research assistant and 2) a clinical assessment by a child and adolescent psychiatrist. The course of bipolar disorder in 57 subjects also was assessed with the *life charting method*. This group reported that the average age at first manic episode was 6.7 years and that affected youths developed an average of approximately 5.8 of the 7 symptoms of mania during periods of elevated or irritable mood. In this sample, bipolar I disorder was found to be a cyclic disorder characterized by high rates of rapid cycling (50%) with almost no interepisode recovery. Of these total subjects, 83% also met DSM-IV-TR criteria for another comorbid disorder while euthymic. The authors concluded that these data suggest that the presentation of juvenile bipolar I disorder is a "cyclic and valid clinical condition with manifestations on a continuum with the later-onset forms of this illness."

Barbara Geller, M.D., at Washington University, is one of the leaders in the diagnosis and phenomenology of pediatric bipolar disorder. She developed and validated the Washington University K-SADS, which is an elaboration of the original K-SADS with more age-appropriate items for mania (Geller et al. 1998b). The Washington University K-SADS has been widely used in research involving children and adolescents with mood disorders ("National Institute of Mental Health Research Roundtable on Prepubertal Bipolar Disorder" 2001).

Geller et al. (2000) reported the results of a 4-year longitudinal study of a sample of 93 consecutively ascertained outpatients with bipolar disorder. During the course of this study, the Washington University K-SADS was blindly administered by research nurses to the subjects' mothers and to children or adolescents about themselves. In this study, Geller and colleagues elected to use current DSM-IV-TR mania or hypomania with elated mood and/or grandiosity as their inclusion criterion for bipolar disorder. The caseness criterion was established by consensus conferences that included diagnostic and impairment data, teacher and school reports, agency records, videotapes viewed by Dr. Geller, and medical charts. The mean±SD age of the subjects with bipolar disorder was 10.9±2.6 years. The current episode had lasted an average of 3.6±2.5) years, with an early age at onset (7.3±3.5 years). Subjects with bipolar disorder and comorbid attention-deficit/hyperactivity disorder (ADHD) were more likely to be younger and male. The investigators concluded that their findings supported the existence of a "homogeneous pediatric bipolar phenotype" with elation and grandiosity as cardinal symptoms (Craney and Geller 2003). One problem with selecting pediatric bipolar subjects with elation and grandiosity as cardinal symptoms is that it limits the generalizability of the sample because many patients with bipolar I disorder may not have these symptoms (Biederman et al. 2000; Findling et al. 2001; West et al. 1996).

The Massachusetts General Hospital/Harvard University group led by Wozniak and Biederman studied 86 subjects satisfying DSM-IV-TR criteria for bipolar disorder with and without the proposed cardinal symptom of euphoria (Wozniak et al. 2005). These researchers reported that severe irritability was the predominant abnormal mood (DSM-IV-TR Criterion A) rather than euphoria (94% vs. 51%). They also found that for Criterion B, grandiosity was not uniquely overrepresented in youths with mania, and the rate of grandiosity did not differ regardless of whether irritability or irritability and euphoria were the Criterion A mood symptoms. This finding challenges the notion that euphoria represents a cardinal symptom of mania in children. Instead, the results support the clinical relevance of severe irritability as the most common presentation of mania in their sample.

The Western Psychiatric Institute and Clinic group, in collaboration with two other university centers, University of California, Los Angeles, and Brown University, assessed the clinical presentation and family history of children and adolescents with bipolar I disorder, bipolar II disorder, or bipolar disorder not otherwise specified (NOS) (Axelson et al. 2006). A total of 438 children and adolescents with bipolar I disorder (n=255), bipolar II disorder (n=30), or bipolar disorder NOS (n=153) were assessed. These researchers reported that subjects with bipolar disorder NOS were not given the diagnosis of bipolar I disorder primarily because they did not meet the DSM-IV-TR duration criteria for a manic or mixed episode. No significant differences were found between the bipolar I disorder and the bipolar disorder NOS groups in age at onset, duration of illness, lifetime rates of comorbid diagnoses, suicidal ideation and major depression, family history, and the types of manic symptoms that were present during the most serious lifetime episode. Compared with youths with bipolar disorder NOS, subjects with bipolar I disorder had more severe manic symptoms, greater overall functional impairment, and higher rates of hospitalization, psychosis, and suicide attempts. Elevated mood was present in 81.9% of the subjects with bipolar disorder NOS and 91.8% of the subjects with bipolar I disorder. Subjects with bipolar II disorder had higher rates of comorbid anxiety disorders compared with the other two groups and less functional impairment and lower rates of psychiatric hospitalization than did the subjects with bipolar I disorder.

Table 2–2 summarizes the findings from each of these four studies. The mean age at onset for bipolar disorder was 7.3 years, and the mean episode duration was 3.2 years. Across studies, 58% of the subjects had mixed episodes, 69% experienced rapid cycling, 35% had psychotic symptoms, 75% had comorbid ADHD, and 30% were suicidal during the assessment period. Geller and colleagues (2007) have proposed developmentally specific criteria for "episodes" and "cycling" based on five similar recent data sets. They propose that *episode* be used for the interval between onset and offset of full DSM-IV-TR criteria for bipolar I disorder, and *cycling* be used to describe only daily (ultradian) switching of mood states that occurs during an episode. Geller and colleagues pointed out that in the previous adult bipolar literature, the terms *episode* and *cycle* were used interchangeably, and *rapid cycling* actually referred to multiple episodes per year. To avoid confusing episodes with daily cycling, they proposed to use *episode* for the duration that a patient meets the DSM-IV-TR criteria for mania, to use *cycling* for daily switching phenomena during an episode, and to replace the historical term *rapid cycling* with *multiple episodes per year*. This proposal is consistent with the data from recent studies as summarized earlier and is clinically useful.

Bipolar Spectrum Disorders

Birmaher and colleagues (2006) have reported the results of a longitudinal study of children and adolescents with bipolar spectrum disorders: the Course and Outcome of Bipolar Illness in Youth study (COBY). This study included 152 subjects with bipolar I disorder, 19 with bipolar II disorder, and 92 with bipolar disorder NOS. The current (DSM-IV-TR) criteria for bipolar disorder NOS are too vague to be useful, so bipolar disorder NOS was defined in this study as the presence of clinically relevant bipolar symptoms that did not fulfill the DSM-IV-TR criteria for bipolar I or II disorder. In addition, subjects were required to have a minimum of elated mood plus two associated DSM-IV-TR symptoms or irritable mood plus three DSM-IV-TR associated symptoms, along with a change in the level of functioning, a duration of a minimum of 4 hours within a 24-hour period, and at least 4 cumulative lifetime days during which symptoms met the criteria. These subjects were interviewed, on average, every 9 months for an average of 2 years with the Longitudinal Interval Follow-up Evaluation interview. The mean age at onset for mood symptoms in the COBY study was 8.9±3.9 years, with a mean duration of illness of

Table 2–2. Course of bipolar disorder in adolescents: findings from four studies

	Case Western Reserve University[a]	Washington University[b]	Massachusetts General Hospital/ Harvard University[c]	Western Psychiatric Institute and Clinic[d]	Mean across studies
Number of subjects	90	93	86	255	131
Mean age±SD (years)	10.8±3.5	10.8±2.7	10.3±3.7	12.7±3.2	11
% Male	71	62	78	53	66
Age at onset±SD (years)	6.7±4	7.4±3.5	5.7±3.3	9.5±4	7.3
Duration of episode (years)	NA	3.5±2.5	2.7±2.6	3.3±2.5	3.2
CGAS score	NA	43.2±7.8	45±6.6	54±12	47
Mixed (%)	20	88	89	34	58
Rapid cycling (%)	50	88	NA	NA	69
Psychotic symptoms (%)	17	59	30	35	35
Suicidal ideation and behavior (%)	NA	24	NA	35	30
ADHD (%)	70	86	82	60	75
ODD (%)	47	78	90	41	64
Conduct disorder (%)	17	13	51	13	23
Anxiety disorders (%)	14	17	55	37	31

Note. ADHD=attention-deficit/hyperactivity disorder; CGAS=Children's Global Assessment Scale; NA=not applicable; ODD= oppositional defiant disorder; SD=standard deviation.
[a]Findling et al. 2001. [b]Geller et al. 2004. [c]Wozniak et al. 2005. [d]Axelson et al. 2006.

4.2±2.9 years. Birmaher and colleagues reported that approximately 70% of the subjects with bipolar disorder recovered from their index episode, and 50% had at least one syndromal recurrence, particularly a depressive episode. Analyses of weekly mood symptoms showed that 60% of the follow-up time, subjects had syndromal or subsyndromal symptoms, with numerous changes in symptoms and shifts of polarity, and 3% of the time, they had psychosis.

It is important to note that in this longitudinal study, 20% of the bipolar II subjects converted to bipolar I disorder, and 25% of the bipolar disorder NOS subjects converted to bipolar I or II disorder. Early-onset bipolar disorder, bipolar disorder NOS, long duration of mood symptoms, low socioeconomic status, and psychosis were associated with poorer outcomes and rapid mood changes. The COBY subjects showed a continuum of bipolar symptom severity from subsyndromal to full syndromal with frequent mood fluctuations.

The COBY, the first longitudinal study of pediatric subjects with bipolar spectrum disorders, is very important because many pediatric patients first present with "bipolar spectrum" symptoms (Masi et al. 2007). The criteria that were developed in this study for bipolar disorder NOS are more specific than the current DSM-IV-TR criteria and identified a group of patients who were likely to develop full bipolar disorder. A secondary analysis comparing the bipolar I subjects in Birmaher et al.'s study with the bipolar I adults in the Judd et al. (2002) 20-year longitudinal study showed that the pediatric subjects with bipolar I disorder spent significantly more time symptomatic with mood symptoms and had more mixed or cycling episodes, mood symptom changes, and polarity switches than did adults with bipolar disorder.

The developmental course of bipolar disorder in children that is emerging from these longitudinal studies is that many prepubertal patients begin their illness with chronic mood symptoms and that clear "episodes" of mania or depression appear 4–5 years after these initial symptoms.

The Problem of Comorbidity

Children and adolescents with pediatric bipolar disorders frequently have comorbid diagnoses that complicate their presentation and treatment response. These comorbid disorders most often include ADHD, anxiety disorders, oppositional defiant disorder, and conduct disorder (Kovacs and Pollock

Table 2–3. Common comorbid disorders found in patients with pediatric bipolar disorder

Disorder	Prepubertal (%)	Adolescent (%)
Attention-deficit/hyperactivity disorder	70–90	30–60
Anxiety disorders	20–30	30–40
Conduct disorder	30–40	30–60
Oppositional defiant disorder	60–90	20–30
Substance abuse	10	40–50
Learning disabilities	30–40	30–40

1995; West et al. 1995; Wozniak et al. 1995). ADHD is the most common comorbid disorder among pediatric bipolar patients, with leading research groups finding rates of comorbidity as high as 98% (Wozniak et al. 1995) and 97% (Geller et al. 1998a). The comorbidity between these two disorders may be problematic because symptoms of distractibility, irritability, and increased talkativeness and risk-taking behaviors may be seen in ADHD. However, these features of ADHD typically are not as severe as those in a manic or hypomanic episode and do not occur within discrete episodes. One must also carefully differentiate between mood swings associated with the development of personality disorders and those that occur purely in the context of medication or substance use. Common comorbid disorders found in patients with pediatric bipolar disorders are listed in Table 2–3.

Table 2–4. Features for which a higher level of suspicion about possible bipolar disorder should be considered

Family history of mood disorders

Episodes of aggressive behavior in the context of other manic symptoms

Early age at onset for depression

Mood disorder with psychotic features

Recurrent depressive episodes resistant to treatment

Episodic presentation of attention-deficit/hyperactivity disorder

Mood destabilization secondary to stimulants or antidepressants

Conclusion

The inherent nature of pediatric bipolar disorder is one of rapidly changing mood states affected by development, the environment, and the context in which the behaviors occur. It is also important to recognize that in some children with mood and behavior problems, the phenomena of the disorder are developing and will "show themselves" in time. Table 2–4 lists features of patients for which a higher level of suspicion about the possible diagnosis of bipolar disorder should be considered. Many children whose symptoms do not initially meet the full criteria for bipolar I or II disorder may develop the full illness as they mature. A spectrum of bipolar disorders exists in children and adolescents with varying degrees of symptom expression, and the initial presentation and course differ in children and adults.

References

Akiskal HS, Downs J, Jordan P, et al: Affective disorders in referred children and younger siblings of manic-depressives: mode of onset and prospective course. Arch Gen Psychiatry 42:996–1003, 1985

American Psychiatric Association: Diagnostic and Statistical Manual of Mental Disorders, 4th Edition, Text Revision. Washington, DC, American Psychiatric Association, 2000

Axelson D, Birmaher B, Strober M, et al: Phenomenology of children and adolescents with bipolar spectrum disorders. Arch Gen Psychiatry 63:1139–1148, 2006

Biederman J, Mick E, Faraone SV, et al: Pediatric mania: a developmental subtype of bipolar disorder? Biol Psychiatry 48:458–466, 2000

Birmaher B, Axelson D, Strober M, et al: Clinical course of children and adolescents with bipolar spectrum disorders. Arch Gen Psychiatry 63:175–183, 2006

Craney JL, Geller B: A prepubertal and early adolescent bipolar disorder-I phenotype: review of phenomenology and longitudinal course. Bipolar Disord 5:243–256, 2003

Dilsaver SC, Benazzi F, Akiskal HS: Mixed states: the most common outpatient presentation of bipolar depressed adolescents? Psychopathology 38:268–272, 2005

Findling RL, Gracious BL, McNamara NK, et al: Rapid, continuous cycling and psychiatric co-morbidity in pediatric bipolar I disorder. Bipolar Disord 3:202–210, 2001

Geller B, Sun K, Zimerman B, et al: Complex and rapid-cycling in bipolar children and adolescents: a preliminary study. J Affect Disord 34:259–268, 1995

Geller B, Cooper TB, Sun K, et al: Double-blind and placebo-controlled study of lithium for adolescent bipolar disorders with secondary substance dependency. J Am Acad Child Adolesc Psychiatry 37:171–178, 1998a

Geller B, Warner K, Williams M, et al: Prepubertal and young adolescent bipolarity versus ADHD: assessment and validity using the WASH-U-KSADS, CBCL and TRF. J Affect Disord 51:93–100, 1998b

Geller B, Zimerman B, Williams M, et al: Diagnostic characteristics of 93 cases of a prepubertal and early adolescent bipolar disorder phenotype by gender, puberty and comorbid attention deficit hyperactivity disorder. J Child Adolesc Psychopharmacol 10:157–164, 2000

Geller B, Tillman R, Craney JL, et al: Four-year prospective outcome and natural history of mania in children with a prepubertal and early adolescent bipolar disorder phenotype. Arch Gen Psychiatry 61:459–467, 2004

Geller B, Tillman R, Bolhofner K, et al: Proposed definitions of bipolar I disorder episodes and daily rapid cycling phenomena in preschoolers, school-aged children, adolescents, and adults. J Child Adolesc Psychopharmacol 17:217–222, 2007

Judd LL, Akiskal HS, Schettler PJ, et al: The long-term natural history of the weekly symptomatic status of bipolar I disorder. Arch Gen Psychiatry 59:530–537, 2002

Kovacs M, Pollock M: Bipolar disorder and comorbid conduct disorder in childhood and adolescence. J Am Acad Child Adolesc Psychiatry 34:715–723, 1995

Masi G, Perugi G, Millipiedi S, et al: Clinical implications of DSM-IV subtyping of bipolar disorders in referred children and adolescents. J Am Acad Child Adolesc Psychiatry 46:1299–1306, 2007

National Institute of Mental Health research roundtable on prepubertal bipolar disorder. J Am Acad Child Adolesc Psychiatry 40:871–878, 2001

West SA, McElroy SL, Strakowski SM, et al: Attention deficit hyperactivity disorder in adolescent mania. Am J Psychiatry 152:271–273, 1995

West SA, Strakowski SM, Sax KW, et al: Phenomenology and comorbidity of adolescents hospitalized for the treatment of acute mania. Biol Psychiatry 39:458–460, 1996

Wozniak J, Biederman J: Childhood mania: insights into diagnostic and treatment issues. J Assoc Acad Minor Phys 8:78–84, 1997

Wozniak J, Biederman J, Kiely K, et al: Mania-like symptoms suggestive of childhood-onset bipolar disorder in clinically referred children. J Am Acad Child Adolesc Psychiatry 34:867–876, 1995

Wozniak J, Biederman J, Kwon A, et al: How cardinal are cardinal symptoms in pediatric bipolar disorder? An examination of clinical correlates. Biol Psychiatry 58:583–588, 2005

Course and Outcome

Robert L. Findling, M.D.

It has long been known that bipolar disorder in adults is a chronic, serious, protracted illness that is frequently associated with pronounced disability, serious mood symptomatology, and human suffering. Only relatively recently has it become more commonly recognized that children and adolescents also experience this serious illness. Youths diagnosed with bipolar disorder often have increased suicide rates, school failure, aggression, risk-taking behaviors such as sexual promiscuity and substance abuse, and other impairments in psychosocial functioning (Carlson and Kelly 1998; Geller et al. 2004). Unfortunately, many youths endure the symptoms of bipolar disorder for years before their illness is diagnosed (Findling et al. 2001; Geller and Luby 1997).

In adults, data support the assertion that bipolar disorder is a chronic condition that is associated with a progressive course (Post et al. 1996). Because growing evidence shows that this condition exists in children and adolescents, it is important to examine the course of bipolar disorders throughout the life span, for several reasons. In youths with bipolar disorders, research about the course of illness and patient outcomes can provide evidence-based information to youngsters, their families, and their treating clinicians about what to expect over time. In addition, when we have the means to identify accurately the first harbingers of bipolar illness, effective early interventions can be developed that might improve the long-term prognosis of patients while preventing substantial human suffering.

Unfortunately, compared with what is known about the outcome of bipolar disorder in adults, relatively little is known about the longitudinal course of bipolar disorder in the young. Currently, only a few prospective, longitudinal studies of bipolar disorder in the child and adolescent population have been published. The purpose of this chapter is to review what is known about the course and outcome of pediatric bipolar disorder. After a discussion of the course of bipolar illness in adults, I review the results of prospective studies in children and adolescents.

Course of Bipolar Illness in Adults

Bipolar illness causes adult patients to experience fluctuating levels of severity of manic and depressive symptoms interspersed with symptom-free (euthymic) periods. As patients fluctuate between episodes that meet full diagnostic symptom criteria for mania and major depression, it is well recognized that adult patients also experience subsyndromal mood periods (Judd et al. 2002, 2003; Miller et al. 2004). For this reason, it is helpful to consider bipolar disorder as a condition characterized by a continuum of various mood states that are interspersed with periods of euthymia. For the sake of completeness, it also should be noted that symptoms of mania and depression can occur together in what are referred to as *mixed states* or *mixed episodes*.

By definition, bipolar illness is distinguished from depressive disorders by the presence of periods of mania and hypomania. However, it has been recognized recently in adults that not only is the most problematic mood state in bipolar disorder usually depression but also the severity of depression is likely worse than previously appreciated (Perlis et al. 2006). For instance, Judd et al. (2002) found that adults with bipolar disorder (ages 17–79) had three times as many depressive symptoms as manic symptoms over the course of approximately 20 years. In addition, the depressive symptoms in adults with bipolar disorder are often treatment resistant and there is a low recovery rate from them (Nierenberg et al. 2006).

Earlier age at onset of bipolar disorder has been reported to be associated with greater illness severity. Adults who report bipolar symptom onset during childhood or adolescence also report a more chronic and pernicious course when compared with adults with onset after adolescence. Compared with patients with adult-onset bipolar disorder, patients who had onset of bipolar illness during childhood and adolescence experienced faster cycling, a greater number of days depressed, more manic and depressive episodes, an increased risk of substance abuse, more comorbid diagnoses, and a greater risk of suicide attempts over their lifetimes (Henin et al. 2007; Leverich et al. 2007; Perlis et al. 2004). In addition, early age at illness onset has been associated with poorer response to lithium, more psychotic features during affective episodes, more mixed episodes, and greater comorbidity with panic disorder (Bellivier et al. 2001; Leverich et al. 2007; Perlis et al. 2004). Overall, early age at onset points toward greater overall severity and a poorer outcome for adults with bipolar illness (Leverich et al. 2007; Perlis et al. 2004).

Progression of Bipolar Disorders

Evidence from adult literature suggests that bipolar disorder is a progressive illness characterized by worsening symptoms with more rapid mood fluctuations over time (Post et al. 1996). For example, a retrospective study found that adults with bipolar illness frequently had less severe mood disorders and symptoms during childhood and adolescence (Manzano and Salvador 1993). Evidence also has emerged suggesting that more modest expressions of the illness, bipolar disorder not otherwise specified (NOS) and cyclothymia, may precede the development of bipolar I disorder and bipolar II disorder (Birmaher et al. 2006; Leverich et al. 2007; Lewinsohn et al. 2000; Manzano and Salvador 1993). Specifically, Akiskal and colleagues (1985) found that cyclothymia evolved into bipolar I or II disorder in adolescents and adults during a follow-up period of approximately 3 years.

Additional evidence that bipolar illness might be a progressive disorder comes from the observation that mood episodes may increase in severity over time as patients spend increasingly more time symptomatic rather than eu-

Table 3–1.   Evidence that bipolar illness may be a progressive disorder

Episode severity increases over time.

As illness progresses, patients spend more time symptomatic than euthymic.

Although episodes may be initially brought on by psychological stress, over time episodes may begin without being precipitated by stressors.

Tolerance to effective treatments can occur over time.

Patients being discontinued from an effective treatment may not experience the same effectiveness if the medication is reinitiated.

Rapid fluctuations in mood appear to develop in the later stages of mood disorders.

Source.   Post et al. 1996.

thymic (Post et al. 1996). Although episodes may be initially brought on by psychological stress, eventually episodes may begin without being precipitated by stressors (Leverich et al. 2007; Post et al. 1996). Additionally, nonresponse to once-effective treatments can develop throughout the course of illness. Furthermore, when an effective treatment is discontinued, the patient may not receive the same benefit from the same medication and dose as previously experienced if the treatment is reinitiated (Post et al. 1996). It also has been observed that bipolar disorders appear to change: rapid fluctuations in mood appear to develop in the later stages of mood disorders. Therefore, different treatment plans may be necessary for those individuals in the early phase and those in the later phase of the mood disorder (Post et al. 1996). These phenomena that characterize the progressive nature of bipolar illness highlight the need for early intervention in patients with mood symptoms. Table 3–1 summarizes these key points.

Prospective Studies of Bipolar Illness in Youths

Only a handful of prospective, longitudinal studies of bipolar I disorder, bipolar II disorder, and bipolar disorder NOS in the child and adolescent population have been published. As will be seen, what is known is that pediatric or juvenile bipolar I disorder is a chronic disorder characterized by few euthymic periods and far more manic or mixed episodes than depressed episodes. Also notable about pediatric or juvenile bipolar I disorder is its rapid, continuous cycling pattern with mixed states and absence of interepisode recovery (Findling et al. 2001; Geller et al. 2004; Kramlinger and Post 1996). Furthermore, if and when these young patients with bipolar disorder are euthymic, the euthymic periods are not sustained for a long time. As a result, children and adolescents with bipolar I disorder suffer substantially as a result of their mood disorder.

What follows is a succinct review of selected prospective studies that examined the course of juvenile bipolar illness. These studies are summarized in Table 3–2.

Lewinsohn et al. 2000

This first report of a large-scale epidemiological study of adolescents with bipolar disorders described results similar to epidemiological data in adult samples. Lewinsohn and colleagues (2000) conducted the Oregon Adolescent Depression Project, which consisted of a cohort of 1,709 high school students, ascertained between 1987 and 1989. In this cohort, the prevalence and clinical characteristics of bipolar disorders and manic symptoms in adolescents were examined. In addition, use of mental health services in this population was reviewed. As part of this study, Lewinsohn and colleagues sought to explore the stability and consequences of adolescent bipolar disorder in young adulthood, determine the rate of switching from major depressive disorder (MDD) to bipolar disorder, and evaluate the significance of subsyndromal bipolar disorder.

The adolescents, ranging in age from 14 to 18 years, were interviewed at three time points: the first interviewing "wave" (T_1) occurred between 1987 and 1989 and consisted of 1,709 students. The second "wave" (T_2) occurred approximately 1 year after the first interview (mean interval between T_1 and T_2 was 13.8 months) and consisted of 1,507 students of the original sample of 1,709. Subsequently, participants who had been given a psychiatric disorder diagnosis and a random selection of participants with no psychiatric diagnosis were invited to be interviewed for a third time (T_3) when they reached age 24 years. Of the 1,507 interviewed at T_2, 893 participants returned for the interview at T_3.

Table 3–2. Selected prospective, longitudinal studies of the course and outcome of pediatric bipolar disorder

Study	Age range (years)	N	Diagnosis	Length of follow-up	Key findings
Lewinsohn et al. 2000	14–18	1,507	Bipolar I disorder, bipolar II disorder, cyclothymic disorder, subsyndromal bipolar disorder, MDD	1. 1 year after first interview 2. At age 24	1. Elevated mood occurred more frequently than irritable mood 2. High rate of suicide attempts in syndromal and subsyndromal bipolar disorder groups 3. High rates of illness progression (see Figure 3–1)
Strober et al. 1995	13–17	54	Bipolar I disorder	5 years	1. Only two patients did not meet recovery criteria at some point during 5-year follow-up 2. Patients with manic episodes recovered much more quickly than did patients who were depressed 3. Mixed episode and cycling between mood states at index episode associated with multiple relapses
Srinath et al. 1998	11–16	30	DSM-III-R bipolar disorder	4–5 years	1. High rates of relapse (67%) after recovery from index episode 2. All patients recovered during study follow-up
Jairam et al. 2004	9–16	25	Bipolar I disorder	4–5 years	1. All patients recovered from index episode 2. More than half of the patients had least one relapse
Geller et al. 2004	8–13	86	Bipolar I disorder, manic or mixed	4 years	1. Long time to recovery from mania or "mixed mania" 2. Large percentage of follow-up time spent in bipolar episode

Table 3–2. Selected prospective, longitudinal studies of the course and outcome of pediatric bipolar disorder (*continued*)

Study	Age range (years)	N	Diagnosis	Length of follow-up	Key findings
Birmaher et al. 2006	7–17	263	Bipolar I disorder, bipolar II disorder, bipolar disorder NOS	2 years	1. Recovery from mood symptoms at some point in time achieved by approximately two-thirds of cohort 2. Half of the two-thirds who recovered experienced a new mood episode during follow-up 3. Approximately 20% of bipolar II disorder patients converted to bipolar I disorder during follow-up; 30% of bipolar disorder NOS patients converted to bipolar I disorder or bipolar II disorder
DelBello et al. 2007	12–18	71	Bipolar I disorder, manic or mixed	1 year	1. Large percentage of syndromic recovery, but lower rates of symptomatic and functional recovery 2. Only 20% of patients achieved both symptomatic and functional recovery at some point in time 3. Adolescent-onset bipolar disorder associated with "poor medication adherence, persistent affective symptoms, and functional impairment"

Note. MDD=major depressive disorder; NOS=not otherwise specified.

The most frequent lifetime mood disorder found at the first two time points was MDD ($n=316$). Additionally, 18 cases of bipolar disorder were identified across T_1 and T_2. The subjects with bipolar disorder included 2 subjects with bipolar I disorder; 11 subjects with a history of a major depressive episode who also met criteria for a manic episode, with the exception of marked impairment or hospitalization, and who had bipolar disorder NOS (DSM-III-R; American Psychiatric Association 1987); and 5 subjects who met criteria for cyclothymia. It should be noted that those individuals who were given the diagnosis of bipolar disorder NOS according to DSM-III-R criteria at T_1 and T_2 would have met DSM-IV-TR (American Psychiatric Association 2000) criteria for bipolar II disorder (Lewinsohn et al. 1995). However, most of the subjects reporting manic symptoms in this large sample did not meet criteria for bipolar disorder. For instance, 97 additional participants were identified who did not meet criteria for bipolar I or II disorder or cyclothymia but had experienced elevated, expansive, or irritable mood for a distinct period; these participants were described as having *subsyndromal* symptoms.

The mean age at onset of a mood episode in the first 18 patients with a bipolar disorder was 11.75 years. Among youths receiving a diagnosis of a bipolar disorder, 1 experienced onset with a manic or hypomanic episode, 11 experienced onset with major or minor depression, and 6 reported onset episodes that could not be determined. At the time of the assessment, 11 of the 18 participants diagnosed with a bipolar disorder were currently symptomatic. This currently symptomatic group experienced longer episode duration (median duration=39.7 months) and more time ill (median duration of illness=69.0 months) than the currently asymptomatic group (median episode duration= 13.1 months; median duration of illness=13.2 months).

By T_3, 11 of the 18 participants with bipolar disorder identified at either the first or the second interview had recovered from their initial mood episode at some time point by age 19, prior to the third interview. Three of these 11 experienced relapse into another mood episode by age 24. Additionally, 6 participants with bipolar disorder had not yet recovered from their initial mood episode by age 19, and 2 of those 6 still had not recovered by age 24. Thus, 2 participants had not yet met criteria for recovery at any time by the third interview.

Looking at the T_3 sample as a whole, 23 participants were identified as having a bipolar disorder. These 23 participants met DSM-IV-TR diagnostic criteria for bipolar I disorder ($n=8$), bipolar II disorder ($n=13$), or cyclothymia

(n=2). Within this group, 1 participant evolved from bipolar II disorder to bipolar I disorder between T_2 and T_3, and 3 progressed from cyclothymic disorder to bipolar II disorder between T_2 and T_3. Six of these 23 participants were given a new bipolar disorder diagnosis at T_3. Three of the 6 were given the diagnosis of bipolar I disorder, whereas the other 3 were given the diagnosis of bipolar II disorder. Furthermore, 3 of those newly diagnosed with a bipolar disorder had been given a diagnosis of MDD at the previous time points. These results are summarized in Figure 3–1.

Several notable trends were described by both the participants with bipolar disorder and the patients with subsyndromal symptoms in this study. First, these two groups reported elevated mood more frequently than irritable mood. This trend was consistent with other data that indicated that the dominant mood state in early-onset bipolar disorder is mania or hypomania, compared with depression in patients with adult-onset bipolar disorder (Miller et al. 2004; Perlis et al. 2004). Second, the subsyndromal group and the group with any bipolar disorder reported higher rates of lifetime comorbid anxiety disorders—especially separation anxiety and panic disorder—and the highest rates of disruptive behavior disorders and attention-deficit/hyperactivity disorder (ADHD) when compared with those patients with no history of mood symptoms. The subsyndromal participants had higher rates of overanxious, obsessive-compulsive, conduct, and oppositional defiant disorders; substance use disorders; and eating disorders than did the rest of the cohort—both participants with a bipolar disorder and those with no diagnosis.

In discussing their results, the investigators noted several key findings. Only 11% of the participants who received a bipolar disorder diagnosis during the first two interviews had experienced "full-blown mania"; therefore, it was anticipated that these adolescents might eventually experience a worsening course of illness over time. Furthermore, the subjects with syndromal and subsyndromal bipolar disorders had high rates of suicide attempts. Approximately 44% of the subjects with bipolar disorder reported a history of a suicide attempt. In addition, a suicide attempt was reported in 17.6% of those subjects with a subsyndromal bipolar disorder (Lewinsohn et al. 2003).

Strober et al. 1995

Another prospective, longitudinal study examined 54 adolescents ages 13–17 years with a bipolar I disorder diagnosis over the course of 5 years (Strober et

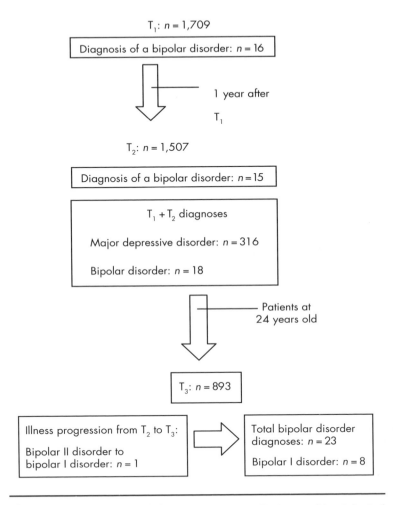

Figure 3–1.   Oregon Adolescent Depression Project: epidemiological study of adolescents with bipolar disorder (Lewinsohn et al. 2000).

Note. T_1 = first interviewing "wave" (1987–1989; n = 1,709); T_2 = second "wave" (approximately 1 year after the first interview; n = 1,507 students of the original sample of 1,709); T_3 = participants interviewed for a third time when they reached age 24 years; n = 893.

al. 1995). The objectives of this study were to document the course of recovery and relapse during study follow-up and to identify variables of predictive importance.

Mood episode at study entry included mania ($n=20$ adolescents), depression ($n=14$), a mixed state ($n=10$), and cycling between mood states ($n=10$). Study results suggested that these patients might have a good prognosis for recovery because only 2 patients failed to achieve criteria for recovery at any time during the 5-year follow-up. The time to euthymia was influenced by polarity of symptoms at study entry; those patients who had mania or a mixed state recovered more quickly than did the depressed patients. These results were consistent with adult data obtained from a prospective study (Bromet et al. 2005).

When subjects achieved recovery from their initial mood episode, they were likely to relapse into another episode within 2–5 years of study enrollment. More specifically, the highest probability of experiencing a mood episode after achieving "recovery" (no less than 8 consecutive weeks with no more than two affective symptoms of mild intensity) was in those patients who were cycling at study entry (60%), followed by those who entered in a manic episode (42%), depression (38%), and a mixed episode (40%). These rates of relapse into a mood episode after recovery are lower than relapse rates seen in adult samples from three different studies: the National Institute of Mental Health (NIMH) Collaborative Study (Keller et al. 1993), a 4-year prospective study of 75 adults with an index episode of mania (Tohen et al. 1990), and a 4-year prospective study of 123 first-admission adults (Bromet et al. 2005). However, despite the low rates of relapse in Strober et al.'s (1995) prospective study of children and adolescents, during the course of follow-up, 23 participants relapsed: 12 relapsed once, 7 relapsed twice, and 4 relapsed three times. According to the authors, these multiple relapse cases were associated with mixed and cycling index episodes. Therefore, it has been hypothesized that mixed and cycling states may be associated with poorer outcome in children and adolescents with bipolar disorders.

Srinath et al. 1998

A prospective study of children and adolescents with bipolar disorder was initiated in India to document the rates and identify the predictors of recovery and relapse and to assess the rates of comorbid conditions during 4–5 years of follow-up. Thirty ill children, ages 11–16, whose symptoms met the DSM-III-R criteria for bipolar I disorder, composed this cohort. At intake, 25 children were given the diagnosis of bipolar disorder. Subsequently, during the study period, 5 additional patients developed bipolar I disorder—2 who had entered the study with MDD, 2 who were initially diagnosed with psychosis NOS, and 1 who was initially diagnosed with schizophrenia.

All 30 patients with a diagnosis of bipolar I disorder achieved recovery (minimum of 2 months without symptoms) at some point during the course of follow-up. The most common relapse state after recovery from the index episode was mania, followed by depression, cycling between mood states, and mixed state. Twenty patients relapsed during study follow-up; all relapses occurred within 3 years of study entry. During the course of follow-up, two patients were not reevaluated; one committed suicide and another was hospitalized for deliberate self-harm.

A positive finding of this study was the high rate of recovery at some point from index episodes. Thus, although bipolar disorder has a chronic course, these data suggest that children and adolescents who have bipolar illnesses have a good chance of remitting.

Jairam et al. 2004

In another effort to assess the course and outcome of pediatric bipolar disorder, the group of investigators from the Srinath et al. (1998) study described above conducted a second 4- to 5-year prospective, longitudinal study of 25 children and adolescents ages 9–16 years (mean = 14.1 years) with symptoms meeting criteria for a manic or mixed affective episode (Jairam et al. 2004). Assessments at baseline, 3 months, and 6 months were made with DSM-III-R criteria; subsequent assessments throughout study follow-up were made with DSM-IV-TR criteria. At the 6-month follow-up, 24 patients (96%) had recovered (absence of symptoms for a minimum of 2 months) from their index episode; the remaining patient did not recover within 6 months but did subsequently recover. The total duration of the index episode, from onset to recovery, ranged from 1.7 to 28.6 weeks. The investigators noted that patients who had had an earlier onset of mood episodes before study entry tended to have episodes of longer duration than did those patients whose first episode occurred at enrollment. This finding is consistent with Post and colleagues' (1996) observation that over time, episode length increases.

Of the 24 patients who recovered from their index episode, 9 (38%) never relapsed (experienced a new affective episode after a period of recovery) during the longitudinal study period once they had achieved remission. Seven patients (29%) had a single relapse, and 9 others (38%) had multiple relapses: 5 patients had two relapses, 2 had three relapses, and 2 had four relapses during follow-up. In all relapsing patients, the most common relapse was to a manic state (58%), followed by depressive (23%), mixed affective (16%), and hypomanic (3%) states. These data duplicate results from Srinath et al. (1998), who noted that the most common relapse state in children and adolescents with bipolar disorder is mania or hypomania.

The authors noted that this cohort had a high rate of recovery and hypothesized that early intervention in this study contributed to the substantial initial recovery rate because the patients entered this study early in their index episodes. Comorbid ADHD is generally associated with poor recovery (Consoli et al. 2007); the low rate of comorbid ADHD (limited to one patient) in this sample likely contributed to the high rate of recovery. Finally, the authors suggested that because this sample consisted of mainly adolescents, the data indicate that adolescents may have better recovery rates compared with children.

Geller et al. 2004

A 4-year prospective, longitudinal study of 86 children (ages 8–13 years at baseline) who had an episode of mania at the start of study participation was initiated to investigate the chronicity and severity of early-onset bipolar disorder (Geller et al. 2004). Age at illness onset was, on average, 6.9 years. Throughout the 4 years of study follow-up, 11 patients did not recover (8 consecutive weeks symptom-free) from mania. The patients who did recover during the study experienced their initial recovery at a mean time point of 60.2 weeks after study ascertainment. The children who recovered at some point spent, on average, slightly more than half of the follow-up period with mania or hypomania (56.9% of total weeks) and slightly less than half of the follow-up period with depressive symptoms (47.1% of total weeks). Results such as these support earlier findings that children with bipolar disorders experience most of their mood episodes as manic. Additionally, the length of time to recovery here validates previous data on the long durations of episodes of mania in children (Srinath et al. 1998; Strober et al. 1995).

Birmaher et al. 2006

As observed in Lewinsohn and colleagues' (2000) epidemiological study, it appears that the most common manifestations of bipolarity in children and adolescents are likely bipolar disorder NOS and cyclothymia. Recently, these conditions have become of particular interest for study. The Course and Outcome of Bipolar Illness in Youth (COBY) study, funded by the NIMH, is a multisite, prospective study of the clinical presentation and family psychiatric history of children and adolescents with bipolar spectrum disorders designed to build on and extend the existing scientific database of the cross-sectional presentation and longitudinal course of pediatric bipolar disorder (Axelson et al. 2006; Birmaher et al. 2006). The 263 children and adolescents enrolled in the study were 7–17 years of age (mean age = 13.0 years). At baseline, 152 participants received a diagnosis of bipolar I disorder, 19 of bipolar II disorder, and 92 of bipolar disorder NOS. Results of this study described a 21% (4 of 19) conversion of bipolar II to bipolar I disorder, a 20% (18 of 92) conversion of bipolar disorder NOS to bipolar I disorder, and a 10% conversion (9 of 92) of bipolar disorder NOS to bipolar II disorder (Birmaher et al. 2006). Thus, such data indicate the diagnostic evolution and possible illness evolution of both bipolar II disorder and bipolar disorder NOS in children and adolescents with a bipolar illness and point toward the necessity of early intervention.

During the course of 2-year follow-up, approximately two-thirds of the patients recovered from their index episode at some point in time, experiencing few to no affective or psychotic symptoms for 8 consecutive weeks. However, half of those who recovered experienced at least 1 week with mania or hypomania or 2 weeks with depression (a syndromal recurrence) at some point during the follow-up period, subsequent to recovery. The authors noted that the patients had, on average, 1.5 syndromal recurrences (particularly depressive episodes) per year. Patients with bipolar I and II disorder both recovered from their index episode and experienced recurrence more frequently than did those with bipolar disorder NOS. Although patients with bipolar disorder NOS had subsyndromal symptoms for a longer time, after recovery they took longer to relapse than did those patients with bipolar I or II disorder.

Overall, the entire cohort spent approximately two-thirds of the study follow-up in a symptomatic condition. Additionally, these youths showed numerous changes in mood symptom intensity and frequent changes in affective polarity. In comparison with adults with bipolar I disorder (Judd et al. 2002), the COBY study patients spent more time symptomatic and had more mixed episodes, mood symptom changes, and polarity switches, thus indicating a more severe illness course.

DelBello et al. 2007

DelBello et al. (2007) followed up a cohort of 71 adolescents (ages 12–18 years) with a bipolar I diagnosis for 1 year after the patients were discharged from the hospital. This study found that only 20% of the patients experienced total recovery—syndromic, symptomatic, and functional—from mania or a mixed episode.

Sixty (85%) of the patients achieved 8 consecutive weeks without symptoms or with subsyndromal symptoms at some point during the first year after hospitalization. The investigators found that the mean episode duration (time from index episode to no longer having mood symptoms) after a patient's manic or mixed episode was 27 weeks. Additionally, the mean time to first achieving a subsyndromal mood state or no symptoms (syndromic recovery) was found to be 20 weeks after initial hospitalization. Comorbid disorders such as anxiety disorders, disruptive behavior disorders, and ADHD and medication nonadherence were associated with lower rates of syndromic recovery.

Of the 60 patients who achieved syndromic recovery, 31 had at least one recurrence of either 1 week of mania or 2 weeks of depression during the course of follow-up. The mean length of recurrent episodes was 8 weeks. The investigators noted that alcohol use disorders and lack of psychotherapeutic intervention following hospitalization were associated with the development of a new mood episode. Also of note, antidepressant treatment was associated with shorter time to syndromic recurrence.

Overall, these patients had at least a moderate degree of symptomatology for 84% of the first year after hospitalization. Specifically, patients spent 38% of follow-up with a mood episode and an additional 46% of the time with subsyndromal symptoms.

The investigators also considered symptomatic and functional recovery in this cohort. Twenty-eight patients, at some point, achieved symptomatic recovery with no mood symptoms being present, with a mean time to recovery of 35 weeks. Additionally, at some point, 28 other patients reported that they were doing as well as or better than they were during the period before onset of bipolar disorder symptoms, with a mean time to recovery of 38 weeks. The authors called such recovery "functional recovery."

As mentioned earlier, only 20% of this cohort experienced syndromic, symptomatic, and functional recovery at some point. Thus, despite at least partial recovery from mood episodes, younger populations with bipolar disorders spend a great deal of time not well.

High-Risk Offspring Studies

Bipolar disorder is a highly heritable condition (Faraone et al. 2003); therefore, evaluating the offspring of bipolar parents in a longitudinal fashion may allow for the early identification of symptoms that precede a diagnosis of bipolar disorder. A meta-analysis of 17 high-risk offspring studies found that offspring of parents with bipolar disorder showed elevated rates of risk for developing affective and other psychiatric illnesses during childhood and adolescence (Lapalme et al. 1997). In their meta-analysis of studies of child and adolescent offspring of bipolar parents, DelBello and Geller (2001) found results similar to those from the Lapalme et al. (1997) meta-analysis.

Another study of high-risk offspring has identified and described subsyndromal bipolar disorders in this patient population (Findling et al. 2005). Analogous to the construct of schizotaxia in schizophrenia, the term *cyclotaxia* has been coined by Findling and colleagues (2005) to characterize this putative early expression of bipolar disorder in high-risk offspring. The key distinguishing features of cyclotaxia are elevated mood with irritability and rapid mood fluctuation. Although these children of parents with a bipolar disorder may not fulfill criteria for bipolar I or II disorder, evidence indicates that these young people may have substantial mood symptoms that cause psychosocial dysfunction (Findling et al. 2005; Mao and Findling 2007). This population offers further support of the need for effective early identification of and intervention in bipolar disorder.

As mentioned earlier, less malignant mood symptoms, ADHD symptoms, and anxiety symptoms commonly precede the onset of bipolar I disorder. Despite the knowledge that these symptoms precede bipolar onset, it is difficult to predict who will eventually develop bipolar I disorder on the basis of the presence of these symptoms. In short, it may be important not only to examine those offspring who are reporting psychiatric symptoms but also to examine those at-risk youths who are not currently experiencing psychiatric symptoms. Examining the illness evolution of symptomatic youths over time may provide a better understanding of the course of bipolar disorders. By studying the nonsymptomatic high-risk offspring who never develop psychiatric symptoms, it may be possible to identify resiliency factors.

Conclusion

In addition to genetic high-risk studies, studies of youths with subsyndromal bipolar illnesses are being conducted to better ascertain the longitudinal course of these disorders. It is not completely clear if all children and adolescents with a bipolar spectrum disorder will eventually develop bipolar I or II disorder. Additionally, problems in accurately ascertaining this population are a result of more modest mood symptom expression, high rates of comorbid psychiatric diagnoses such as ADHD (Findling et al. 2001; Geller et al. 2000; Wozniak et al. 2002), symptom overlap with other conditions, and difficulty distinguishing these mood states from extremes of normal childhood temperament. The chronic and evolving nature of bipolar disorder in adults further supports the importance of assessing the disorder's longitudinal course in children and adolescents. Because adults with bipolar disorder have been studied more extensively than youths, the existing data in adults serve as a benchmark against which to compare children.

Pediatric bipolar I disorder is a chronic disorder that appears to be characterized by few euthymic periods and substantially more manic or hypomanic episodes than depressed episodes. These phenomena distinguish pediatric bipolar disorder from adult-onset bipolar disorder because the latter is characterized by greater difficulties with depression and more distinct mood episodes punctuated by euthymic epochs. Whether pediatric bipolar illness evolves such that it resembles the clinical characteristics of this condition in adults remains unclear and thus is an important area of future research.

Important clinical implications are associated with the observation that bipolar disorder, whether it occurs in children, adolescents, or adults, is a chronic, potentially serious illness. As a result of its chronicity, bipolar disorder generally requires that it be vigilantly managed throughout a person's lifetime.

However, one key opportunity in preventing human suffering might be to accurately identify the earliest manifestations of this condition, thereby providing a means by which early intervention can be pursued. Retrospective studies in adults historically have been used as a means to identify these earliest manifestations. However, meticulous examination of genetically at-risk youths over time may prove to be the most effective way to delineate the earliest manifestations of bipolar disorders. This avenue of investigation may one day allow clinicians to intervene earlier in the course of illness, thereby achieving the ultimate goal: the prevention of human suffering.

References

Akiskal HS, Downs J, Jordan P, et al: Affective disorders in referred children and younger siblings of manic-depressives. Arch Gen Psychiatry 42:996–1003, 1985

American Psychiatric Association: Diagnostic and Statistical Manual of Mental Disorders, 3rd Edition, Revised. Washington, DC, American Psychiatric Association, 1987

American Psychiatric Association: Diagnostic and Statistical Manual of Mental Disorders, 4th Edition, Text Revision. Washington, DC, American Psychiatric Association, 2000

Axelson D, Birmaher B, Strober M, et al: Phenomenology of children and adolescents with bipolar spectrum disorders. Arch Gen Psychiatry 63:1139–1148, 2006

Bellivier F, Golmard JL, Henry C, et al: Admixture analysis of age at onset in bipolar I affective disorder. Arch Gen Psychiatry 58:510–512, 2001

Birmaher B, Axelson D, Strober M, et al: Clinical course of children and adolescents with bipolar spectrum disorders. Arch Gen Psychiatry 63:175–183, 2006

Bromet EJ, Finch SJ, Carlson GA, et al: Time to remission and relapse after the first hospital admission in severe bipolar disorder. Soc Psychiatry Psychiatr Epidemiol 40:106–113, 2005

Carlson GA, Kelly KL: Manic symptoms in psychiatrically hospitalized children—what do they mean? J Affect Disord 51:123–135, 1998

Consoli A, Bouzamondo A, Guile JM, et al: Comorbidity with ADHD decreases response to pharmacotherapy in children and adolescents with acute mania: evidence from a metaanalysis. Can J Psychiatry 52:323–328, 2007

DelBello MP, Geller B: Review of studies of child and adolescent offspring of bipolar parents. Bipolar Disord 3:325–334, 2001

DelBello MP, Hanseman D, Adler CM, et al: Twelve-month outcome of adolescents with bipolar disorder following first hospitalization for a manic or mixed episode. Am J Psychiatry 164:582–590, 2007

Faraone SV, Glatt SJ, Tsuang MT: The genetics of pediatric-onset bipolar disorder. Biol Psychiatry 53:970–977, 2003

Findling RL, Gracious BL, McNamara NK, et al: Rapid, continuous cycling and psychiatric co-morbidity in pediatric bipolar I disorder. Bipolar Disord 3:202–210, 2001

Findling RL, Youngstrom EA, McNamara NK, et al: Early symptoms of mania and the role of parental risk. Bipolar Disord 7:623–634, 2005

Geller B, Luby J: Child and adolescent bipolar disorder: a review of the past 10 years. J Am Acad Child Adolesc Psychiatry 36:1168–1176, 1997

Geller B, Zimmerman B, Williams M, et al: Diagnostic characteristics of 93 cases of a prepubertal and early adolescent bipolar disorder phenotype by gender, puberty and comorbid attention deficit hyperactivity disorder. J Child Adolesc Psychopharmacol 10:157–164, 2000

Geller B, Tillman R, Craney JL, et al: Four-year prospective outcome and natural history of mania in children with a prepubertal and early adolescent bipolar disorder phenotype. Arch Gen Psychiatry 61:459–467, 2004

Henin A, Biederman J, Mick E, et al: Childhood antecedent disorders to bipolar disorder in adults: a controlled study. J Affect Disord 99:51–57, 2007

Jairam R, Srinath S, Girimaji SC, et al: A prospective 4–5 year follow-up of juvenile onset bipolar disorder. Bipolar Disord 6:386–394, 2004

Judd LL, Akiskal HS, Schettler PJ, et al: The long-term natural history of the weekly symptomatic status of bipolar I disorder. Arch Gen Psychiatry 59:530–537, 2002

Judd LL, Akiskal HS, Schettler PJ, et al: A prospective investigation of the natural history of the long-term weekly symptomatic status of bipolar II disorder. Arch Gen Psychiatry 60:261–269, 2003

Keller MB, Lavori PW, Coryell W, et al: Bipolar I: a five-year prospective follow-up. J Nerv Ment Dis 181:238–245, 1993

Kramlinger KG, Post RM: Ultra-rapid and ultradian cycling in bipolar affective illness. Br J Psychiatry 168:314–343, 1996

Lapalme M, Hodgins S, LaRoche C: Children of parents with bipolar disorder: a metaanalysis of risk for mental disorders. Can J Psychiatry 42:623–631, 1997

Leverich GS, Post RM, Keck PE Jr, et al: The poor prognosis of childhood-onset bipolar disorder. J Pediatr 150:485–490, 2007

Lewinsohn PM, Klein DN, Seeley JR: Bipolar disorders in a community sample of older adolescents: prevalence, phenomenology, comorbidity, and course. J Am Acad Child Adolesc Psychiatry 34:454–463, 1995

Lewinsohn PM, Klein DN, Seeley JR: Bipolar disorder during adolescence and young adulthood in a community sample. Bipolar Disord 2:281–293, 2000

Lewinsohn PM, Seeley JR, Klein DN: Bipolar disorders during adolescence. Acta Psychiatr Scand 108:47–50, 2003

Manzano J, Salvador A: Antecedents of severe affective (mood) disorders: patients examined as children or adolescents and as adults. Acta Paedopsychiatr 56:11–18, 1993

Mao AR, Findling RL: Growing evidence to support early intervention in early onset bipolar disorder. Aust N Z J Psychiatry 41:633–636, 2007

Miller IW, Uebelacker LA, Keitner GI, et al: Longitudinal course of bipolar I disorder. Compr Psychiatry 45:431–440, 2004

Nierenberg AA, Ostacher MJ, Calabrese JR, et al: Treatment-resistant bipolar depression: a STEP-BD equipoise randomized effectiveness trial of antidepressant augmentation with lamotrigine, inositol, or risperidone. Am J Psychiatry 163:210–216, 2006

Perlis RH, Miyahara S, Marangell LB, et al: Long-term implications of early onset in bipolar disorder: data from the first 1000 participants in the Systematic Treatment Enhancement Program for Bipolar Disorder (STEP-BD). Biol Psychiatry 55:875–881, 2004

Perlis RH, Ostacher MJ, Patel JK, et al: Predictors of recurrence in bipolar disorder: primary outcomes from the Systematic Treatment Enhancement Program for Bipolar Disorder (STEP-BD). Am J Psychiatry 163:217–224, 2006

Post RM, Weiss SRB, Leverich GS, et al: Developmental psychobiology of cyclic affective illness: implications for early therapeutic intervention. Dev Psychopathol 8:273–305, 1996

Srinath S, Janardhan Reddy YC, Girimaji SR, et al: A prospective study of bipolar disorder in children and adolescents from India. Acta Psychiatr Scand 98:437–442, 1998

Strober M, Schmidt-Lackner S, Freeman R, et al: Recovery and relapse in adolescents with bipolar affective illness: a five-year naturalistic, prospective follow-up. J Am Acad Child Adolesc Psychiatry 34:724–731, 1995

Tohen M, Waternaux CM, Tsuang MT: Outcome in mania: a four-year prospective follow-up of 75 patients utilizing survival analysis. Arch Gen Psychiatry 47:1106–1111, 1990

Wozniak J, Biederman J, Monuteaux MC, et al: Parsing the comorbidity between bipolar disorder and anxiety disorders: a familial risk analysis. J Child Adolesc Psychopharmacol 12:101–111, 2002

4

Diagnosis

Stephanie Danner, Ph.D.
Mary A. Fristad, Ph.D., A.B.P.P.

A key component in diagnosing bipolar spectrum disorders is documenting a cycle of moods ranging from too high or explosively irritable to too low
or pervasively irritable. Gathering information about onset of different
symptoms is critical to determine whether current symptoms can be accounted
for by one disorder or several disorders. Comorbidity of bipolar spectrum
disorders with behavioral, developmental, anxiety, and other disorders is
discussed in Chapter 9 ("Comorbidity") in this volume. Recently, researchers
have advocated approaching bipolar spectrum disorders from a developmental psychopathology perspective, framing the presentation and emergence
of symptoms with the child's developmental stage (Miklowitz and Cicchetti
2006). In brief, careful elicitation of various symptom onsets and offsets helps
to clarify both differential diagnosis and patterns of comorbidity. For example,
a child who has been oppositional since he was 3 years old and develops periods
of alternating low mood and grandiosity with accompanying depressive and

manic symptoms at age 6 probably should be given a diagnosis of both oppositional defiant disorder (ODD) and a bipolar spectrum disorder. If symptoms of oppositional behavior and mood disturbance develop at the same time, ODD and bipolar spectrum disorders cannot both be diagnosed because a diagnosis of ODD requires that the child show oppositional behavior in the absence of a mood disorder.

In this chapter, we illustrate how to use a lifeline history approach to systematically collect longitudinal information about a child's current diagnoses and how to obtain a family history of mental illness. Table 4–1 summarizes information needed for the lifeline history. Figure 4–1 provides a lifeline form, which can be used to asssemble the information as it is gathered. A case example illustrating the use of this lifeline is presented in Figure 4–2. In the following section, we describe the case example illustrated in Figure 4–2. In the second section of the chapter, we focus on how to develop a family genogram and, in the third section, on how to use the genogram to gather a comprehensive family history of mental health diagnoses and symptoms.

Using the Lifeline to Assess Pediatric Bipolar Disorder

General Background

Ashley, an 8-year-old white girl, attends the interview with her mother, Ms. Miller. During the interview with Ms. Miller, Ms. Miller is asked about who lives in the home (see Figure 4–4 later in this chapter for Ashley Miller's family tree; family history assessment is described in the section "Collecting Family History of Mental Illness"). Ashley lives with her biological mother; stepfather, Mr. Miller; full biological brother Matthew (age 7); and two maternal half-siblings, a brother Alec (age 3) and a sister Brianna (age 1). Because Ashley does not live with both of her biological parents, Ms. Miller is asked about Ashley's contact and relationship with her biological father. Ashley has not seen her biological father since age 2.5 years, when he left the family and divorced Ms. Miller.

The following information can now be placed on the lifeline: Ashley's date of birth, the date of interview, Ashley's age, calendar years, birth of siblings, and the divorce of Ashley's biological parents. Incorporating both the child's age in

- **Above line:** pregnancy, labor and delivery, age in years, calendar years, moves, life stressors, child care arrangements, school placement
- **Below line:** physical health (onset, offset) and treatment, mental health (onset, offset, mood and comorbid diagnosis) and treatment, current functioning (home, school, peers)

Pregnancy

L & D

DOB _____ DOI

Sx Hx

Tx HX

School: Peers:

Home:

Figure 4–1. Blank lifeline.

Note. DOB=date of birth; DOI=date of interview; L&D=labor and delivery; Sx Hx=symptom history; Tx Hx=treatment history.

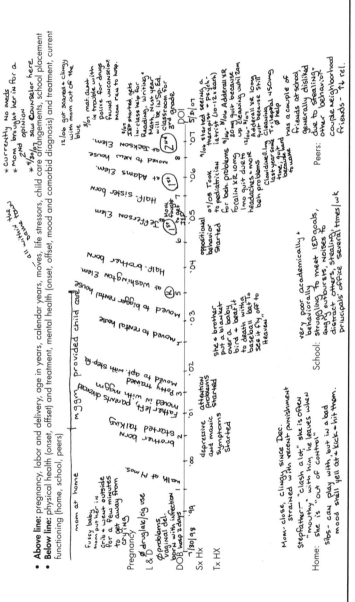

Figure 4–2. Case example lifeline.

Note. DOB=date of birth; DOI=date of interview; IEP=individualized education plan; L&D=labor and delivery; mggm=maternal great-grandmother.

Table 4–1.   Lifeline background questions

Date of birth and age

Pregnancy
Drug or alcohol and cigarette use or abuse during pregnancy
Pregnancy and labor and delivery complications

Developmental milestones and history
Walking, talking, toilet training (On time? Delays? Age reached?)
What was he or she like as an infant?

Child care
If parents are employed, who took care? After-school care?
Who lives in the household? Any changes in caregivers? Why?

School
Did the child attend preschool?
At what age did child attend kindergarten?
Grades completed? Any repeated? Why?
School district(s) and school name(s)
School transitions? Why?
General functioning and problems in school—behavioral or academic
Services (individualized education plan, tutoring)

Moves
What age(s)? From where and to where?

Major life events
Deaths, domestic violence, jail, alcohol or drug abuse, physical or
    sexual abuse, accidents, parental divorce or separation, changes in
    household members

Physical health
Major or chronic illnesses, hospitalizations, surgeries, injuries
Medications

Table 4–1.   Lifeline background questions *(continued)*

Mental health

Why was treatment first sought?

What interventions were tried (medication, therapy)?

When did these symptoms begin? (Try to get onset of each problem separately.)

Peer relationships

Number of friends

Best or closest friends

Quality of friendships

Activities involvement (e.g., Cub Scouts, sports teams)

Frequency of spending time with friends

Family relationships

How do you get along with _____?

What kinds of activities do you enjoy doing with _____?

Ask about mother, father, siblings, other household members, important adults, and any visits with noncustodial parent, if applicable

years and the calendar years helps the interviewer place information provided by the parents onto the timeline documents. Because parents often vary in how information is presented (e.g., "We moved when Ashley was 3." "Her brother was born in 2004."), establishing several sets of time markers minimizes confusion in the subsequent interview.

Pregnancy and Early Development

Next, the interviewer works through a chronological history of various events, starting with pregnancy and working toward the date of the interview. Important areas to consider are included in Table 4–1. Ms. Miller reports no drug, alcohol, or cigarette use during pregnancy. She acknowledges that her pregnancy with Ashley was easy. Labor took 13 hours, and Ashley was born via vaginal delivery with no complications. She had an infection at birth, but this cleared with a few days of antibiotics, and Ashley was released from the hospital within 2 days of birth. Ashley was a very fussy baby and cried most of the day. Ms. Miller reports times when she had to leave Ashley safely in her crib and sit on the porch to get away from her crying. Ms. Miller initially reports that Ashley was late for all of her developmental milestones; however, when asked specifically, she stated that Ashley walked at 14 months, talked at age 2 years, and was toilet trained at age 3 years.

This brief history of early development provides relevant information about disorders resulting from prenatal teratogen exposure, problems resulting from birth complications, temperament, and developmental milestones. Prenatal exposure to drugs (prescription and illicit), alcohol, and cigarettes has been associated with limited attention span, fetal alcohol syndrome, low birth weight, failure to thrive, and many other conditions (Ridgeway and Clarren 2005). In this case, substance use was denied; therefore, problems stemming from substance use could be ruled out unless there was reason to disbelieve the mother's report (which was not the case for Ms. Miller). Parents are not always honest about prenatal substance use, given the stigma about harming an unborn child and potential legal concerns. Birth complications, including anoxia, ingestion of meconium, and infections, also can contribute to associated health problems for the infant (Ridgeway and Clarren 2005). Again, in this case, birth complications appeared to be minimal.

When asked about Ashley's temperament as an infant, Ms. Miller describes Ashley as quite fussy and difficult. Some parents describe their children with mood disorders as temperamentally difficult children who become moodier or more anxious as they mature. Others describe colicky children who "grow out of it" but develop mood symptoms at a later date. Still other parents describe their children as being easy babies who started having problems at a specific age. Research is under way to study the link between early temperament and early-onset bipolar spectrum disorder (Akiskal et al. 2006). Regardless, such information is helpful to have when considering parent-child interactions from an early age, attachment, and the attitude of the parent toward the referred child.

In assessment of a child to determine whether he or she met developmental milestones on time, the interviewer's developmental knowledge base is critical. In this case, Ms. Miller underestimates her child's abilities, stating that all of her developmental milestones were significantly delayed, when in reality, only speech development was later than expected. The background inquiries include questions about walking, talking, and toilet training because these are milestones parents usually can remember and reflect motor, language, and psychophysiological development. Children typically take their first steps and say their first words around age 1 year (Ollendick and Schroeder 2003). Most children can walk steadily and combine two- to three-word sentences between 18 and 21 months (Ollendick and Schroeder 2003). Toilet training is usually accomplished by age 4 for bowel movements and age 5 for urination (American Psychiatric Association 2000). Approximately 5%–7% of children experience problems with encopresis, with four to five times as many boys as girls having this problem (Ollendick and Schroeder 2003). Approximately 7% of boys and 3% of girls have enuresis at age 5 (Ollendick and Schroeder 2003). In addition to encopresis and enuresis, there are other disorders associated with delayed development (e.g., language delays with pervasive developmental disorders). In this case, the late development of language was a symptom to keep in mind as the interview continued.

Psychosocial Stressors

When Ms. Miller was pregnant with her first son, Ashley's biological father left, and Ms. Miller moved into her great-grandmother's home. Ms. Miller reports having been at home with Ashley until a few months after her brother was born, when Ashley was 2 years old. Ashley's great grandmother took care of Ashley when Ms. Miller returned to work. When Ashley was about 3, the family moved into an apartment with Ashley's stepfather. They moved twice when she was 4, to a rental house and then a larger rental house, where they stayed until just before Ashley started second grade. Other than the moves and the births of Ashley's siblings, Ms. Miller describes only one other stressful life event. In March 2007, the police came to the house looking for Ms. Miller's sister, who uses drugs. Later, Ms. Miller's sister was found unconscious on the street, and Ms. Miller quickly left the house to see her sister at the hospital. Ms. Miller reported that Ashley was concerned about her aunt and worried while she was in the hospital.

Major psychosocial stressors often exacerbate behavior or emotional problems in children or trigger the onset of disorders (Johnson and McMurrich 2006). Parents often have not linked the stressors experienced by the child with the child's symptoms until being interviewed by the clinician. For example, a parent may describe inattention and hyperactivity that became problematic in preschool, around age 4. If, during the lifeline, the parent tells the interviewer about the child observing severe domestic violence around that age, then the attention problems might be better accounted for by acute stress disorder or posttraumatic stress disorder than by attention-deficit/hyperactivity disorder (ADHD). In this case, noting the ages at the moves, changes in who was living in the home and caregivers, and the birth of siblings may be helpful in understanding the development of Ashley's difficulties.

Medical History

Ashley's physical health has been good all of her life, with no major illnesses, injuries, head traumas, or accidents.

A brief medical history provides information about possible causes of current diagnoses and general impairment. For instance, a child who fell in a pool and was deprived of oxygen for several minutes may have a limited attention span as a result of brain damage rather than ADHD.

School History and Current Functioning

Understanding a child's functioning in school, with peers, and at home is essential to evaluate adequately the extent to which mood symptoms might cause impairment. Thus, reviewing a child's history in school settings as well as his or her current functioning in school is crucial.

Ashley did not attend preschool. She started kindergarten shortly after she turned 5 at Washington Elementary School, a public school in her local school district. Ms. Miller reports that Ashley's teachers did not talk with Ms. Miller about any behavior problems or academic concerns. The school district reformulated school boundaries, so the following year, Ashley attended first grade at Jefferson Elementary School, where she had difficulty focusing and was held back, although Ms. Miller was not informed of Ashley's lack of satisfactory progress until the last quarter of the school year. When Ashley was held back, Ms. Miller spent a great deal of time advocating for the school to complete a multifactor evaluation (MFE) and to develop an individualized education plan (IEP) for Ashley (see Chapter 11, "The Bipolar Child and the Educational System," in this volume for more details about these procedures).

During the summer after Ashley's first-grade year, the school district reorganized again because of financial concerns. Following this reorganization, all the first-graders in the district attended one school, and all the second-graders attended another school, and so forth. Therefore, Ashley attended Adams Elementary School, her third school in as many years, for her repeated first-grade year. At the time of the assessment, she is about to complete her second-grade year at Jackson Elementary School. Despite Ms. Miller's verbal request, the MFE and IEP were not completed until winter of her second-grade year. Results indicated that Ashley was functioning in the borderline range (Wechsler Intelligence Scale for Children Full-Scale IQ=72) and that she was behind in reading, writing, and mathematics. Ashley received extra tutoring in these areas after her IEP was completed. Next year, Ashley will be in a third-grade special education classroom for these subjects. Ms. Miller states that Ashley has done very poorly in school this year and has struggled to meet the goals of her IEP, which were lower than what is expected of most second-grade students. She also has been having angry outbursts, has been sent to the principal's office several times per week, has stolen from other children, and has generally been disruptive and unfocused in class. Ashley enjoys one-on-one attention and praise from her teacher; however, when her teacher has been unable to provide this, Ashley becomes disruptive.

This academic history provides much important information. Symptoms mentioned by Ms. Miller during the course of presenting Ashley's school history provided the interviewer with many areas about which to inquire during the mental health portion of the lifeline.

Current Functioning With Peers and at Home

Finally, before reviewing Ashley's mental health history in more detail, the interviewer asks Ms. Miller about Ashley's functioning with peers and at home. Ms. Miller reports that Ashley has a few friends at school with whom she plays only at school, although some live in her neighborhood. Overall, Ashley does not get along well with her classmates because of her stealing from them and other disruptive behaviors.

All of Ashley's relationships at home are strained by her frequent angry outbursts, defiant behavior, and "bad moods." Ms. Miller describes her relationship with Ashley as "pretty close." About 6 months prior to the interview, Ashley became very anxious about being away from her mother. Ms. Miller reports that the frequent corrections and punishments recently required as a result of Ashley's bad behavior have strained their relationship. Ashley and her stepfather "clash a lot." When Ashley has gotten "mouthy" with him, which he refers to as Ashley's being "out of control," Mr. Miller has left the house for a break, leaving his wife to handle Ashley's behavior alone. This has led to marital strain. Ashley can get along with her siblings if she is in a good mood, but she often hits them and yells at them when she is in a bad mood.

Understanding Ashley's current functioning in school, with peers, and at home provides information about her level of impairment at the time of the interview. Furthermore, the information about Ashley's relationships with her stepfather and siblings provides insight about the family environment and how Ashley's behavior affects other members of the household.

Using the Lifeline to Collect Mental Health History

Assessing symptoms in children and adolescents requires knowledge of the child's previous behavior, developmental norms, and how to assess important areas of functioning. A behavior can be considered pathological when it represents a change from the child's baseline behavior, is inappropriate for the situation, and is functionally impairing (Geller et al. 2002). General guidelines about when a behavior change meets criteria for a mood disorder can be remembered with the acronym FIND (see Table 4–2 for FIND general guidelines, as discussed in Kowatch et al. 2005, p. 215):

- Frequency
- Intensity
- Number of occurrences
- Duration

Finally, practitioners need to ask about functioning at school, in the home, and with peers at school and in the neighborhood—three important domains that can be affected differentially by psychopathology or situational change.

The description of Ashley's current functioning provides many leads from which to proceed with collection of mental health information. Ms. Miller talked about irritability, defiant behavior, concentration problems, stealing,

Table 4–2.   FIND guidelines

Frequency	Symptoms occur most days in a week
Intensity	Symptoms are severe enough to cause extreme disturbance in one domain (home, school, or peers) or moderate disturbance in two or more domains
Number	Symptoms occur three to four times per day
Duration	Symptoms occur 4 or more hours a day, total, not necessarily contiguously

Source.   Reprinted from Kowatch RA, Fristad MA, Birmaher B, et al.; Child Psychiatric Workgroup on Bipolar Disorder: "Treatment Guidelines for Children and Adolescents With Bipolar Disorder: Child Psychiatric Workgroup on Bipolar Disorder." *Journal of the American Academy of Child and Adolescent Psychiatry* 44:213–239, 2005, p. 215. Used with permission.

moodiness, separation anxiety, cognitive limitations, and speech delays. Following these leads, the clinician can begin by inquiring further about these symptoms, then methodically following up with a sufficient number of questions to cover all the behavior, anxiety, mood, and other disorder (BAMO) diagnoses (Cerel and Fristad 2001; see Table 4–3). This allows for a flexible format that is clinically sensitive by attending to the information perceived as most germane by the parent first, while still allowing for a careful determination of differential diagnoses and comorbid conditions.

Mood Symptoms

When asked about Ashley's irritability, Ms. Miller reports that Ashley is mad two-thirds of every day and that she frequently gets mean and aggressive. When asked about separate periods of explosive irritability, Ms. Miller describes "rages" during which Ashley is explosively angry, breaks and throws things, and does not seem to know what she is doing or care about punishment. One occasion Ashley tried to turn over the kitchen table. Ashley broke all of the keys off Ms. Miller's new computer when she was "raging" about a request from her mother. These episodes occur three times per week and can last a few minutes to an hour. Ms. Miller states that Ashley has had both grumpy moods and "rages" since she was 2 years old.

Table 4–3. BAMO: behavior, anxiety, mood, and other disorders

Behavior	Attention-deficit/hyperactivity disorder
	Oppositional defiant disorder
	Conduct disorder
	Cigarette dependence
	Drug abuse
	Alcohol abuse
Anxiety	Generalized anxiety disorder
	Separation anxiety disorder
	Social phobia
	Panic disorder
	Phobia
	Obsessive-compulsive disorder
	Acute or posttraumatic stress disorder
Mood	Major depressive disorder
	Dysthymia
	Mania
	Hypomania
	Cyclothymia
Other	Anorexia
	Bulimia
	Enuresis
	Encopresis
	Psychosis
	Somatization disorder
	Tic or Tourette's disorder
	Pervasive developmental disorders

Source. Summarized from Cerel and Fristad 2001.

When asked about elated or very silly moods, Ms. Miller describes periods of 1–2 hours that occur up to three to four times per day when Ashley cannot be calmed, is overactive, makes funny noises, talks nonstop, is very silly, laughs at inappropriate things, and thinks she is smarter than other children. Once, when Ashley was feeling really energetic and silly, she propped an inflatable bed up on the bunk beds and used it as a slide into the room, and on another occasion she had a snowball fight on the second-story porch. Ashley reports having high-energy moods and talks about feeling much smarter than other kids at those times. Ms. Miller also reports that Ashley constantly makes rude and loud noises when she is in a high-energy, silly mood.

When asked about hypersexuality, Ms. Miller reports that Ashley has always been more "sexual" than other children her age. When Ashley is in her "too happy mood," she will ask people to touch her buttocks and sing "I like big butts." Ashley has pulled her pants down to let the dog lick her private parts, and she has taken the diaper off her baby brother (not to change it). She and her 7-year-old brother have touched each other's private parts under blankets at their grandma's house. Ashley's history does not suggest that she has ever been sexually abused or exposed to sexual material inappropriate for her age (e.g., pornographic magazines, X-rated movies).

In the 2 weeks prior to the assessment, Ashley has had 4–5 nonconsecutive days during which she was explosive or elated more often than not during the day. Ms. Miller reports that Ashley's "too happy moods" never last more than 2 days at a time, and she has breaks of a few days to a week between periods of mood lability. Ashley does not have rages at school, but she does have the really silly, hyperactive moods there.

This information provides the interviewer much detail about depressive and manic symptoms. The depressive symptoms include possible irritable mood, and the manic symptoms include explosive irritability, elevated mood, inflated self-esteem, increased talking, and excessive involvement in pleasurable activities that have a high potential for painful consequences. These symptoms appear to be causing impairment in Ashley's functioning at school, at home, and possibly with peers.

Next, the interviewer asks about other associated symptoms not yet described. For example, manic symptoms that have not yet been addressed are decreased need for sleep, racing thoughts, distractibility, and an increase in goal-directed activity or psychomotor agitation. When asked about sleep,

Ms. Miller describes problems nearly every night. When Ashley has difficulty going to sleep, she either lies in bed for at least an hour worrying or gets out of bed and cleans or rearranges her room. On the latter nights, it takes Ashley 2–3 hours to fall asleep. Frequently, Ashley reports waking up in the middle of the night, at which time she stays in bed awake for 30–45 minutes worrying. Also, Ms. Miller reports that Ashley wakes up 2–3 hours before she needs to be up several days per week. Ashley is not tired on many days after having lost significant sleep. Ms. Miller notes that on some days, however, Ashley seems very tired, just wants to lie on the couch, and is sad and cranky after having difficulty sleeping. Thus, it appears that Ashley experiences a mixture of manic decreased need for sleep not associated with fatigue and possible depressive or anxious insomnia associated with worrying and fatigue. In addition, Ashley describes racing thoughts, a jittery feeling that manifests as psychomotor agitation, and an increase in distractibility during her "high" mood states.

From this information, Ashley meets all criteria for a manic episode except for duration. Failing to meet the duration criteria (feeling manic more often than not for 7 days for a manic episode or 4 days for a hypomanic episode) is common in children and adolescents. Children and adolescents frequently meet criteria for a few hours a day for 2–3 days in a row (Kowatch et al. 2005).

To review depressive symptoms other than irritability and insomnia, the interviewer asks about dysphoric mood, anhedonia, appetite or weight change, psychomotor agitation or retardation associated with low mood, fatigue, feelings or worthlessness or guilt, difficulty with concentration, and recurrent thoughts of death or suicide. Ashley's mood is always either very high or very low, according to Ms. Miller. Ms. Miller describes periods of very sad mood during which Ashley is tearful without knowing why. These occur nearly every day for 20 minutes or longer, sometimes lasting an entire day. They average about half of a day. During these times, Ashley seems to have no energy, moves and talks in slow motion, is not interested in her usual activities, and wants to be left alone to lie on the couch and watch television. Ms. Miller notes that on these days, Ashley does not feel like eating. Neither Ms. Miller nor Ashley endorses any increase in difficulty concentrating during her low mood, morbid or suicidal ideation, or feelings of worthlessness or guilt. Ashley does talk about feeling down and sad on some days, but she does not endorse the level of severity that Ms. Miller describes. Ms. Miller says that the low moods have been happening since Ashley was 2 years old and that Ashley has never had a period of 2 consecutive months without regular episodes of sadness, grumpiness, "rage," or elevated mood. Ms. Miller also reports that Ashley's mood swings cause the most trouble for her at home and at school. With all of this information about depressed mood and manic episodes, we can be fairly confident in a diagnosis of bipolar disorder not otherwise specified.

Non-Mood-Related Concerns

Following up on the other symptoms described by Ms. Miller that are not captured with the bipolar diagnosis is the next concern. Ms. Miller mentioned Ashley's difficulties with concentration, stealing, oppositional behavior, and separation anxiety. Ms. Miller described nearly all of the inattentive and hyperactive-impulsive symptoms of ADHD as having been present since Ashley was 3 years old. She noted that regardless of Ashley's mood, Ashley has had difficulty focusing and has switched activities much more often than her other three children would. Ms. Miller also endorsed nearly every symptom of ODD, and these symptoms appeared when Ashley was 6 years old. Before a diagnosis of ODD is given, however, conduct disorder needs to be ruled out because Ms. Miller noted that Ashley steals from other children, a conduct disorder symptom.

Ms. Miller described the following conduct disorder symptoms. Ashley has stolen money and other items from children at school, including, on several occasions, items of significant value. She has lied to other children many times to get things from them. She left school on one occasion to avoid going to her classes. She has frequently initiated physical fights with her siblings. Ashley set fire to a piece of paper and burned a hole in her mother's linoleum floor a few months ago. When angry, Ashley has left the house and wandered around the neighborhood and backyard for as long as 15–20 minutes. She has done this four or five times in the past year. Ashley and her brother, at ages 4 and 3, respectively, put a blanket over a baby bird and beat it to death with a baseball bat. When Ms. Miller asked why they did it, Ashley replied that they "wanted to see it fly off to Heaven." Ashley's brother recently pointed out to Ms. Miller that the family cats run away from Ashley, and when she does catch them, she squeezes them until they meow loudly. This year, Ashley chased her brother and sister with scissors and threatened them with a butcher knife. She stabbed her brother through the cheek with a pencil. Ashley's brother has repeatedly told Ms. Miller that Ashley has taken off her younger brother's diaper; Ms. Miller is not sure whether Ashley has touched him inappropriately. Ashley's behavior clearly meets the criteria for conduct disorder, childhood onset, with the first symptom occurring at approximately age 4.

The final disorder suggested by Ms. Miller's timeline information is separation anxiety disorder. Ms. Miller reported that about 6 months prior to the interview, Ashley became very clingy and did not want to go anywhere without her mother. Ashley was very afraid something bad was going to happen to her mother. She also started having nightmares about her mother leaving and started having difficulty sleeping by herself. Ashley began sleeping with her sister whenever possible. Symptoms have declined since then but are still problematic. Ms. Miller reported that several times in the past month, Ashley has complained of stomachaches in an effort to avoid school and stay home with her mother. When asked whether Ashley follows her through the house, Ms. Miller reported that for the last 4 months, Ashley has rarely left her mother alone, and Ms. Miller has even left the bathroom door open a little so that Ashley could feel she would be able to reach her mother if she needed to. Thus, Ashley's behavior also meets criteria for separation anxiety disorder.

Finally, to capture any other disorders that have not been discussed thus far, the parent should be asked about key symptoms of other BAMO diagnoses (see Table 4–3). A few questions help ensure that a key element of the diagnostic picture is not missed. This review can be particularly important when working with a highly impaired child with a variety of concerns, one of which may be overshadowed by the others.

In summary, systematically gathering a psychosocial and symptom history organized by the lifeline gives the clinician context to 1) understand current concerns; 2) obtain information essential for differential diagnosis, including various emotional and behavior problems, in a coherent manner that allows the parent or guardian to tell the child's story in a meaningful way; 3) assess level of functioning in the critical domains of home, school, and peer relationships; 4) integrate the possible role of psychosocial stressors and family environment in the child's problems; and 5) develop a relevant treatment plan that acknowledges the history of treatment attempts and their outcomes. Overall, a single sheet conveys most of the pertinent clinical information necessary for diagnosis and individualized treatment planning influenced by the family's perspective and history. In addition, this format can be translated easily into a narrative report for sharing with other clinicians.

Collecting Family History of Mental Illness

Collecting information about a child's first- and second-degree relatives' history of mental illness is a key aspect of evaluating for bipolar spectrum disorders. These disorders are some of the most heritable brain disorders. In general, the risk for bipolar spectrum disorder in relatives of people with bipolar spectrum disorder is significantly elevated (Faraone et al. 2003). The younger the age at onset, the more familial loading will be noted. Childhood-onset bipolar spectrum disorder is associated with a higher percentage of first-degree family history of depression, anxiety, ADHD, conduct disorder, and substance dependence and second-degree family history of depression and ADHD than is adolescent-onset bipolar spectrum disorder (Rende et al. 2007).

Gathering a family history of mental illness is a sensitive, multistep process. First, the interviewer has to determine who the relevant relatives are without the reporter feeling judged. Second, the interviewer must ascertain whether these relatives have psychiatric symptoms and possibly diagnoses. Third, the interviewer should document whether the informant is knowledgeable about family members on both the mother's and the father's sides of the family. The interviewer should gather both social and genetic history of the family. For example, one may begin by eliciting a brief narrative about the mother's and father's upbringing (e.g., "Could you tell me in a nutshell, what was growing up like for you?"). This generic prompt should be followed up with specific questions, as needed, to document the parents' educational levels obtained; the parents' general level of functioning at school, in their family, and with peers; and how they were parented. The information elicited from these questions can be particularly important in understanding what natural parenting skills each parent brings to the family system. Next, the interviewer should explain his or her attempt to better understand the child's problems by learning about each parent's genetic history, given the genetic contributions to many disorders.

When the interviewer is gathering a complete family mental health history, it is helpful first to generate a three-generation genogram, which then can be used as a reference point for the parent and the interviewer. To generate the genogram, the interviewer begins by asking about the biological mother's and father's families of origin (i.e., their biological parents, any stepparents, full and half siblings). Next, he or she documents all the relationships the mother and father have had and the children produced in each of these relationships. Finally, the interviewer circles the family members currently living together in one household. Figure 4–3 provides a key to family genogram symbols, indicating how to record various types of relationships. To maintain convention, fathers should be placed on the left-hand side of the parent and grandparent relationships, and siblings should be listed in chronological order, left to right, oldest to youngest. Figure 4–4 is the generated genogram for our case example.

Some areas about which the interviewer will inquire can be sensitive topics for the informant (e.g., whether couples were married or lived together, how much is known about a former partner's family, and the current relationships of a former partner). Parents may be reluctant to admit to having had multiple partners or to not knowing about the other parent's siblings or parents if they were not in a long-term relationship. In extreme cases, the child may be the result of stranger rape, and the parent may know nothing about the child's other parent and prefer not to think about circumstances surrounding the child's conception. If this occurs, discomfort can be minimized by reminding the parent that you are trying to get a picture of the child's genetic history because there are genetic contributions to many disorders. Collecting this information is further complicated when talking with legal guardians or adoptive parents with limited knowledge about the child's biological family.

When the genogram has been completed, the interviewer should clarify that the remaining questions pertain to only first- and second-degree relatives, reminding the parent that the purpose of these questions is to determine genetic, rather than social, explanations of the child's behavior. For example, information about the mother's adopted sister will not be relevant to the genetic history of the son, even if that aunt takes care of him on a regular basis and has a close relationship with him. However, in circumstances such as this, it is useful to document the quality of the child's relationship with such a caregiver on the lifeline, as previously discussed. When the parent and interviewer have agreed on which family members are of interest for this part of the as-

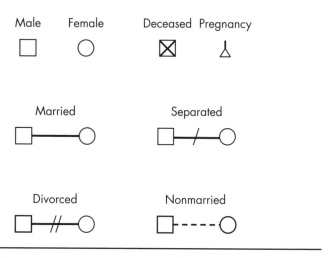

Figure 4–3.   Key to family genogram symbols.

sessment and how they are related to the child, then the interviewer can focus on reviewing possible diagnoses and symptoms of those relatives.

For several reasons, simply asking about the *diagnoses* of family members is not an adequate assessment of the mental health history. First, the reporter may not know about a diagnosis another family member has received (e.g., his sister-in-law may have never told the referred child's father about the postpartum depression she experienced before he joined the family). Second, the reporter may report only a "label" that is incorrect (e.g., the child's uncle may have been hospitalized because he had hallucinations, and the family assumed that he had schizophrenia, when, in fact, he had a psychotic mania). Third, the family member may not have received a disorder diagnosis because that person never sought help because of concerns such as stigma, job security, or a belief that treatment would not help. Cultural and generational norms about mental illness can be important to keep in mind here. For instance, Asian Americans and people who grew up during the Great Depression are unlikely to seek help outside of their families for mental health concerns (Hillier and Barrow 1999; Sattler 1998). Thus, inquiring about the presence of specific symptoms of mental illness will provide more accurate data than will simply asking about diagnoses.

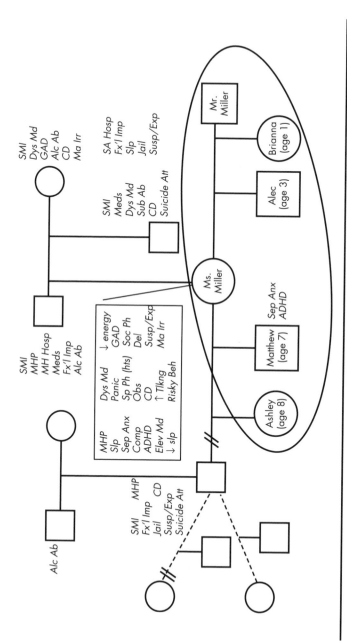

Figure 4–4. Generated genogram for family in case example.

See Table 4–4 for abbreviations.

Interviewers should ask about symptoms and their treatment (see Table 4–4 for recommended areas of inquiry and questions). A structured interview to collect family mental health history, the Weissman Family History Screen (Weissman et al. 2000), provides a comprehensive instrument to collect family history information. Recommended areas of assessment and questions to use are modeled after the Family History Screen (Table 4–4). A logical first step is to inquire about mental illness diagnoses in relatives, with follow-up questions about what has been diagnosed for each endorsed relative. Next, the interviewer should ask about treatment for mental or emotional problems that anyone has received. Then, he or she must systematically ask about the presence of BAMO symptoms without referring to the disorder specifically. Doing this provides more confidence about the information gathered. For example, a mother may report that she has been given a bipolar disorder diagnosis. However, in the symptom review, she denies ever having experienced any bipolar symptoms during her lifetime. This calls into question the veracity of the diagnosis or possibly the parent's ability to report and may suggest possible reporting bias that requires further inquiry. When the symptoms and diagnoses do not agree, the interviewer should be careful about drawing conclusions regarding genetic predisposition for a disorder.

Family history data can be summarized on the genogram next to each relative. Some families have a striking amount of pathology noted on one or, more often than not, both sides of the family tree. Patterns also may be discernible concerning classes of disorders noted in different groupings of family members. For instance, a family may have depression endorsed for most of the women and alcohol or drug abuse endorsed for all of the men.

Conclusion

Taken together, the lifeline and genogram with family mental health history provide a comprehensive encapsulation of the patient. These two tools can summarize a wealth of knowledge about the child and his or her family and can clarify the clinical description in a way that standard written reports cannot do concisely. The system for collecting lifeline and family mental health history data expedites the process of gathering relevant information, maintains rapport with the parents or guardians by letting them present information from their perspective, provides sufficient depth and breadth for differential diagnosis, and supplies the clinician with a succinct, comprehensive illustra-

Table 4–4. Family history areas of inquiry

Topic	Possible wording; "Has anyone…"	Abbreviations[a]
Severe mental illness	Been diagnosed with a mental illness or emotional or behavior problem?	SMI
	What illnesses?	
	Attempted suicide?	suicide att
	Completed suicide?	suicide
Treatment	Seen a mental health professional (e.g., psychiatrist, psychologist, social worker) or his or her family physician because of emotional or behavior problems?	MHP
	Been hospitalized for mental illness?	MH Inpt
	Been hospitalized for substance abuse?	SubAb Inpt
	Taken medication for emotional or behavior problems?	Meds
ADHD	Gotten into trouble because he or she could not sit still or pay attention much more compared with peers when he or she was young?	ADHD
ODD or CD	Broken rules or skipped school more than peers?	CD
	Been suspended or expelled from school?	Susp/Exp
	Been arrested or convicted of a crime?	Jail
Substance abuse	Had a problem with illegal drugs or prescription drugs?	**Sub Ab**
	Had a problem with alcohol?	Alc Ab

Table 4–4. Family history areas of inquiry *(continued)*

Topic	Possible wording; "Has anyone…"	Abbreviations[a]
Depressive symptoms		
Functional impairment	Had difficulty meeting responsibilities such as working or taking care of children for several days or more (not related to physical illness)?	Fx'l Imp
Insomnia	Had trouble falling asleep, been waking up in the middle of the night, or been waking up too early in the morning?	Slp
Dysphoric mood	Felt sad or down most of the time for 2 weeks or longer (not related to a death)?	Dys Md
Fatigue	Had a lot less energy than usual or lost interest in his or her usual activities for 2 weeks or longer?	↓Energy
Manic symptoms		
Elevated mood	Had times when he or she felt really happy or energetic for no reason or out of proportion to his or her circumstances?	Elev Md
Manic irritability	Had times when he or she was so irritable that even little things made him or her out-of-control angry?	Ma Irr
Excessive talking	Talked a lot more or a lot louder than usual?	↑Tlkng
Racing thoughts	Seemed to have more thoughts running through his or her head than he or she could handle?	↑Th
Risky behavior	Taken a lot more risks than usual or spent more money than he or she had?	Risky Beh
Decreased need for sleep	Seemed like he or she could sleep a lot less than usual and not feel tired?	↓slp

Table 4–4. Family history areas of inquiry *(continued)*

Topic	Possible wording: "Has anyone…"	Abbreviations[a]
Anxiety symptoms		
Generalized anxiety	Worried about a lot of different things so much that it interfered with his or her life?	GAD
Panic	Felt very scared all of a sudden (e.g., heart racing, sweating, tense muscles) without a major cause?	Panic
Separation anxiety	Become really nervous when he or she had to be away from his or her family when he or she was young or worried a lot about something bad happening to a family member or himself or herself?	Sep Anx
Social phobia	Had a really hard time doing things in front of others or being around new people?	Soc Ph
Specific phobia	Been really scared of something so much that he or she worked hard to avoid it (e.g., crowds, certain animals, bugs, needles, blood, heights)?	Sp Ph
Compulsions	Felt like he or she had to do something over and over again even though it seemed silly to him or her (such as counting or checking things, washing his or her hands, cleaning even when things were already clean)?	Comp
Obsessions	Had annoying or disturbing thoughts that he or she could not get out of his or her head (such as that everything was covered in germs; did he or she turn off the stove or lock the door)?	Obs

Table 4–4. Family history areas of inquiry (continued)

Topic	Possible wording: "Has anyone…"	Abbreviations[a]
Anxiety symptoms (continued)		
Acute or posttraumatic stress	Had an experience in which he or she or someone he or she loved was in danger of being seriously hurt or killed, and had a hard time not thinking or dreaming about that experience?	A/PTSD
Eating disorder symptoms		
Anorexia nervosa	Become so thin that people worried about him or her?	↓wt
Bulimia nervosa	Eaten a lot of food all at once and felt like he or she could not control his or her eating?	Binge
Psychosis		
Hallucinations	Seen things that other people could not see or heard things others could not hear?	Hall
Delusions	Had strange ideas that were not true, such as that someone was out to get him or her, he or she was somebody famous or really important, the television had special messages for him or her?	Del

Note.   ADHD=attention-deficit/hyperactivity disorder; CD=conduct disorder; ODD=oppositional defiant disorder.
[a]Abbreviations used in the example of a family genogram shown in Figure 4–4.
Source.   This table summarizes the topics of the items on the Family History Screen; see Weissman et al. 2000.

tion of the case that can be reviewed quickly before the family's return visits. The information also can be transcribed into a written report for ease of communicating with other clinicians involved in care of the child.

References

Akiskal HS, Kilzieh N, Maser JD, et al: The distinct temperament profiles of bipolar I, bipolar II and unipolar patients. J Affect Disord 92:19–33, 2006

American Psychiatric Association: Diagnostic and Statistical Manual of Mental Disorders, 4th Edition, Text Revision. Washington, DC, American Psychiatric Association, 2000

Cerel J, Fristad MA: Scaling structured interview data: a comparison of two methods. J Am Acad Child Adolesc Psychiatry 40:341–346, 2001

Faraone SV, Glatt SJ, Tsuang MT: The genetics of pediatric-onset bipolar disorder. Biol Psychiatry 53:243–256, 2003

Geller B, Zimerman B, Williams M, et al: Phenomenology of prepubertal and early adolescent bipolar disorder: examples of elated mood, grandiose behaviors, decreased need for sleep, racing thoughts, and hypersexuality. J Child Adolesc Psychopharmacol 12:3–9, 2002

Hillier SM, Barrow GM: Aging, the Individual, and Society, 7th Edition. New York, Wadsworth, 1999

Johnson SL, McMurrich S: Life events and juvenile bipolar disorder: conceptual issues and early findings. Dev Psychopathol 18:1169–1179, 2006

Kowatch RA, Fristad MA, Birmaher B, et al; Child Psychiatric Workgroup on Bipolar Disorder: Treatment guidelines for children and adolescents with bipolar disorder. J Am Acad Child Adolesc Psychiatry 44:213–239, 2005

Miklowitz DJ, Cicchetti D: Toward a life span developmental psychopathology perspective on bipolar disorder. Dev Psychopathol 18:935–938, 2006

Ollendick TH, Schroeder CS (eds): Encyclopedia of Clinical Child and Pediatric Psychology. New York, Kluwer Academic/Plenum, 2003

Rende R, Birmaher B, Axelson D, et al: Childhood-onset bipolar disorder: evidence for increased familial loading of psychiatric illness. J Am Acad Child Adolesc Psychiatry 46:197–204, 2007

Ridgeway JJ, Clarren SK: Prenatal factors affecting the newborn, in Pediatrics. Edited by Osborn LM, De Witt TG, First LR, et al. Philadelphia, PA, Elsevier Mosby, 2005, pp 1238–1244

Sattler JM: Clinical and Forensic Interviewing of Children and Families: Guidelines for the Mental Health, Education, Pediatric, and Child Maltreatment Fields. San Diego, CA, Jerome M Sattler, 1998

Weissman MM, Wickramaratne P, Adams P, et al: Brief screening for family psychiatric history: the Family History Screen. Arch Gen Psychiatry 57:675–682, 2000

5

Etiology

Robert M. Post, M.D.

Causes and Mechanisms of Bipolar Illness

Although the precise causes and mechanisms involved in the onset and progression of bipolar illness have not been conclusively identified, much evidence is accumulating about the general processes involved. We know that bipolar illness has a strong familial origin, with positive family history documented in approximately 50% of the adult patients with bipolar illness. Genetic vulnerability likely plays an even greater role in childhood-onset bipolar disorder because the incidence of positive family histories is increased as a function of an earlier age at onset. However, a substantial number of patients with bipolar illness do not have a family history of bipolar illness in their first-degree relatives, so other nonhereditary mechanisms such as psychosocial adversity also must be considered.

The occurrence of early stressors may increase sensitivity to subsequent stressors that precipitate initial episodes of mania or depression. In those who are highly genetically predisposed or who have experienced many affective episodes, bouts of illness may begin to occur even in the absence of psychosocial stressors. In adult bipolar illness, clear evidence now shows biochemical, physiological, and structural abnormalities in the brain (Post 2007b; Post et al. 2003). These generally reflect decreased neural activity in the frontal cortex and increased activity in deeper limbic areas of the brain, which are thought to be most intimately involved in the regulation of emotion. To the extent that the illness tends to be recurrent, and neurobiological alterations associated with each episode further increase the vulnerability to recurrences, the importance of the early institution of long-term prophylactic treatment becomes increasingly clear.

Some of the potential mechanisms by which stresses and episodes of illness may alter the brain and produce vulnerability to further episodes have now been identified. One example is a substance that is necessary for neuronal growth and survival and for making new synaptic connections that are important for long-term learning and memory. This substance is called *brain-derived neurotrophic factor* (BDNF). Stresses can decrease BDNF, and BDNF also decreases in the serum of patients with both depression and mania as a function of the severity of the episode (Post 2007a, 2007b). To the extent that these decreases in BDNF reflect what is happening in the brain, BDNF alterations could affect brain function and increase neural changes in the brain that make someone even more vulnerable to further episodes.

However, countering this potential are the new observations that a host of medications can increase BDNF and prevent stress from decreasing it (Chuang 2004; Manji et al. 2003). Moreover, medications could prevent episode-related decrements in BDNF and, indirectly, protect the brain. Thus, all of the details have not been determined, but we are beginning to see how both genetic and environmental mechanisms can interact in producing illness vulnerability and that episodes themselves can lead to further illness progression (Post 2007a). This process is definitely not inevitable because the brain is highly plastic and adaptable, and with the help of medications, illness progression can be halted or prevented, and patients could achieve and sustain long-term remission.

Genetic Mechanisms in Bipolar Illness Onset

Genetic alterations that convey disease risk have two major categories: 1) the *genetic mutation* is very rare and occurs in less than one in a million instances, and 2) the *single nucleotide polymorphism* (SNP: pronounced "snip") occurs commonly in the general population. The SNP results from a single nucleotide variation in the DNA that causes a single amino acid substitution in a given protein that may have many hundreds or thousands of amino acids strung together.

A series of SNP variations have now been delineated in the illness of schizophrenia, and, interestingly, many of these now are also candidate vulnerability genes for bipolar illness. One of the most striking examples of a vulnerability factor that has been replicated multiple times in bipolar disorder is that involving BDNF. A single amino acid substitution at the 66 position of a normal valine (Val) for a methionine (Met) makes BDNF function less efficiently in cells. Animals that have the Val66Met allele of the BDNF gene, compared with those with the Val66Val allele, have deficient long-term potentiation, a good model of learning and memory (Egan et al. 2003). In parallel to these findings, nonbipolar adults who have the Val66Met version of the BDNF gene have smaller hippocampal and frontal cortical volumes and have minor deficits in specific declarative memory tasks (Pezawas et al. 2004; Szeszko et al. 2005).

Surprisingly, several studies have indicated that the better-functioning Val66Val allele is associated with bipolar illness in general or its early-onset or rapid-cycling variants (Geller et al. 2004; Green et al. 2006; Lohoff et al. 2005; Müller et al. 2006; Neves-Pereira et al. 2002; Post 2007b; Skibinska et al. 2004; Sklar et al. 2002). Why this might be the case is not entirely clear, but one can speculate that it also might be related to the finding of increased creativity that consistently has been noted to be associated with the illness. Also, in the manic phase, rapid and pressured speech with hyperassociativity and a profusion of ideas is present. This symptomatology is also paralleled by increases in connectivity in the brain that can be seen on functional brain imaging (Benson et al., in press), and one could ultimately evaluate whether these types of abnormalities are, in fact, more common in bipolar patients who have the better-functioning Val66Val allele of the BDNF gene compared with the Val66Met version.

Gene-Environment Interactions

It seems very likely that this BDNF variant will be one of many different SNPs that might act as either vulnerability or protective factors in the risk for bipolar illness and other psychiatric illness onsets (Craddock 2007). Moreover, considerable evidence indicates that gene-environment interactions play an extremely important role in illness vulnerability and onset. Some evidence for this is found in the area of BDNF itself, but the most clear-cut evidence is seen in instances of unipolar depression. In this disorder, there is a common variation in the serotonin transporter (the site at which the selective serotonin reuptake inhibitors [SSRIs] act)—that is, the short form appears to be less efficient than the long form. In the absence of environmental adversity, individuals with either variation have about the same risk for illness onset. However, when there is a history of early childhood adversity and a current adult stressor, individuals with the short form of the serotonin transporter are at double the risk of depressive onset (60% compared with 30% for those with the long version; Caspi et al. 2003; Kaufman et al. 2006). This kind of gene-environment interaction is likely to be important in relation to a whole host of these common gene variants or SNPs, in which each conveys small effects but, together and in association with environmental circumstances, may aggregate and play a more fundamental role in illness onset and course.

The genetic vulnerability associated with bipolar illness is most evident from studies of identical twins compared with fraternal twins. Identical twins share the same genes and thus have the same illnesses, to the extent that genetically mediated factors are involved. Identical twins are highly concordant for bipolar illness (both having the illness between 40% and 70% of the time; i.e., a rate much higher than for other psychiatric illnesses), whereas the concordance is less than half this rate for fraternal twins (who do not share the same genes but do share the same environment) (Craddock and Jones 1999).

These data for identical twins are supported by familial studies indicating that when a positive family history of bipolar illness is found in first-degree relatives, risk in their children increases considerably, from about 1% of the nonbipolar population to about 10%–20% (Craddock and Jones 1999). Thus, one in five children is likely to develop bipolar illness on the basis of this type of vulnerability. However, when there is a positive history of bipolar illness on one side of the family and either unipolar or bipolar illness is present on the other side, the lifetime risk of developing some type of affective illness (either unipolar or bipolar) then increases to about 70% (Lapalme et al. 1997). This is because the risks appear to be additive or multiplicative because of what is thought to be a very complex and polygenic (multicausal) basis of the hereditary vulnerability, as well as an environmental influence. Thus, several vulnerability genes may come from one side of the family and converge with other vulnerability genes from the other side of the family.

The risk is evident not only from family studies but also from the opposite direction. That is, if one studies first-degree relatives of children with early-onset bipolar disorder, more relatives are affected than in those with adolescent-onset or, especially, adult-onset bipolar disorder (Pavuluri et al. 2006). These data suggest that a greater background of genetic vulnerability is associated with the increased risk of childhood-onset bipolar illness.

Cohort (Year of Birth) Effects

The *cohort* effect has been described: each generation born since World War I appears to have an increased rate as well as an earlier age at onset of unipolar and bipolar illness than the previous generation (Gershon et al. 1987; Lange and McInnis 2002; Weissman and Klerman 1978). There has been much speculation about the potential mechanisms involved in the increased rate and earlier onset of mood disorders in the general population.

Whatever reasons emerge to account for this dramatic trend, it has been a factor in a very considerable change in recognizing affective illness in children. Some 20–30 years ago, it was argued that childhood-onset depression may not exist, and mania in children was almost unheard of. Today, both depressive and manic mood states are common, and recurrent depressions and bipolar illness can begin in the very first years of life in highly predisposed individuals (Figure 5–1).

Some people have wondered whether the increased recognition of rapid mood fluctuation in children is partially attributable to the increasing use of psychomotor stimulants for the treatment of attention-deficit/hyperactivity disorder (ADHD) (Reichart and Nolen 2004). This is of some concern because many investigators have noted a high rate of comorbidity between ADHD and bipolar illness (Biederman et al. 1996), and the comorbid ADHD cannot be treated adequately until the bipolar illness is first treated with a

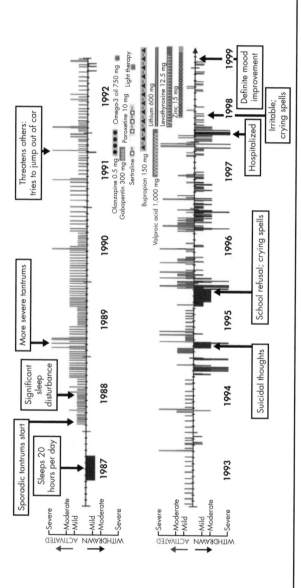

Figure 5–1. "Kiddie" Life Chart of a 13-year-old child with bipolar disorder diagnosed at age 10 (1997), but with severe affective dysregulation since age 2 years.

The diagnosis would have been bipolar disorder not otherwise specified (BPNOS) in the early 1990s, bipolar disorder II in 1994, and bipolar disorder I in 1995. However, the illness was not recognized and treated until 1997. It took several years of clinical trials to find the combination of medications effective for her mood stabilization. The drugs used are listed above the charting of activated and inhibited behaviors 1997 to 1999, and symbols indicate the timing and duration of treatment (see Post and Leverich 2008, Chapter 67, for details).

mood stabilizer (Kowatch et al. 2005). In the potentially bipolar child, if one uses stimulants or antidepressants alone, without a mood stabilizer or atypical antipsychotics, mood fluctuations could be exacerbated.

Anticipation (Generational) Effects: Potential Genetic and Environmental Mechanisms

A large generational effect of about 10 years also appears to affect the onset of childhood bipolar illness. For example, if a parent with bipolar illness onset at age 25 has a child who develops bipolar illness, the onset may be at about age 15 in that child. There are both genetic and nongenetic explanations for such observations (DePaulo 2004; Lange and McInnis 2002).

Genetic anticipation refers to the findings in some genetic illnesses that a decrease in the age at onset may occur in successive generations. This has been found to be true for neurological illnesses characterized by single genetic mutations such as Huntington's disease, spinal cerebellar degeneration, fragile X syndrome, and other neurodegenerative disorders (Li and el Mallakh 1997). In the case of Huntington's disease, the defect that causes this illness (associated with progressive dementia and involuntary motor movements) is in a single protein called huntingtin. The genetic code for this protein has multiple triple-repeat sequences in a row that code for the amino acid glutamine. If an individual has fewer than 40 of these triple-repeat sequences, Huntington's disease does not occur. If an individual has about 47 or more, he or she will develop Huntington's disease late in life. With a very large number of triple repeats (e.g., 60 or 70), the illness may be associated with a very early onset (even in childhood).

When the sperm and egg cells of individuals with the Huntington's disease gene reproduce themselves, the number of triple-repeat sequences tends to expand. Thus, people who might be destined to develop Huntington's disease relatively late in life because they were born with about 50 triple-repeat sequences may have children with 60–70 triple repeats in a row, rendering the huntingtin protein highly dysfunctional and associated with a very early onset of the illness in these individuals' children.

This expansion of the triple-repeat sequence is referred to as *genetic anticipation* and indicates that mechanisms within the replication of an individual's reproductive cells (egg or sperm) can increase the degree of defect in some single-gene illnesses from one generation to the next. Although this effect has not been consistently shown, several investigative groups have suggested that triple-repeat sequences are associated with bipolar illness.

Regardless of whether this proves to be the case, considerable evidence indicates an anticipation-like mechanism whereby the next generation may have an illness onset 10 years earlier than did their parents (DePaulo 2004; Mendlewicz et al. 1997). However, an earlier onset of illness in the children of a parent with bipolar illness may be only a manifestation of the general cohort effect or could be associated with a variety of other factors that are not necessarily related to genetic inheritance (Lange and McInnis 2002).

Multiple Genetic Vulnerability Factors

Over the past decade, there has been an increasing effort to identify the genetic changes that may increase vulnerability to bipolar illness. One of the most promising leads involves a marker on the short arm of chromosome 18, as initially demonstrated by Berrettini et al. (1994), whose findings were replicated and extended by DePaulo and colleagues (McMahon et al. 1997; Stine et al. 1995). These investigators noted that inheritance with a marker on chromosome 18 was associated with bipolar II illness on the father's side of the family and that maternal transmission of the illness was not associated with such a vulnerability factor on this chromosome. These findings suggest that one should search further in this region of chromosome 18 to identify precisely the nature of the molecular alteration involved. However, even when the general area of the short arm of chromosome 4 was found to convey vulnerability to Huntington's disease (which shows a much simpler pattern of genetic inheritance involving a single gene), it was not until almost a decade later that the actual protein defect was isolated and found to be the huntingtin protein. Moreover, even though the exact defect has been known for more than a decade, it has not so far led to new approaches to therapeutics.

Thus, in the case of bipolar illness, it will likely take as long or longer for this possible gene defect on chromosome 18 to be identified, and it is highly likely to be one of a great many vulnerability factors (Craddock 2007), much like those now evident in diabetes and in cancer. For example, in the development of colon cancer, increased proliferation and cell multiplication occur in the initial stages, and with further evolution, a cancerous tumor may develop in a single location characterized by more aggressive cell types that are clearly abnormal on microscopic examination. In later stages, the tumor cells may metastasize and break away from the primary site and, with this transition, become relatively resistant to treatment. This progression, in terms of colon cancer, involves a series of mutations that not only increase cellular proliferation but also disable normal tumor suppressor factors. If an individual is born into a family that already has a genetic vulnerability, for example, as a result of loss of a tumor suppressor factor, he or she may be at particularly high risk for earlier onset of the disorder because fewer somatic mutations occurring in precancerous cells are necessary to produce the full-blown malignancy.

We believe that many different types of gene changes are involved in the stages of illness progression that occur in bipolar disorder, with a certain number of alterations in gene expression occurring as a result of heredity and another group occurring on the basis of life experiences, stresses, and the experience of multiple episodes of affective dysregulation (Figure 5–2). However, instead of these environmental events causing irreversible mutations in a cell-replicating factor or tumor suppressor factor, as in cancer, in bipolar illness, the changes are not mutations but only changes in what genes are expressed and to what degree. Therefore, when the vulnerability factors for bipolar illness are ultimately identified, they are not likely to provide the same definitive information that comes with knowing whether one has inherited the single gene defect of Huntington's disease. In that case, one knows with a fair degree of certainty whether one will eventually acquire the illness.

In contrast, in the case of multiply determined or polygenic illnesses such as heart disease or bipolar illness, the inheritance of a given susceptibility gene would have only a small effect and would not necessarily mean that an individual will become ill. However, the identification of a series of small-effect susceptibility genes for bipolar illness may not only help to understand the mechanisms of illness generation and progression but also eventually help identify the treatments to which a patient may best respond.

Importance of Stressors in the Onset and Progression of Bipolar Illness

Stress Sensitization

Kraepelin (1921) first observed that initial episodes of mania or depression are often precipitated by psychosocial stressors but that with sufficient num-

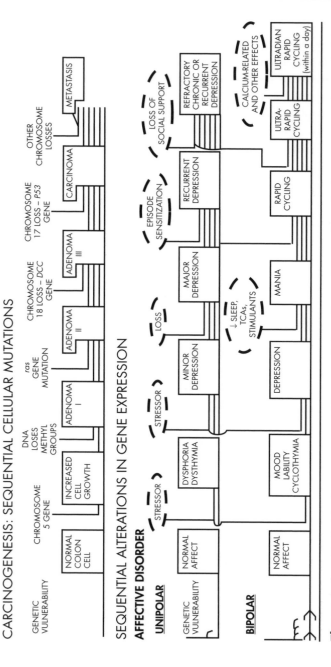

Figure 5–2. Similarities between sequential accumulation of somatic mutations altering gene expression underlying carcinogenesis and the accumulation of environmentally induced changes in gene expression observed in unipolar and bipolar affective disorder. TCA=tricyclic antidepressant.

bers of recurrences, lesser degrees of stress are required, and episodes begin to emerge more spontaneously or autonomously. In a meta-analysis, we found that a substantial literature has validated this concept (Post 1992). New data are highly supportive of this stress sensitization perspective. Data in the Stanley Foundation Bipolar Network are also consistent with an important role of early stressful life events in conveying a long-lasting vulnerability to stressors and their ability to trigger episodes. In a study of more than 600 patients in the Stanley Foundation Bipolar Network, those with a history of early extreme environmental adversity (i.e., physical or sexual abuse in childhood or adolescence) had an earlier onset of bipolar illness; a more pernicious course; and more Axis I, II, and III comorbidities (Leverich et al. 2007).

Leverich et al. (2001) also reported an interaction between familial or genetic vulnerability and environmental adversity. Adults with bipolar illness who had neither of these vulnerability factors had the latest ages at onset, whereas those who had both a positive history of bipolar illness in the family and early life adversities had the very earliest age at onset of their bipolar illness.

Data in laboratory animals have indicated that early severe life stressors can alter biochemistry and behavior in a long-lasting fashion. For example, animals exposed to repeated stressors may show a lifelong anxious phenotype in association with secretion of high levels of corticosterone (the rodent version of the human stress hormone cortisol) (Duman and Monteggia 2006; Kuma et al. 2004; Roceri et al. 2002, 2004). Other studies have now reported that this kind of neonatal adversity can produce long-lasting changes in brain levels of BDNF and lower the set point for the production of new neurons (neurogenesis) throughout an animal's lifetime. Thus, adverse experiences occurring in specific periods of the developmental window may lead to lifelong alterations in neurobiology and behavior.

Preliminary evidence indicates that a similar process could occur in humans subjected to early adverse experiences. These individuals show long-lasting endocrine abnormalities, and a recent study by Kauer-Sant'Anna et al. (2007) found that in patients with bipolar disorder, those with a history of early traumatic life events had lower levels of BDNF in their serum. Whether alterations in serum actually reflect those occurring in the brain has not been definitively established, but these results are at least suggestive of long-term changes in biological processes as a result of early life experiences in some circumstances.

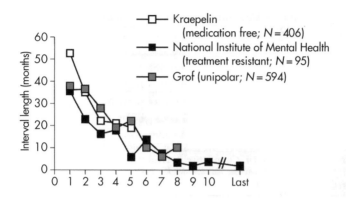

Figure 5–3.   Decreasing "well intervals" between successive episodes or cycle acceleration in recurrent affective illness in three different study samples.

Kindling and Episode Sensitization

Again, Kraepelin was among the first to document that the "well interval" between the first and the second episodes tends to be longer than the interval between the second and the third and other successive episodes (Figure 5–3). However, this finding, which has now been well validated in the literature, does not imply that the tendency for progression cannot be stopped with successful treatment. Rather, the general course of untreated or inadequately treated illness, even given its extreme varieties of cyclic presentation, tends to go in the direction of cycle acceleration.

Kessing and associates (Kessing and Andersen 2004; Kessing et al. 1998) in Denmark have provided the best documentation of this phenomenon (i.e., that "episodes beget episodes"; Figure 5–4). They observed that in both unipolar and bipolar hospitalizations, the best predictors of the incidence of and time course to relapse were the number of previous episodes. These data were observed in 20,350 patients carefully tracked in the Danish case registry and provide further confirmation of Kraepelin's original formulation of cycle acceleration as a function of episode recurrence (Kessing et al. 1998).

These kinds of data have been synthesized in the concept that both recurrent stressors and episodes can predispose an individual to an increased vulnerability to future episodes in a long-lasting fashion (Figure 5–5). For either

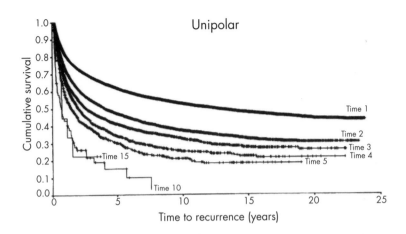

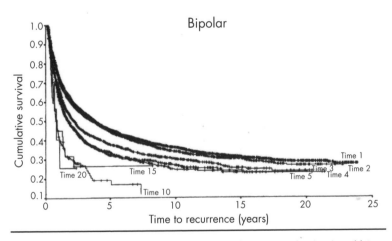

Figure 5–4. Recurrence of successive episodes in unipolar (top) and bipolar (bottom) mood disorder.

Cumulative survival (probability of remaining well) was calculated with the Kaplan-Meier method for estimation with censored observations. For both unipolar and bipolar patients, time to recurrence (labeled Time 1, Time 2, etc.) decreased with the number of previous episodes.

Source. Reprinted from Kessing LV, Andersen PK, Mortensen PB, et al.: "Recurrence in Affective Disorder, I: Case Register Study." *British Journal of Psychiatry* 172:23–28, 1998. Used with permission.

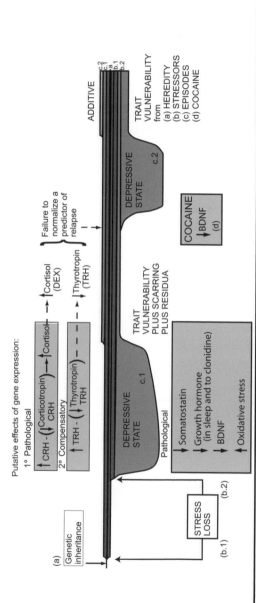

Figure 5–5.   Accumulating experiential genetic vulnerability in recurrent affective illness.

Initial stressors (b.1) that might not be sufficient to trigger the full neurobiological concomitants of a depressive episode (STATE) may nonetheless leave behind biological (TRAIT) vulnerabilities (shaded center line) to subsequent events and stressors (b.2). The state of depression with its associated peptide and hormonal increases (top) and decreases (bottom) then may leave behind additional trait vulnerabilities and residua. Brain-derived neurotrophic factor (BDNF), which supports cell survival and long-term memory, decreases during each episode (see Figure 5–6). Oxidative stress, which generates substances that endanger cells, increases with each episode. Cocaine and other substances of abuse also alter BDNF, such that there can be more or less genetic vulnerability from heredity (a) that remains constant, but vulnerability from (b) psychosocial stressors, (c) episodes, and (d) substance abuse can progressively accumulate. CRH=corticotropin-releasing hormone; DEX=dexamethasone; TRH=thyrotropin-releasing hormone.

stressor or episode sensitization to occur, some kind of underlying memory-like mechanism must convey these long-term changes. Given these general tendencies for the course of bipolar illness to accelerate over time and move from psychosocially triggered to spontaneous episodes, we became very interested in the phenomena of sensitization and kindling in animals as models of neuronal learning and memory that had certain parallels with the evolution of affective illness.

Kindling Model

In kindling, repeated intermittent subthreshold electrical or chemical stimulation of a given region of the brain in rodents eventually leads to full-blown seizures (Goddard et al. 1969; Racine 1978), and with sufficient numbers of these triggered seizures, the seizures begin to occur spontaneously (i.e., the animal begins to have seizures even when its brain is not stimulated) (Post 2007a, 2007b). The neurobiology of this neuronal learning process is beginning to be identified at the level of long-term changes in gene expression of neurotransmitters, receptors, and nerve growth or neurotrophic factors, as well as in the microstructure of the synapse and nerve cell survival and cell death. These alterations probably occur as a result of changes in gene transcription (Post 1992). That is, whatever one's genetic inheritance, genes continue to be turned on and off not only throughout the development of the nervous system but also in response to stressors, life events, and even normal processes of learning and memory.

The kindling formulation also has helped us to conceptualize that some of the changes in gene transcription are related to the primary pathophysiology of kindling (i.e., the "bad guys" mediating the long-term-kindled memory trace), whereas others are secondary, compensatory, transient anticonvulsant adaptations (i.e., the "good guys" trying to prevent further seizures) (Post 2007a; Post and Weiss 1992, 1996).

It is of some interest that thyrotropin-releasing hormone (TRH) is not only a likely endogenous antidepressant in affective illness but also an anticonvulsant substance in the kindling model. In both instances, TRH increases are driven by increases in gene transcription (i.e., a cellular signal arrives at the nucleus, which turns on the gene for TRH) (Figure 5–5). A messenger RNA (mRNA) is read off the DNA portion encoding TRH, and the mRNA for TRH then instructs the cell to synthesize more TRH peptide. It

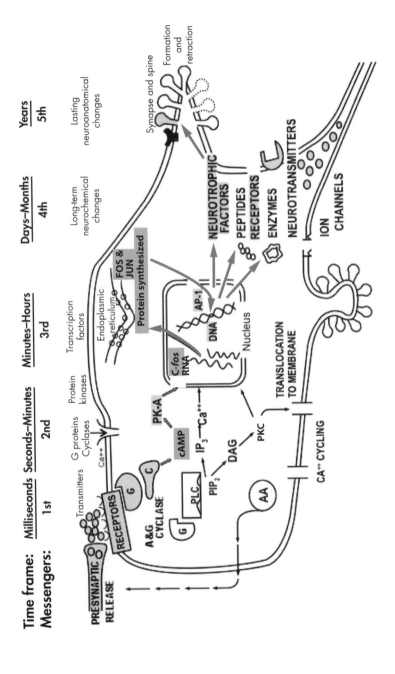

Figure 5–6. *(opposite)* Neural mechanisms of synaptic plasticity and short- and long-term memory.

This schematic of a cell illustrates how transient synaptic events induced by external stimuli (top, left) can exert longer-lasting effects on neuronal excitability and the microstructure of the brain (right side) via a cascade of effects involving alterations in gene transcription (of DNA) and translation (of messenger RNA [mRNA]) of new proteins and peptides. Neurotransmitters activate receptors and second-messenger systems, which then induce immediate early genes (or transcription factors) such as c-*fos* and c-*jun*. Fos and Jun proteins are synthesized in the cell cytoplasm on the endoplasmic reticulum and then translocate (migrate) back into the nucleus and bind to DNA to further alter the transcription of other late effector genes and other regulatory factors, the effects of which could last for months or years. Simple types of learning and memory involve these types of changes in gene expression in hundreds of thousands to millions of neurons in forming the long-term memory trace.

AA=arachidonic acid; A&G=adenylate and guanylate cyclase; AP-1=activator protein–1 (binding site on DNA); cAMP= cyclic adenosine monophosphate; DAG = diacylglycerol; IP_3=inositol 1,4,5-triphosphate; PIP_2=phosphatidylinositol 4,5-biphosphate; PK-A=protein kinase A; PKC=protein kinase C; PLC = phospholipase C.

does this by stringing together in the correct sequence the appropriate amino acid building blocks that constitute the TRH peptide. Thus, transient episode-induced increases in TRH and other anticonvulsant neuropeptides may help reestablish equilibrium and prevent further seizures from occurring.

Pathological Versus Adaptive Changes in Gene Expression

The repeated occurrence of seizures in the kindling process or, by analogy, affective episodes may be not only propelling the animal or human toward easier triggering of further episodes but also engendering the body's own adaptations in attempts at preventing future episodes. However, these endogenous adaptations (such as TRH) tend to be relatively short-lived. As TRH peptide levels return to normal, the kindled animal or recurrent depressed patient (Figure 5–5) is again more highly vulnerable to recurrences (Figure 5–6).

It is important to reemphasize that kindling is not a literal model of mood disorder, because motor seizures are not a manifestation of the illness (Post 2007a; Post and Weiss 1992, 1996; Weiss and Post 1994). However, the development and regular occurrence of seizures in the amygdala kindling model, as well as their becoming spontaneous, provide an easily identifiable and studied end point. We can examine some of the general conceptual principles underlying this type of illness progression and ask whether they are pertinent to the mood disorders. This may be the case even if seizures and affective episodes are mediated via different neurochemical systems in the brain.

It is of some interest that BDNF actions via its receptor called TrkB are necessary to kindle seizure progression. If animals are created that do not have the TrkB receptor, they do not kindle (He et al. 2004). These data suggest that BDNF-related mechanisms may, in part, account for some of the elements of illness progression in the kindling model, as well as in affective illness (Post 2007b).

Role of BDNF in
Defeat-Stress Depression-Like Behaviors in Animals

If animals are subjected to defeat stress, BDNF increases in the dopamine pathway to an area of brain mediating motivation activity and reward. If intruder rodents are introduced into the environment of the home cage of another animal, they are readily defeated and may even be killed if not adequately protected in the experimental situation. Such defeat-stressed animals show many depression-like behaviors, but these do not occur if the BDNF increases in this dopamine pathway are prevented either directly through genetic manipulations or indirectly via antidepressant treatment.

At the same time, defeat-stressed animals show decreases in BDNF in the hippocampus, and this effect also can be prevented by increasing BDNF directly or by protecting animals with antidepressant treatment that prevents the hippocampal decrements (Berton et al. 2006). Thus, defeat stress causes opposite change in BDNF—decreases in the hippocampus and increases in the ventral tegmental area/nucleus accumbens dopamine pathway, each of which appears causally involved in producing the associated depressive behaviors (Tsankova et al. 2006).

Episode-Related Decrements in Serum BDNF

Several investigators from different laboratories have found that episodes of depression and of mania (Cunha et al. 2006; Machado-Vieira et al. 2007) are both associated with decrements in serum BDNF in association with severity of symptomatology (Cunha et al. 2006; Gonul et al. 2005; Karege et al. 2002; Shimizu et al. 2003). In both unipolar and bipolar depressed patients, BDNF is decreased during depressive episodes and tends to increase toward normal with treatment.

Similarly, episodes of mania also have been associated with decrements in BDNF as a function of episode severity, and these decrements are not apparent during euthymia or treatment in the well state. Most recently, Pandey et al. (2008) reported that BDNF (the levels of both protein and its messenger RNA) were also very significantly (*P*<.001) reduced in the platelets of children with bipolar disorder.

In addition to these episode-related decrements in BDNF, the group headed by Kapczinski and colleagues (2008) also has reported that white blood cells show evidence of oxidative stress during each affective episode (Andreazza et al. 2007). Oxidative stress generates free radicals and other cellular toxins that are destructive to cell functioning and, potentially, cell survival.

In this fashion, one can envision these dual mechanisms for cellular dysfunction occurring with each affective episode. Decrements in the cell survival factor BDNF and increases in toxic products together may endanger cellular functioning and either exacerbate previous alterations or produce new ones.

These new data provide plausible mechanisms for considering how episodes may increase vulnerability to future episodes via both active and learned processes of sensitization potentially mediated by BDNF changes in the hippocampus and the nucleus accumbens, as well as passive or general deficits in cellular functioning caused by a loss of neuroprotective factors and increases in oxidative stress. In either instance, the new findings again emphasize the importance of effective treatment and episode prevention, not only to ameliorate the many severe educational, social, and employment dysfunctions associated with manic and depressive episodes but also to protect the brain. Adolescents who commit suicide have lower levels of BDNF in prefrontal cortex than do comparison subjects (Pandey et al. 2007). These results parallel those of Dwivedi et al. (2005), who found that individuals who committed suicide had low levels of BDNF in frontal cortex and hippocampus.

Cocaine-Induced Behavioral Sensitization

Another potential complication of adolescent- and adult-onset bipolar illness is that of substance abuse. Wilens et al. (2004) estimated that adolescents with bipolar illness are seven to nine times more likely than are those in the general population to engage in substance abuse. Problematically, use of illicit substances has been shown to alter brain functions in a variety of damaging ways. For example, abuse of the psychomotor stimulant cocaine causes pro-

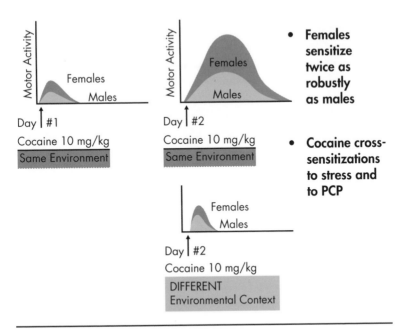

Figure 5–7.   Behavioral effects of cocaine increase (sensitize) with repetition.

The effects are context dependent because animals are more active after cocaine administration in the same environment (top right) but not when the same dose is given in a different environment (bottom right). Females sensitize to cocaine more rapidly than do males. Animals sensitized to cocaine are more responsive to stress (and vice versa) and also more responsive to other drugs of abuse, such as amphetamine or phencyclidine (PCP or "angel dust").

gressive increases in behavioral reactivity and stereotypy in animals (called *behavioral sensitization;* Post et al. 1987) (Figure 5–7) . This behavioral sensitization may have some parallels to effects that occur in humans as well. Initial experiences with cocaine are often pleasant and associated with euphoria and mild increases in sociability. However, with repeated use and dose escalation, more dysphoric, frantic, and frenetic activity may occur, and, ultimately, a full-blown paranoid psychosis can develop.

This behavioral sensitization phenomenon has been associated with dopaminergic alterations in the pathway to the reward area of the brain (nucleus accumbens) and, most interestingly, is associated with increases in BDNF in the same pathway (Figure 5–8). Thus, defeat stress, behavioral sensitization, and cocaine-induced behavioral sensitization appear to have mechanisms in common because each makes the other more likely to occur and each appears to involve BDNF increases in this same dopaminergic pathway (Figure 5–9). If the BDNF increases are prevented, behavioral sensitization does not occur (Berton et al. 2006; Tsankova et al. 2006).

Thus, there appears to be the potential for interaction and facilitation among stressors, substances of abuse, and episodes of affective illness. Each can increase the likelihood of the occurrence of the other. Moreover, as noted earlier, evidence indicates that each phenomenon can show sensitization or increased reactivity on repetition of the stressors, substances of abuse, or episodes of mood disorder (Figure 5–10).

Cross-Sensitization Among Stressors, Episodes of Affective Illness, and Substances of Abuse

In addition to the potential vicious circle interactions described in the previous sections is the possibility that each type of vulnerability shows not only sensitization to itself but also cross-sensitization to the others. Because BDNF is implicated in all three instances of stress sensitization, episode sensitization, and cocaine-induced behavioral sensitization, this could represent a common mechanism conferring this increasing degree of cross-vulnerability.

From a clinical standpoint, this suggests the great importance of attempting to ameliorate each of these aspects of illness that can lead to disease progression. One cannot, at this time, alter one's genetic inheritance vulnerability (e.g., whether you have a better or worse functioning version of BDNF), but one can clearly change the balance of BDNF and other related neurochemical alterations associated with occurrences in the environment, namely, stressors, episodes, and substances of abuse (Figure 5–10). Each of these then becomes an important target of clinical therapeutics, and this emphasizes the importance of early intervention to prevent increasing biochemical changes that confer increasing vulnerability to episode recurrence.

Because the chances of adopting substance abuse are so high in adolescents with bipolar illness, it would appear prudent to begin a treatment process of attempting primary prevention of substance abuse in any adolescent who has onset of bipolar illness and who has not yet begun to abuse drugs. In

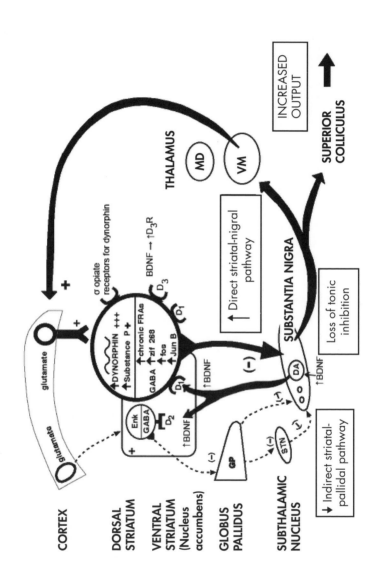

Figure 5–8. *(opposite)* Chronic cocaine administration, which leads to increased responsivity to cocaine and stress, is associated with changes in transmitter release and in gene expression.

Increased dopamine (DA) release and increased brain-derived neurotrophic factor (BDNF) in the ventral striatum (nucleus accumbens) lead to greater reactivity in this important dopamine pathway involved in motivation, reward, activity, and emotional memory. Increases in dynorphin and its σ opiate receptors also occur. Because dynorphin is dysphorogenic and psychotomimetic, this could help to explain the progressively more prominent degrees of anxiety and dysphoria seen with chronic cocaine use. It is noteworthy that increases in BDNF in the nucleus accumbens also occur, in repeated defeat stress depressive-like behaviors in animals and in autopsy specimens of humans with depression.
D_1, D_2, D_3 = dopamine receptors; DM = dorsomedial nucleus of the thalamus; enk = enkephalin; FRAs = Fos-related antigens; GABA = γ-aminobutyric acid; STN = subthalamic nucleus; VM = ventromedial nucleus of the thalamus.

addition, psychotherapeutic maneuvers aimed at instilling stress coping mechanisms and stress immunization techniques would appear particularly important in addition to cognitive and behavioral focuses on symptom recognition and medication adherence (see Chapters 10, "Working With Patients and Their Families," and 12, "Special Treatment Issues"). Such work then would enhance the likelihood of long-term consistent use of therapeutic agents that may either increase BDNF and other neurotrophic factors in their own right or prevent their episode-induced decreases.

Most troubling, however, is that such early conservative treatment is not necessarily either standard procedure or readily available in many instances in the United States. Studies in the National Institutes of Health–sponsored Systematic Treatment Enhancement Program for Bipolar Disorder (STEP-BD) network (Perlis et al. 2004) and in our own Bipolar Collaborative Network (BCN; originally sponsored by the Stanley Foundation) (Leverich et al. 2007) have both found that a very high proportion of adults with bipolar illness had their onset in childhood or adolescence. This ranged from 50% of the subjects in the BCN to 66% in the STEP-BD outpatient program. In both patient populations, those with earliest ages at onset had the most difficult courses of illness throughout early life and into adulthood. In the BCN, we verified these find-

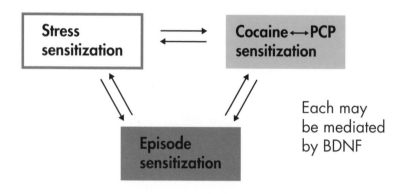

Figure 5–9.   Repeated stress, cocaine, and affective episodes each increase reactivity not only to themselves (sensitization) but also to the others (cross-sensitization).

Alterations in brain-derived neurotrophic factor (BDNF) may be involved in each type of sensitization because BDNF decreases in hippocampus of animals and serum of humans with stress and affective episodes. Interestingly, both defeat stress and cocaine sensitization in animals increase BDNF in the ventral tegmental area (VTA)–ventral striatal–dopamine pathway (see Figure 5–8). Preventing the BDNF decreases in the hippocampus (with antidepressants or other means) or the BDNF increases in the VTA–ventral striatal–dopamine pathway prevents the occurrence of defeat-stress depression-like behaviors in rodents. PCP = phencyclidine.

ings and showed that those with the earliest age at onset had more difficulties at an average age of about 40, when they were treated naturalistically by experts and rated prospectively by clinicians.

Sensitization Phenomena Emphasizing the Need for Early Treatment

Association of Early-Onset Bipolar Illness With Long Delays to First Treatment

We found that those with the earliest age at onset of bipolar illness had the longest delays to first treatment (Leverich et al. 2007; Post and Kowatch 2006; Post et al. 2008). Those with childhood onset (i.e., before age 13) had average

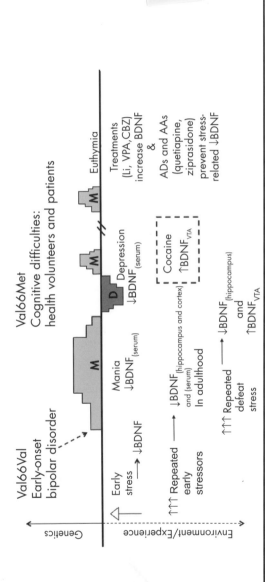

Figure 5–10. Brain-derived neurotrophic factor (BDNF) is involved in each phase of bipolar illness vulnerability, episode recurrence, and comorbid cocaine abuse, and in many of the treatments of bipolar illness.

Vulnerability to illness onset may include a combination of both hereditary genetic and environmental stress-mediated BDNF alterations (i.e., gene-environment interactions). Stressors (up arrows) decrease BDNF in brain, and manic (M) and depressive (D) episodes decrease BDNF in serum in proportion to the severity of symptoms. Mood stabilizers and atypical antipsychotics (AAs) can directly increase BDNF or prevent its decrease by stress (in animals) and prevent the decreases in BDNF caused by manic and depressive episodes (in humans) with successful long-term prophylaxis.

AD = antidepressant; CBZ = carbamazepine; Li = lithium; VPA = valproate; VTA = ventral tegmental area.

delays of about 15 years from first symptoms of the illness to first treatment for either mania or depression (Leverich et al. 2007; Post and Kowatch 2006). Those with adolescent onset experienced an average of a 10-year delay before first treatment, whereas those with early and late adult onset experienced much shorter delays from symptom onset to first treatment: about 5 and 2 years, respectively. Thus, it would appear that about 20 years ago, when these adults (average age $N=40$) were youngsters, their affective symptomatology was ignored and not treated for an extraordinarily long time. During this untreated interval, symptoms, episodes, and severe dysfunction occurred, and many began to use substances and develop other secondary psychiatric and medical comorbidities (Kapczinski et al. 2008).

Thus, it would be hoped that with earlier recognition and effective treatment, these individuals not only would have had more positive childhood and adolescent experiences in social and educational development but also could have changed their course of illness in a more positive direction and prevented the otherwise more impairing course of illness that typically occurs with childhood onset compared with adult onset.

Differences in Incidence and Vulnerability Factors for Childhood-Onset Bipolar Illness in the United States Compared With Some European Countries

Problems of treatment access are particularly difficult in the United States compared with some European countries in which medical care is available to all. In addition, it appears that childhood-onset bipolar illness is notably more common in the United States compared with in the Netherlands and Germany (Figure 5–11). In our BCN, we had sites in Los Angeles, CA; Dallas, TX; Cincinnati, OH; and Bethesda, MD; as well as three European sites—in Utrecht, the Netherlands, and Freiburg and Munich, Germany. Of our adult patients in the United States, 22% had onset of their bipolar illness before age 13, compared with only 2% of those from the European sites. This difference was seen but less pronounced in the adolescents, such that child and adolescent onsets together were twice as likely to occur in the U.S. patients compared with the Europeans (Post et al. 2008).

This difference in onset between the United States and other countries is not likely to be an artifact, because it emerged from both patient question-

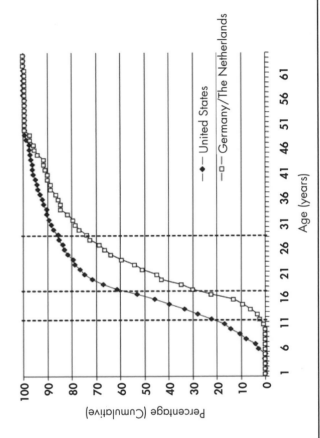

Figure 5–11.   Childhood- and adolescent-onset bipolar illness is more commonly reported by adult outpatients (average age = 42) in the United States than by those in two European countries (Germany and the Netherlands) (Post et al. 2008). This was seen both with self-reported age at onset and during a systematic interview by clinicians. It is noteworthy that a high incidence of early-onset bipolar illness is now being reported in Spain, Italy, Turkey, and Norway, but not the British Isles.

naire data and formal clinician interviews with the Structured Clinical Interview for DSM-IV. If one assumes that these differences were not an artifact, one would begin to look for potential vulnerability factors in the United States and protective factors in the Netherlands and Germany. In fact, the very first factors examined provided striking differences. Along with twice the incidence of childhood- and adolescent-onset bipolar illness in the United States was an approximate doubling in the percentage of patients with positive family histories of bipolar and unipolar disorder in first-degree relatives in the United States compared with the European cohorts. At the same time, the incidence of early adversity in the form of childhood physical or sexual abuse doubled in the United States compared with European bipolar outpatients. Therefore, it appeared that two of the major vulnerability factors for bipolar onset—genetic or familial background and the occurrence of severe psychosocial adversity—were both much more prevalent in the U.S. bipolar patient cohort than in the Europeans. Thus, either or both of these factors interacting could, in part, explain the much higher incidence of childhood- and adolescent-onset bipolar illness in the United States.

Why there might be an increased genetic or familial background for bipolar illness in the United States compared with the Netherlands and Germany is not readily ascertained. A variety of possibilities deserve to be mentioned for further exploration, however. These include the possible increased migration of those with bipolar vulnerability genes from Europe to the United States; a higher rate of assortative mating (those with bipolar illness marrying other patients with mood disorder, which we did, in fact, observe in the United States compared with Europe); and the possibility of increased genetic background occurring in the United States because of greater incidence of vulnerability genes caused by shorter reproductive cycles, as suggested by David Comings (1996).

Likewise, multiple potential explanations exist for the increased incidence of childhood adversity, including an increased incidence of substance abuse, higher divorce rates, and a generally more stressful lifestyle with less time for vacations. Also, environmental variables such as diet or exposure to potentially toxic substances cannot be excluded as possibilities. Whatever the mechanisms turn out to be, they may provide not only new targets for therapeutic intervention but also the potential for public health preventive measures to attempt to ameliorate some of the risk factors that appear to be heightened in the United States and lessened in at least some European countries (Post et al. 2008).

Recognition of Bipolar Illness and Early Treatment

Somehow, we must begin to do a better job in recognizing and treating bipolar illness in children and adolescents to help ameliorate their suffering and potentially prevent the illness from further progressing or deteriorating. One means of achieving this goal is to pay greatest attention to those at high risk by virtue of having a positive history of bipolar illness on one side of the family or those at very high risk because of a positive family history for bipolar illness on both sides of the family. Greater attention to the potential early difficulty of some of these children may allow earlier and more effective intervention, much like that achieved in many other areas of medicine. We treat mild to moderate levels of high blood pressure in the hope of preventing not only more extreme increases but also heart attacks, strokes, and kidney dysfunction, with which hypertension is associated.

Clinicians often ignored early phases of affective dysregulation, even when they were associated with considerable dysfunction, for fear of stigmatizing the child; now it would appear that the opposite perspective is more cogent and prudent. That is, we should not ignore these early signs of mood disorder in children any more than we would the early signs of heart disease, cancer, epilepsy, or diabetes in children. To put the mood disorders in a different category would appear in itself to be the result of misunderstanding the seriousness and consequences of bipolar illness and bowing to stigma.

Do Treatments Differ as a Function of Stage of Illness?

In the development and progression of kindled seizures, different drugs are effective in the early, middle, and late phases. Will this also be the case for the development and progression of bipolar illness? The different phases of kindling evolution are 1) the first or developmental stage, in which minor seizures progress to more major ones; 2) the middle or completed stage of full seizure episodes triggered by brain stimulation; and 3) the late or spontaneous phase, in which seizures occur in the absence of stimulation, different neural substrates are involved, and different drugs are effective in different stages. For example, some drugs that are effective against fully expressed kindled seizures do not prevent their early phase development. Other drugs show the opposite pattern (Post and Weiss 1992, 1996). Remarkably, some drugs that are ineffective against the fully triggered seizures are effective against the sponta-

	Dynamic	Interpersonal	Psychoeducation (PE)	Cognitive-behavioral	Supportive/Rehabilitative
Severity: (Mania / Depression)					
Stressor:					
Episode pattern:		Intermittent	Continuous/Regular	Irregular → Chaotic	Autonomous
Frequency:			Rapid 4/year	Ultrarapid 4/week	Ultradian >1/day
Psychotherapy:	Dynamic	Interpersonal	PE / Cognitive-behavioral		Supportive/Rehabilitative
Medications*					
ADs, SSRIs, MAOIs	+++	++	±	±	
Lithium		++	+++	++	+
Lamotrigine		++	+++	++	+
Carbamazepine		++	+++	++	+
Valproate		++	+++	++	+
Atypical antipsychotics		++	+++	++	+
Calcium channel blockers				±	+

Figure 5–12. *(opposite)* Phases in the evolution of mood cycling; hypothetical relation to treatment response.

In an analogous fashion to kindling, episodes of affective illness may progress from triggered (arrows) to spontaneous and show different patterns and frequencies (top) as a function of the stage of syndrome evolution. Just as different neural substrates and anticonvulsant treatments are involved in different phases of kindling evolution, a similar principle is postulated in affective illness; these phases also might be responsive to different types of pharmacotherapies or psychotherapies. Although systematic and controlled studies have not examined the relation of phase of illness to treatment response, anecdotal observations provide suggestive data that some treatments may be differentially highly effective (+++), moderately effective (++), possibly effective (+), or equivocal (±) as a function of course of illness (* = all ratings are highly preliminary and provisional). Note that the pharmacological dissociations and the specific anticonvulsant drugs that are effective in the model of kindling are different from those postulated in mood disorders; nonetheless, the principle of differential response as a function of stage of syndrome evolution may be useful and deserves to be specifically examined and tested in the clinic. The need to use multiple agents in combination as a function of late or severe illness stage is standard in many medical illnesses, and this requirement is also apparent both in the late and the rapid-cycling phases of bipolar illness, as well as in childhood-onset illness (Findling et al. 2005, 2006; Kowatch et al. 2005). If one were attempting to achieve primary prophylaxis (i.e., heading off the illness before it even starts) in a child at very high risk, the best medications for treating full-blown affective episodes may or may not be effective in preventing the illness from the outset.
AD = antidepressant; MAOI = monoamine oxidase inhibitor; SSRI = selective serotonin reuptake inhibitor.

neous variety, whereas other drugs show the opposite (i.e., are effective for triggered seizures but do not prevent spontaneous seizures from occurring). In a similar fashion, we believe that different stages of development and progression of affective illness may also require different treatment interventions (Figure 5–12).

In the kindling model, Weiss and Post (1994) observed that animals treated with effective anticonvulsants earlier (compared with later) in the course of repeated full-blown seizures were more likely to remain seizure-free and less likely to lose responsivity via a tolerance mechanism (Post 2007a). In a parallel way, we believe that early effective treatment of a recurrent mood

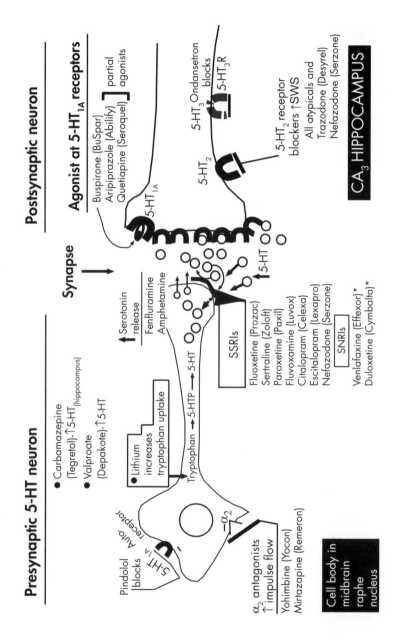

Figure 5–13.   *(opposite)* Mechanisms of antidepressant action.

The selective serotonin reuptake inhibitors (SSRIs) increase the amount of synaptic serotonin by blocking reuptake of serotonin into the presynaptic terminal. This serotonin synapse between the presynaptic ending of a serotonergic raphe neuron and the postsynaptic cell body or dendrite of another neuron in the hippocampus is typical of that occurring throughout the brain (see Figure 5–15). The role of SSRIs and other types of antidepressants in the treatment of bipolar depression in adults has not yet been adequately defined and is even more controversial in children.
*Also blocks NE reuptake.
5-HT=serotonin; 5-HTP=5-hydroxytryptophan; SNRI=serotonin-norepinephrine reuptake inhibitor; SWS=slow-wave sleep; o =5-HT molecules; ∩=5-HT receptors; ∩=antagonists block receptors.

disorder will result in patients more readily entering and maintaining remission. A modicum of data now supports this proposition. Those with more previous episodes have a more difficult course of illness (Kupka et al. 2005; Nolen et al. 2004; Post et al. 2003).

The crucial question is which agents should be used to intervene most effectively in the initial stages of affective dysregulation in childhood and adolescence. The same drugs that are highly effective in treating and preventing full-blown manic and depressive episodes may not be the best ones for preventing the initial stages of affective illness development. Effective preventive treatment (pharmacoprophylaxis) would have many obvious benefits. Children would be saved from not only the considerable pain and suffering of mood swings and manic and depressive episodes (see Figure 5–1 earlier in this chapter) but also their adverse social and educational consequences. Untreated bipolar illness often has a dramatic effect on friends, family, and schooling. The extent to which these factors can be lessened by appropriate pharmacotherapy would be of significance in its own right.

It is also possible (as the kindling and stress sensitization models predict) that effective early treatment intervention could prevent the increased vulnerability to subsequent recurrences and actually change the predicted course of illness. Adolescents are recognized to be at risk for suicide with severe mood disorders, and suicide is rising most rapidly in this population. Moreover, the occurrence of bipolar illness appears to be a particularly high risk factor for

In ●● Mania Drug efficacy ●● In Depression

Antimanics

Benzodiazepines ↑Cl⁻ influx potentiate GABA
- ○ Clonazepam
- ○ Lorazepam

Indirect
- ○ Levetiracetam

Typical antipsychotics Block D_2 receptors
- ●● Trifluoperazine –
- ●● Haloperidol –
- ●● Molindone –

Atypical antipsychotics (AA) ●● to ○ to ●●
Block mesolimbic dopamine D_1, D_2, D_4 and 5-HT$_2$ receptors
Clozapine, Risperidone, Olanzapine, Quetiapine, Ziprasidone
Partial agonist at D_1, D_2, D_3 & $5HT_{1A}$-R
Aripiprazole

Atypical antipsychotics?
- ●● Clozapine ○
- ●● Risperidone ○
- ●● Olanzapine ●
- ●● Quetiapine ●●
- ●● Ziprasidone ○
- ●● Aripiprazole ●

Mood Stabilizers,* Anticonvulsants, Others

↓ 2nd messengers, G proteins ↓ Ca⁺⁺ influx
- ●● Lithium ●*
- ●● Carbamazepine ●*
- ●● Oxcarbazepine ○
- ●● Valproate ●*

↑ Brain GABA
- ●● (Valproate) ●*
- –– (Gabapentin) ○
- – (Tiagabine) ○
- – (Topiramate) ○

↓ Glutamate release (via ↓ Na⁺)
- ●● Carbamazepine ●*
- ● Lamotrigine ●●*
- – (Topiramate) ○
- ● Zonisamide ○

↓ Glutamate (AMPA-R)
- – (Topiramate) ○

(Dihydropyridine) ↓ L-type Ca⁺⁺ channels
- ● Nimodipine ●
- ○ Isradipine ○
- ○ Amlodipine ○

(Phenylalkylamine)
- ● Verapamil –

Thyroid: Augmentation
- ○ T_3 ○

Suppression
High dose
- ○ T_4 ○

Antidepressants

Dopamine (DA)
- – Bupropion ●●
- – Pramipexole ●

Serotonin (5-HT)
- – Fluoxetine ●●
- – Sertraline ●●
- – Paroxetine ●●
- – Fluvoxamine ●●
- – Citalopram ●●

5-HT Plus
- – Nefazodone ●●
- – Mirtazapine ●●

Norepinephrine (NE)
- – Desipramine ●●
- – Nortriptyline ●●
- – Maprotiline ●●
- – Reboxetine ●
- – Atomoxetine ●

5-HT and NE
- – Clomipramine ●●
- – Venlafaxine ●●
- – Duloxetine ●●

Figure 5–14. *(opposite)* Actions of antimanic agents, antidepressants, and mood stabilizers.

Preliminary grouping of drugs used in affective illness by their general category and presumptive mechanisms of action. The anticonvulsants in parentheses (gabapentin, tiagabine, topiramate) are not mood stabilizers because they have no acute antimanic efficacy. Efficacy in mania is coded on the left and in depression on the right of each drug: ●●=established or marked effects; ●=good effect; o=possible effect; –=no effect; – –= symptom worsening. Efficacy of the unimodal antidepressants (at bottom of figure) in depression is coded only for unipolar depression because efficacy in bipolar depression has not been established.
Ca=calcium; Cl⁻=chloride; GABA=γ-aminobutyric acid; T_3=triiodothyronine; T_4=thyroxine.

the subsequent development of alcohol and substance abuse. Because of these findings, juvenile and adolescent bipolar illness should be considered for early intervention, not only to attempt to prevent the development of full-blown affective episodes but also to prevent many of the secondary adverse consequences of the illness.

It is highly promising that in adult bipolar illness, multiple treatment options are now available (Figures 5–13 and 5–14). Unimodal antidepressants, antimanic medications, and antipsychotic agents, as well as drugs such as lithium, have the ability to be effective in both manic and depressive phases, particularly in the prevention of recurrences. Determining the most effective mood stabilizers in children thus deserves the most careful clinical and research attention.

Neurochemistry of Bipolar Illness and Its Treatments

Serotonin

Serotonin is one of several transmitters in cells that help to convey electrical messages from one cell to the next across a synapse. That is, an electrical impulse releases chemical transmitters such as serotonin into the area (synapse) between cells, and serotonin binds to a receptor site on the second cell (the postsynaptic site), which is then associated with activation and firing of the second neuron. A deficiency of serotonin was postulated as a vulnerability factor in the development of recurrent affective illness (Coppen et al. 1972) and in the increased impulsivity associated with suicide attempts and completed suicide.

The serotonin-permissive theory suggests that a relative deficiency of serotonin can result in depression and also forms the basis for excessive mood and behavioral swings in mania caused by other factors. This theory has had much support with the development of SSRI antidepressants, which increase serotonergic tone in the synapse by preventing the reuptake or inactivation of serotonin, thus making serotonin more available for a longer time to act on the postsynaptic receptors (Figure 5–15). Serotonergic mechanisms have most recently been clearly implicated in unipolar depression, with the use of a tryptophan depletion test. When adult patients who have responded to an SSRI are given a diet of amino acids deficient in tryptophan (which is the precursor to serotonin), their mood is transiently worsened for several hours, indicating that blocking serotonin production (via the deficiency of brain tryptophan) transiently is associated with this lowering of mood.

New data from positron emission tomography (PET) scans have now directly shown that patients with unipolar or bipolar illness have lower numbers of the serotonin type 1A (5-HT_{1A}) receptor in their brains—further suggesting faulty serotonin regulation in these affective illnesses. What is less clear is the extent to which SSRIs and related antidepressants are useful in adult and child bipolar illness (Sachs et al. 2007).

Dopamine and Norepinephrine

Two other transmitters, dopamine and norepinephrine, called *catecholamines,* are in different cells in the midbrain and brain stem and also were postulated by Schildkraut (1965) and Bunney and Davis (1965) more than 30 years ago to be deficient in depression and excessive in mania. In terms of mechanisms of action of drugs, considerable support exists for such a theory. For example, the major tranquilizers or antipsychotic drugs that block the action of dopamine at the receptor are all antimanic agents (Figure 5–16). Moreover, blocking the synthesis of dopamine and norepinephrine also has been associated with antimanic effects. High doses of psychomotor stimulants such as cocaine and

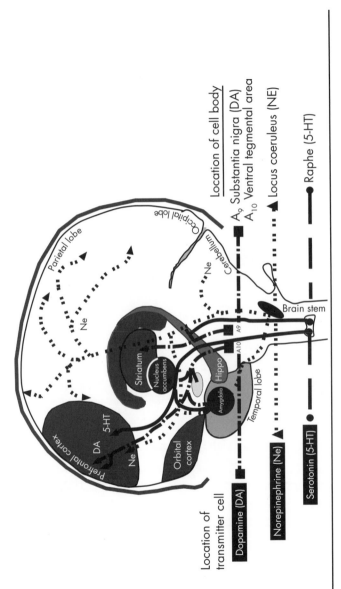

Figure 5–15. Amine systems implicated in mood.

Serotonergic neurons are located in the brain stem raphe nucleus; noradrenergic (norepinephrine, NE) neurons are in the locus coeruleus; and dopaminergic neurons are in the midbrain. Hippo=hippocampus.

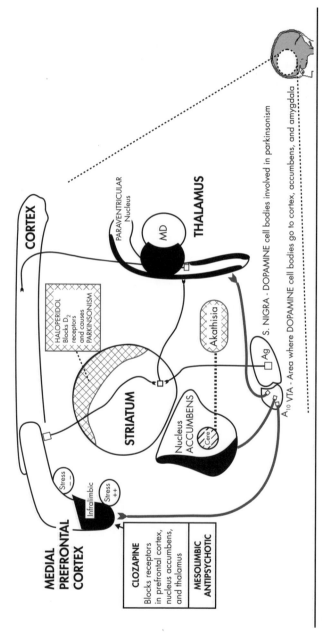

Figure 5–16. Atypical antipsychotic clozapine acts selectively on mesocortical dopamine (dark shading); the neuroleptic (or older typical antipsychotic) haloperidol acts on the striatum and produces parkinsonism and in the core of the nucleus accumbens to produce akathisia (light shading).

Cere=cerebellum; MD=mesocortical dopamine; S. nigra=substantia nigra; VTA=ventral tegmental area.

amphetamine, which increase dopamine and norepinephrine, can cause psychotic symptoms. Excesses in norepinephrine in the spinal fluid have been found in patients during manic episodes (Post et al. 1984).

Neuroendocrine and Peptide Effects

Sachar and other investigators found that depressed patients consistently secreted too much of the adrenal stress hormone cortisol during depressive episodes and that this oversecretion normalized with recovery (Sachar et al. 1973). If one gave a synthetic steroid such as dexamethasone to healthy volunteers, cortisol production in the adrenal glands completely stopped because of the body's feedback messages that there were high levels of the circulating dexamethasone. However, approximately 50% of the severely depressed patients given the same dose of dexamethasone that suppresses cortisol in healthy volunteers failed to suppress cortisol. This has now become one of the most widely replicated findings in the clinical neuroscience of depression and suggests that an increased drive in the hypothalamic-pituitary-adrenal (HPA) axis controls cortisol secretion (Figure 5–17).

Some direct evidence now indicates that corticotropin-releasing hormone (CRH) is hypersecreted in a subgroup of severely depressed patients, as measured indirectly in their spinal fluid (Banki et al. 1992). Thus, an increased amount of CRH in the hypothalamus would increase corticotropin secretion from the pituitary and release cortisol from the adrenal gland (Figure 5–17). When this happens in Cushing's disease, the hypercortisolemia is associated with fatigue, cognitive impairment, and depression in a high percentage of patients.

In a similar manner, the functional endocrine disturbance of depression is thought, at least in part, to be related to such hypercortisolemia driven by increases in CRH. Note that many of the effective antidepressant agents do, in fact, exert mechanisms that reverse this hypersecretion of cortisol. Failure to normalize the dexamethasone suppression test or the CRH hyperactivity is associated with an increased risk of relapse (Kunzel et al. 2003).

In addition to CRH, thyrotropin-releasing hormone, another peptide localized in the hypothalamus, shows evidence of increased secretion in depressive illness. Thyrotropin is released from the pituitary, and the thyroid gland secretes the hormones thyroxine (T_4) and triiodothyronine (T_3). Depressed

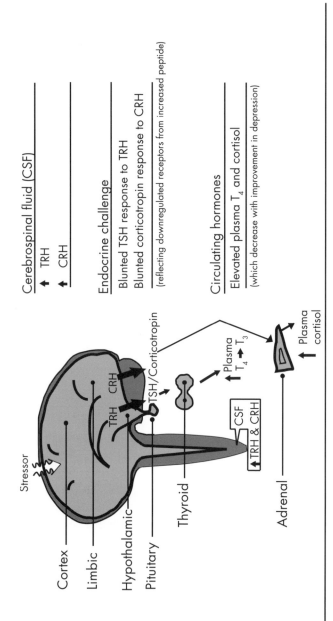

Figure 5–17.   Corticolimbic hypothalamic-pituitary-adrenal (HPA) and hypothalamic-pituitary-thyroid (HPT) axis activity is increased in depression.

CRH=corticotropin-releasing hormone; CSF=cerebrospinal fluid; T_3=triiodothyronine; T_4=thyroxine; TRH=thyrotropin-releasing hormone; TSH=thyroid-stimulating hormone.

patients also tend to hypersecrete these thyroid hormones, which normalize with improvement in the depression. Such hypersecretion is also identified by a blunted thyrotropin response to an intravenous injection of TRH (presumably because the thyrotropin receptor is downregulated secondary to the TRH excesses).

In contrast to CRH, which is thought to be intimately involved in the symptoms of depression as noted earlier, TRH secretion (Figures 5–5 and 5–17) may represent one of the body's compensatory mechanisms that attempt to restabilize the patient and act as an internal (or endogenous) antidepressant. We think that this is the case because studies of intravenous TRH have suggested that it has antidepressant effects (Prange et al. 1972). Moreover, when we injected TRH directly into patients' spinal fluid to allow sufficient quantities to reach the brain, we found that TRH had antidepressant, antianxiety, and antisuicidal effects in a small group of highly treatment-refractory patients studied at the National Institute of Mental Health (Callahan et al. 1997; Marangell et al. 1997).

Thus, because these two peptides (CRH as a representative of an endogenous "bad guy" and TRH as a representative of an endogenous "good guy") with apparently opposite effects on depression are both hypersecreted during episodes, it is thought that their relative ratio might account for the periods of illness or well intervals between episodes (Figure 5–5). That is, when CRH and other pathological factors are hypersecreted out of proportion to compensatory mechanisms, depression occurs. However, when the adaptive factors typified by TRH predominate, periods of wellness may emerge (Post and Weiss 1992).

This formulation not only helps to conceptualize why the illness may fluctuate with periods of illness and recovery between episodes but also provides a new set of targets for therapeutics. One would want not only to inhibit the "bad guys" (CRH and cortisol hypersecretion) but also to enhance the "good guys" (such as TRH and certain other alterations associated with an affective episode that may be helpful in ending it). Some effort in this direction of boosting TRH is being pursued by Winokur and associates at the University of Connecticut (Gary et al. 2003).

Evidence also shows that the peptide somatostatin (Figure 5–5) is decreased during periods of depression and returns to normal with recovery (Rubinow et al. 1987). This is of considerable interest because somatostatin is decreased in the brains of patients with Alzheimer's disease in proportion to the severity of cognitive impairment. Thus, some of the cognitive difficulties that depressed patients transiently experience could be related to alterations in this and other critical chemicals involved in cognition, learning, and memory, such as dopamine and norepinephrine. However, in contrast to Alzheimer's disease, in which cells are permanently damaged or gone, the deficit in gene expression of somatostatin in depression is temporary and normalizes when the patient recovers.

Intracellular Ions

Another highly consistent finding in depression is increased intracellular calcium in blood elements of affectively ill patients compared with healthy volunteers (Post, in press). The precise mechanism of this alteration is not known, but it is hoped that its identification in peripheral cells (i.e., those circulating in blood) might lead to the identification of similar mechanisms that could be involved in parallel with the increased intracellular calcium in brain cells (neurons). Some evidence indicates that the defect in intracellular calcium is a marker for the illness (Dubovsky et al. 1989, 1992) because it has been identified in cultured cells from bipolar patients that have undergone immortalization and multiple replications.

Thus, it would appear that something inherent in the genetics of the cells rather than the biochemical milieu in which they circulate accounts for such calcium increases. These data are also of interest in relation to the recent finding that various agents effective in the treatment of affective illness appear to exert effects on blocking calcium influx into neurons in the brain, and these agents include not only the direct voltage-sensitive calcium channel blockers of the dihydropyridine class, such as nimodipine, isradipine, and amlodipine, but also the mood-stabilizing agents, such as lithium, carbamazepine, valproate, and lamotrigine, which slow calcium influx through the N-methyl-D-aspartate (NMDA)–type glutamate receptor (Post and Leverich 2008).

Effect of Lithium and Valproate on Intracellular Messengers and Neurotrophic Factors

With the recognition that the lithium ion was effective in the treatment of bipolar illness, it was hoped that an understanding of its mechanism of action would rapidly lead to a clarification of the pathological mechanisms involved in the illness. Unfortunately, this has not proven to be easy because lithium has a multiplicity of biochemical effects, and which of these is most important to its effects on mood has not been adequately defined. In addition, the absence of a suitable animal model for bipolar illness has clearly hampered such an investigative route. With a variety of mood-stabilizing anticonvulsants now available, such as carbamazepine, valproate, and the second generation of agents such as lamotrigine, one can further hope to identify convergent mechanisms of action. Thus, finding common mechanisms among the mood stabilizers may help identify the biochemical alterations involved in the illness.

Manji et al. (1996) used this process as the basis for treating animals chronically with lithium and valproate in the hope of identifying common biochemical alterations that occur with these two agents and finding commonalities between these two different chemical substances (lithium, an ion; and valproate, a fatty acid) that might provide new clues. They found that lithium and valproate share several actions in common, one of which is the inhibition of a critical intracellular enzyme or second messenger called *protein kinase C* (PKC) (Manji et al. 1996; Zarate et al. 2007).

They went on to test the hypothesis that inhibition of this enzyme might be associated with therapeutic actions by using a PKC inhibitor (tamoxifen) that already had been approved for use in other illnesses. Tamoxifen, in addition to its effects at the estrogen receptor that make it useful in the treatment of breast cancer, is a highly potent PKC inhibitor. Manji and colleagues thus used tamoxifen in acute manic patients and found rapid-onset effects in six of the first seven patients treated (Bebchuk et al. 2000). Two other controlled, double-blind studies have now shown tamoxifen to be more effective than placebo in the treatment of acute mania. These investigators hope to test a more specific PKC inhibitor that does not share the estrogenic effects of tamoxifen to further clarify such a potential new target of therapeutics.

In addition to the PKC mechanisms, lithium and valproate affect a variety of intracellular second- and third-messenger systems, including effects on G proteins (the mechanism that links receptor activation to intracellular processes and calcium). Both of these drugs also increase binding at a specific site on DNA called *activator protein–1*, which alters gene transcription. They also inhibit a critical intracellular regulatory enzyme called *glycogen synthase kinase–3β* (ESK-3β). It is thought that these effects might be associated with the ability of lithium to increase BDNF and the neuroprotective protein BCL2 that prevents cells from undergoing preprogrammed cell death or apoptosis (i.e., a form of cell suicide). Chuang (2004) also found that lithium inhibited cell death factors (BAX and p53) and that it increased survival of neurons in culture and in animal models of stroke and Huntington's disease. These effects could be important in humans because lithium now appears to increase a marker of neuronal integrity, *N*-acetyl aspartate, and the amount of gray matter in humans, as measured by new brain imaging techniques. Whether these actions are critical to lithium's therapeutic effects in bipolar illness remains to be determined.

Convergent Physiology and Biochemistry of Bipolar Illness: Cortical Deficits and Limbic Hyperactivity

Brain Imaging and Autopsy Studies

Dramatic new technical developments have allowed the examination of functional brain activity in an awake, behaving individual. PET can measure metabolism with 18-fluorodeoxyglucose or blood flow with oxygen-15 water and convey precise information about regional brain activity during depression, mania, and normal states. In bipolar illness, considerable evidence supports the overview that the frontal cortex is underactive (and some of its neural and glial cellular elements are deficient) and the limbic system is overactive (Ketter et al. 2001).

Numerous studies have indicated that depressed patients have decrements in activity (either blood flow or metabolism) in the frontal cortex (Post 2000; Figure 5–18), often in proportion to the severity of depression as rated on the Hamilton Rating Scale for Depression. In many instances, this deficit is reported to normalize on recovery from depression. At this time, evidence also shows hyperactivity of the amygdala and nucleus accumbens (ventral striatum) in adults with bipolar illness.

Evidence links affective illness to alterations in the size and activity of structures in the medial part of the temporal lobe or limbic system, such as the amygdala, hippocampus, and parahippocampal gyrus, that are thought to be intimately involved in modulation of emotion and cognition. Thus, these modern brain imaging techniques are beginning to provide confirmatory evidence of limbic dysfunction that has long been postulated on the basis of indirect data from humans or in laboratory studies of emotion in animals. Papez (1937) first suggested that the limbic circuit is associated with modulation of emotion, and this concept has been advanced further by MacLean (1973) and many others. If this part of the brain is stimulated directly with depth electrodes in patients with epilepsy, various emotional and experiential phenomena are induced, including considerable degrees of anxiety.

Ketter et al. (2001) have shown that the local anesthetic procaine is a relatively selective activator of the amygdala and its outflow pathways into the insula, anterior cingulate gyrus, and orbital frontal cortex. The infusion of procaine is associated with either euphoric or dysphoric affects, further supporting the concept of limbic modulation of emotional function. Depressed patients have altered responsivity to procaine, with a decreased response in these crucial areas of the brain (Biederman et al. 1996).

Although multiple groups have reported an increase in the size of the amygdala in adults with bipolar illness (Altshuler et al. 1998; Brambilla et al. 2001), a substantial number of studies have reported that the amygdala is smaller than normal in children and adolescents with bipolar illness (Chang et al. 2005). Together, these studies suggest that the developmental trajectory of amygdala size is faulty in bipolar illness—too small in children, too large in adults (Post et al. 2003), both of which findings could reflect dysregulation of this critical structure. Consistent with this view are PET scan and other brain imaging studies using functional magnetic resonance imaging that suggest hyperreactivity of the amygdala to specific tasks such as recognition of facial emotion (Pavuluri et al. 2008; Rich et al. 2008; Sheline et al. 2001).

We initially observed that adults with bipolar illness had difficulties in recognizing facial emotion. Recent data from several groups now confirm that this symptom exists in very young children with bipolar illness and could represent a trait or vulnerability marker. In particular, children tended to rate more neutral faces as more angry or hostile. This cognitive dysfunction could lead to some of the difficulties that children with bipolar illness have in reading and responding to the affect of others. Thus, it would appear that the illness has not only expressive components in terms of mood and behavior abnormalities but also deficits in receptive emotional processing and signal detection and other subtle aspects of learning and memory. Attending to these

Imaging: Structural and Postmortem

Biochemistry and Function

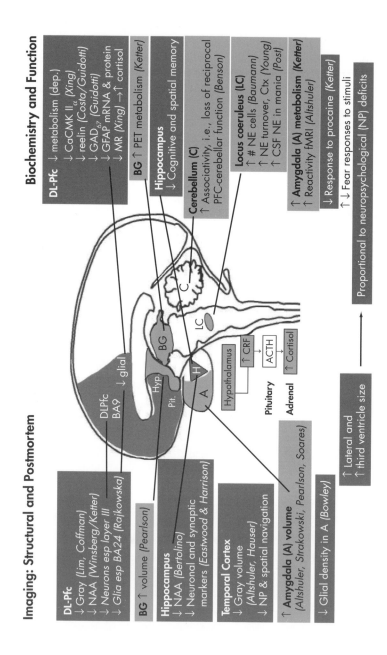

DL-Pfc
→ metabolism (dep.)
↑ CaCMK II$_\alpha$ *(Xing)*
↓ reelin *(Costa/Guidotti)*
↓ GAD$_{67}$ *(Guidotti)*
↓ GFAP mRNA & protein
↓ MR *(Xing)* →↑ cortisol

BG ↑ PET metabolism *(Ketter)*

Hippocampus
→ Cognitive and spatial memory

Cerebellum (C)
↑ Associativity, i.e., loss of reciprocal
PFC-cerebellar function *(Benson)*

Locus coeruleus (LC)
↑ # NE cells *(Baumann)*
↑ NE turnover, Ctx *(Young)*
↑ CSF NE in mania *(Post)*

↑ **Amygdala (A) metabolism (Ketter)**
↑ Reactivity fMRI *(Altshuler)*

↓ Response to procaine *(Ketter)*

↑↓ Fear responses to stimuli

Proportional to neuropsychological (NP) deficits

DL-Pfc
↓ Gray *(Lim, Coffman)*
↓ NAA *(Winsberg/Ketter)*
↓ Neurons esp layer III
↓ Glia esp BA24 *(Rajkowska)*

BG ↑ volume *(Pearlson)*

Hippocampus
↓ NAA *(Bertolino)*
↓ Neuronal and synaptic
markers *(Eastwood & Harrison)*

Temporal Cortex
↓ Gray volume
(Altshuler, Hauser)
↓ NP & spatial navigation

↑ **Amygdala (A) volume**
(Altshuler, Strakowski, Pearlson, Soares)

↓ Glial density in A *(Bowley)*

↑ Lateral and
↑ third ventricle size

Labels in figure: DLPfc BA9 → ↓ glial, Hyp, BG, Pit., Hyp., A, C, LC, Hypothalamus ↑CRF, Pituitary ACTH, Adrenal ↑Cortisol

Figure 5–18. *(opposite)* Consistent changes in bipolar affective illness—anatomy, biochemistry, and physiology: cortical deficits and limbic excesses.

There are convergent findings of decreased numbers and function of neurons and glia in prefrontal cortex (PFC) and hippocampus, whereas functional increases are apparent in adult amygdala, ventral striatum, and cerebellum. In childhood-onset bipolar illness, many investigative groups have seen the amygdala as small compared with that in healthy volunteer control subjects. As such, there appears to be an abnormal trajectory of amygdala volume over the course of bipolar illness—small in children and adolescents and large in adults. Prefrontal deficits and limbic excesses in activity could account for many of the core symptoms of bipolar illness.

ACTH=corticotropin; BA=Brodmann area; BG=basal ganglia; CaCMK II=calcium/calmodulin kinase-II; CRF=corticotropin-releasing factor; CSF=cerebrospinal fluid; ctx=cortex; DL-PFc=dorsolateral prefrontal cortex; FDG = fluorodeoxyglucose; fMRI=functional magnetic resonance imaging; GAD_{67}=glutamic acid decarboxylase; GFAP=glial fibrillary acidic protein; Hypo=hypothalamus; MR=magnetic resonance; NAA=N-acetylaspartate; NE=norepinephrine; PET=positron emission tomography; Pit=pituitary.

deficits and using remedial training techniques may help lessen the effect of such cognitive and emotional-processing deficits.

It is unclear why the amygdala, which apparently begins too small in youths with bipolar illness, ends up larger in adults. A variety of potential explanations are available, but each must be specifically assessed and tested. The amygdala could increase in size because of use-dependent neuroplasticity. For example, it has been found that taxi drivers in Great Britain have an increased size of their hippocampus, an area of brain necessary for spatial navigation. In a similar fashion, use or overuse of amygdala-related emotion modulation mechanisms in the course of the mood disorders may lead to relative hypertrophy of this structure.

Decreases in the number and activity of glial cells have been found in the frontal cortex and related areas of the brain, such as the anterior cingulate gyrus, by several investigators (Rajkowska 2000). Guoqiang Xing in our laboratory found that the enzyme calcium/calmodulin kinase II (which responds to calcium signals and is necessary for long-term memory) was decreased in the frontal cortex of those who had bipolar disorder compared with control subjects (Xing et al. 2002). Such a deficit, along with other changes, could account for some of the difficulties in cognition experienced by bipolar patients. Data also suggest that alterations in the hippocampus and anterior cingulate occur in proportion to the duration of the illness, and increases in the size of the third ventricle are related to the degree of cognitive deficit.

Another potential mechanism is that stressors appear to cause deficits in the volume of hippocampus and cortex in young animals that persist into adulthood, but there appears to be an opposite effect on amygdala and related structures. This could be related to the findings that stress tends to decrease BDNF in the hippocampus but increases it in the amygdala and, as we previously pointed out, in the dopaminergic ventral tegmental area to the nucleus accumbens pathway. Thus, stresses or even substances of abuse could be associated with these changes in the amygdala developmental trajectory.

A third possibility is that the medications used to treat the disorder are affecting amygdala volume. This would be consistent with the view that lithium, valproate, and, likely, carbamazepine all increase BDNF, and initial studies have shown that increased BDNF is associated with increases in gray matter in the cortex. Thus, effects on the amygdala are also possible and remain to be better defined. Likewise, as previously noted, all of the antidepressant modalities appear to increase BDNF, and these also could contribute to alterations in size of limbic structures. Sheline et al. (2003) had already shown that in adult patients with unipolar depression, longer antidepressant treatment compared with shorter treatment was associated with prevention of hippocampal volume losses. These and other data indicate that many of the agents that we are using to treat unipolar and bipolar mood disorders do have effects not only on brain neurochemistry but also, potentially, on the brain's synaptic microstructure and volumetric macrostructure. These drugs also increase BDNF in serum in association with clinical improvement (Aydemir et al. 2005; Gonul et al. 2005; Shimizu et al. 2003).

It is of interest that the atypical antipsychotic quetiapine, which is now approved for monotherapy treatment of not only mania but also bipolar depression in adults, has some effects on BDNF similar to those of other antidepressant modalities. If animals are repeatedly stressed while taking quetiapine (Park et al. 2006) or ziprasidone (Kim et al. 2007), the drug prevents stress from reducing hippocampal BDNF. These and a variety of other data raise the question as to whether BDNF is part of the final common pathway of antidepressant mechanisms, a possibility that requires further study.

Conclusion

Understanding the Neurobiology of Bipolar Illness: Implications for Treatment

We are beginning to have an understanding of some of the alterations in physiology and biochemistry that accompany major fluctuations in mood. The data on genetics; the very well-replicated findings of peptide, endocrine, calcium, and now BDNF alterations in bipolar illness; the consistent deficits in prefrontal cortex activity and biochemistry; and the increases in activity of amygdala and ventral striatal areas of brain (Figure 5–18) place bipolar illness very much in the realm of other medical disorders with not only distinct mood, motor, and vegetative symptoms but also an increasingly well-delineated neurobiology.

Although the "functional" or reversible brain lesions of psychiatry often have been referred to as somehow less consistent or less well documented than those of neurology (such as stroke, tumors, or neural degeneration), the information on the fundamental neurobiology of the mood disorders is beginning to alter this perspective and to place the affective illnesses and schizophrenia in the realm of true brain disorders. In fact, the functional nature of these illnesses suggests that while they may be somewhat more difficult to understand, they are much more amenable to treatment and therefore equally deserving of considerable research efforts and novel attempts at clinical therapeutics. This view is bolstered by the fact that the affective illnesses are potentially lethal medical disorders, with a lifetime incidence rate of suicide between 10% and 20%. Long-term treatment with lithium tends to normalize the suicide rate toward that of the general population, raising the hope that treatment with this agent and others will help ameliorate not only the morbidity and mortality of the mood disorders but also some of their fundamental neural alterations.

Evaluating the Risk-Benefit Ratio for a Given Treatment

The evidence of positive effects of lithium, mood stabilizers, and some atypical antipsychotics on brain neurochemistry, structure, and function puts these classes of drugs in a new perspective when considering the risk-benefit ratio for their use in youngsters with severe mood disorders. These drugs were previously considered as only productive of side effects and other adverse events, but now the potential benefits of these agents have been identified as well and may be helping to ameliorate some of the deficits that have been observed in the brains of patients with bipolar illness (Post et al. 2003) or to prevent their progression.

Such brain-protective effects may be occurring on the basis of the neurotrophic effects of many of these therapeutic agents on a direct basis, or they also may be based indirectly on preventing episodes of mania and depression, which are associated with deficits in BDNF and increases in oxidative stress, which may be further endangering neuronal and glial growth and functioning.

Also changing the risk-benefit ratio for considering the institution of treatments for serious mood disorders in children are the now clear-cut data of the seriousness of these illnesses. The data indicate that those with childhood-onset unipolar or bipolar illness tend to have a more difficult course than do those with early or late adult onsets. Thus, these illnesses are not trivial in terms of their direct consequences on mood, behavior, social functioning, education, and employment, and their indirect adverse consequences make many other psychiatric and medical comorbidities much more common and prevalent. Bipolar illness is associated with the highest incidence of alcohol and substance abuse disorders of the major psychiatric illnesses, and the occurrence and recurrence of depression is a major risk factor for the occurrence of heart attack, stroke, and other medical illnesses in adults.

At this time, it would appear that aggressive effective psychosocial and pharmacological treatment intervention in children with serious unipolar or bipolar affective dysregulation would have many benefits when considering the overall risk-benefit ratio of treatment of this condition in young children. We have underestimated both the severity and the consequences of untreated or inadequately treated childhood-onset bipolar illness, as well as the potential positive and protective effects of some medications on brain structure and functioning.

However, countering these positive impetuses for instituting treatment are other difficult variables that also deserve to be noted. As reviewed in other chapters, the potential adverse consequences of each treatment must be considered. For example, weight gain on some of the atypical antipsychotics can present considerable problems and also be associated with the development of diabetes and other elements of the metabolic syndrome (i.e., high blood pressure, hypercholesterolemia or hypertriglyceridemia, high blood sugar, insulin resistance, and overweight or an increase in waist circumference). Such adverse effects obviously should be avoided if possible, and use of other agents with less adverse side-effect profiles usually is an alternative.

Other problems confounding the early institution of effective treatment in childhood-onset bipolar illness are some of the elements of diagnostic controversy mentioned earlier. However, balanced against this would be the observation that even when the diagnosis is controversial, almost all observers agree about the severe effect of these bipolar-like affective and behavioral dysfunctions on the individual and his or her family (Axelson et al. 2006; Birmaher et al. 2006). Thus, it becomes particularly important to jump over the hurdles of diagnostic controversy and begin to better define the best treatments for those not only with classic presentations of bipolar illness but also with what is considered the broader spectrum of severe mood and irritability (Biederman et al. 1999, 2004) that some have argued is not necessarily part of the evolution to bipolar illness in adulthood (Leibenluft et al. 2003). These children require concerted evaluation and treatment nonetheless.

Some clinicians and investigators consider only bipolar I or II presentations worthy of consideration of true bipolar illness. However, bipolar disorder not otherwise specified is very common, particularly in the youngest children, and as reported by Birmaher and colleagues (2006), it is associated with an extremely difficult course and a much longer time to stabilize than is either bipolar I or II disorder. Moreover, approximately 30% of the children with bipolar disorder not otherwise specified presentations progress to either bipolar I or II characteristics during the time of prospective follow-up. This increased to 50% conversion to bipolar I or II disorder in those with bipolar disorder not otherwise specified on initial presentations if the patient had a positive family history of bipolar illness in first-degree relatives. Thus, even the more controversial bipolar disorder not otherwise specified presentations have a severe effect on behavioral functioning and appear to require even more concerted and long-term treatment to achieve a period of transient remission.

A last consideration complicates the ease of treatment intervention. That is, the database for the efficacy of agents in children is still in its initial stages (Kowatch et al. 2005). Many of the assumptions about treatment have been, by necessity, initially indirectly derived from the adult literature (Post and Altshuler, in press), and whether these assumptions will prove to be entirely accurate remains to be more systematically studied. Obviously, a great need exists for new studies of efficacy, effectiveness, and tolerability of a wide range of agents used alone and in combination in the treatment of childhood-onset bipolar illness. Such studies are not likely to be forthcoming in a timely manner without new infusions of support and funding mechanisms.

The field of adult-onset bipolar illness has similarly experienced for much of the last 30 years a comparative lack of pharmacology-related treatment studies compared with other serious mental illnesses such as schizophrenia (Post 2002). A new perspective is required about the seriousness of affective illness in both children and adults that will allow an acceleration of studies to gain the necessary controlled clinical trials database to make treatment decisions on the basis of evidence-based medicine (Post and Kowatch 2006).

A final difficulty for many children with bipolar illness and their parents is lack of access to expert care in pediatric psychopharmacology. A general deficit is seen in the number of pediatric psychiatrists available in the United States, and in particular those with expertise in the psychopharmacology of bipolar disorder. Thus, many nonspecialists need to help fill this treatment gap, and many of the ambiguities noted earlier are even more problematic for this group of nonspecialist treating physicians.

Obviously, health insurance availability also can be a critical and confounding factor in seeking appropriate care. Against all of these difficulties, it is important to note that all of the authors of this book have seen children with severe bipolar and behavioral dysregulation do extraordinarily well with appropriate treatment. Such psychotherapeutic and psychopharmacological treatment should be pursued by each family, and in this vein, we would highly recommend that parents develop a longitudinal record of their child's mood and behavior dysfunction so that the effects of psychotherapeutic and medication interventions can be systematically assessed (www.bipolarnews.org; see "Life Charting" page). The details of such an approach are discussed in Chapter 10 ("Working With Patients and Their Families") and have much to recommend (Leverich and Post 1998; Post and Leverich 2008). This approach will not only allow systematic evaluation of treatment response but also help facilitate consultation with other treating physicians should the course of illness remain difficult.

Parenting is a difficult enough job in its own right, but parenting and supervising the medical treatment of a child with bipolar disorder can be extraordinarily difficult, frustrating, and confounding. We hope that some of the background information provided about the neurobiology of the illness and its treatment will be helpful in putting the illness in the appropriate perspective and facilitating the institution of the optimal treatment regimens discussed throughout this volume.

References

Altshuler LL, Bartzokis G, Grieder T, et al: Amygdala enlargement in bipolar disorder and hippocampal reduction in schizophrenia: an MRI study demonstrating neuroanatomic specificity (letter). Arch Gen Psychiatry 55:663–664, 1998

Andreazza AC, Frey BN, Erdtmann B, et al: DNA damage in bipolar disorder. Psychiatry Res 153:27–32, 2007

Axelson D, Birmaher B, Strober M, et al: Phenomenology of children and adolescents with bipolar spectrum disorders. Arch Gen Psychiatry 63:1139–1148, 2006

Aydemir O, Deveci A, Taneli F: The effect of chronic antidepressant treatment on serum brain-derived neurotrophic factor levels in depressed patients: a preliminary study. Prog Neuropsychopharmacol Biol Psychiatry 29:261–265, 2005

Banki CM, Karmacsi L, Bissette G, et al: CSF corticotropin-releasing hormone and somatostatin in major depression: response to antidepressant treatment and relapse. Eur Neuropsychopharmacol 2:107–113, 1992

Bebchuk JM, Arfken CL, Dolan-Manji S, et al: A preliminary investigation of a protein kinase C inhibitor in the treatment of acute mania. Arch Gen Psychiatry 57:95–97, 2000

Benson BE, Willis MW, Ketter TA, et al: Altered relationships in rCMRglu associativity in bipolar and unipolar illness. Psychiatry Res (in press)

Berrettini WH, Ferraro TN, Goldin LR, et al: Chromosome 18 DNA markers and manic-depressive illness: evidence for a susceptibility gene. Proc Natl Acad Sci U S A 91:5918–5921, 1994

Berton O, McClung CA, DiLeone RJ, et al: Essential role of BDNF in the mesolimbic dopamine pathway in social defeat stress. Science 311(5762):864–868, 2006

Biederman J, Faraone S, Mick E, et al: Attention-deficit hyperactivity disorder and juvenile mania: an overlooked comorbidity? J Am Acad Child Adolesc Psychiatry 35:997–1008, 1996

Biederman J, Faraone SV, Chu MP, et al: Further evidence of a bidirectional overlap between juvenile mania and conduct disorder in children. J Am Acad Child Adolesc Psychiatry 38:468–476, 1999

Biederman J, Faraone SV, Wozniak J, et al: Further evidence of unique developmental phenotypic correlates of pediatric bipolar disorder: findings from a large sample of clinically referred preadolescent children assessed over the last 7 years. J Affect Disord 82 (suppl 1):S45–S58, 2004

Birmaher B, Axelson D, Strober M, et al: Clinical course of children and adolescents with bipolar spectrum disorders. Arch Gen Psychiatry 63:175–183, 2006

Brambilla P, Harenski K, Nicoletti M, et al: Are amygdala volumes increased in bipolar disorder patients? (abstract) Bipolar Disord 3 (suppl 1):28, 2001

Bunney WE Jr, Davis JM: Norepinephrine in depressive reactions: a review: Arch Gen Psychiatry 13:483–494, 1965

Callahan AM, Frye MA, Marangell LB, et al: Comparative antidepressant effects of intravenous and intrathecal thyrotropin-releasing hormone: confounding effects of tolerance and implications for therapeutics. Biol Psychiatry 41:264–272, 1997

Caspi A, Sugden K, Moffitt TE, et al: Influence of life stress on depression: moderation by a polymorphism in the 5-HTT gene. Science 301(5631):386–389, 2003

Chang K, Karchemskiy A, Barnea-Goraly N, et al: Reduced amygdalar gray matter volume in familial pediatric bipolar disorder. J Am Acad Child Adolesc Psychiatry 44:565–573, 2005

Chuang DM: Neuroprotective and neurotrophic actions of the mood stabilizer lithium: can it be used to treat neurodegenerative diseases? Crit Rev Neurobiol 16:83–90, 2004

Comings DE: The Gene Bomb: Does Higher Education and Advanced Technology Accelerate the Selection of Genes for Learning Disorders, ADHD, Addictive, and Disruptive Behaviors? Monrovia, CA, Hope Press, 1996

Coppen A, Prange AJ Jr, Whybrow PC, et al: Abnormalities of indoleamines in affective disorders. Arch Gen Psychiatry 26:474–478, 1972

Craddock N: The Wellcome Trust Case Control Consortium (WTCCC) Genomewide Association Study of 2000 Cases of Bipolar Depression and 3000 Controls, Seventh International Conference on Bipolar Disorder, Pittsburgh, PA, 2007

Craddock N, Jones I: Genetics of bipolar disorder. J Med Genet 36:585–594, 1999

Cunha AB, Frey BN, Andreazza AC, et al: Serum brain-derived neurotrophic factor is decreased in bipolar disorder during depressive and manic episodes. Neurosci Lett 398:215–219, 2006

DePaulo JR Jr: Genetics of bipolar disorder: where do we stand? Am J Psychiatry 161:595–597, 2004

Dubovsky SL, Christiano J, Daniell LC, et al: Increased platelet intracellular calcium concentration in patients with bipolar affective disorders. Arch Gen Psychiatry 46:632–638, 1989

Dubovsky SL, Murphy J, Christiano J, et al: The calcium second messenger system in bipolar disorders: data supporting new research directions. J Neuropsychiatry Clin Neurosci 4:3–14, 1992

Duman RS, Monteggia LM: A neurotrophic model for stress-related mood disorders. Biol Psychiatry 59:1116–1127, 2006

Dwivedi Y, Mondal AC, Rizavi HS, et al: Suicide brain is associated with decreased expression of neurotrophins. Biol Psychiatry 58:315–324, 2005

Egan MF, Kojima M, Callicott JH, et al: The BDNF val66met polymorphism affects activity-dependent secretion of BDNF and human memory and hippocampal function. Cell 112:257–269, 2003

Findling RL, McNamara NK, Youngstrom EA, et al: Double-blind 18-month trial of lithium versus divalproex maintenance treatment in pediatric bipolar disorder. J Am Acad Child Adolesc Psychiatry 44:409–417, 2005

Findling RL, McNamara NK, Stansbrey R, et al: Combination lithium and divalproex sodium in pediatric bipolar symptom restabilization. J Am Acad Child Adolesc Psychiatry 45:142–148, 2006

Gary KA, Sevarino KA, Yarbrough GG, et al: The thyrotropin-releasing hormone (TRH) hypothesis of homeostatic regulation: implications for TRH-based therapeutics. J Pharmacol Exp Ther 305:410–416, 2003

Geller B, Badner JA, Tillman R, et al: Linkage disequilibrium of the brain-derived neurotrophic factor Val66Met polymorphism in children with a prepubertal and early adolescent bipolar disorder phenotype. Am J Psychiatry 161:1698–1700, 2004

Gershon ES, Hamovit JH, Guroff JJ, et al: Birth-cohort changes in manic and depressive disorders in relatives of bipolar and schizoaffective patients. Arch Gen Psychiatry 44:314–319, 1987

Goddard GV, McIntyre DC, Leech CK: A permanent change in brain function resulting from daily electrical stimulation. Exp Neurol 25:295–330, 1969

Gonul AS, Akdeniz F, Taneli F, et al: Effect of treatment on serum brain-derived neurotrophic factor levels in depressed patients. Eur Arch Psychiatry Clin Neurosci 255:381–386, 2005

Green EK, Raybould R, MacGregor S, et al: Genetic variation of brain-derived neurotrophic factor (BDNF) in bipolar disorder: case-control study of over 3000 individuals from the UK. Br J Psychiatry 188:21–25, 2006

He XP, Kotloski R, Nef S, et al: Conditional deletion of TrkB but not BDNF prevents epileptogenesis in the kindling model. Neuron 43:31–42, 2004

Kapczinski F, Vieta E, Andreazza AC, et al: Allostatic load in bipolar disorder: implications for pathophysiology and treatment. Neurosci Biobehav Rev 32:675–692, 2008

Karege F, Perret G, Bondolfi G, et al: Decreased serum brain-derived neurotrophic factor levels in major depressed patients. Psychiatry Res 109:143–148, 2002

Kauer-Sant'Anna M, Tramontina J, Andreazza AC, et al: Traumatic life events in bipolar disorder: impact on BDNF levels and psychopathology. Bipolar Disord 9 (suppl 1):128–135, 2007

Kaufman J, Yang BZ, Douglas-Palumberi H, et al: Brain-derived neurotrophic factor–5-HTTLPR gene interactions and environmental modifiers of depression in children. Biol Psychiatry 59:673–680, 2006

Kessing LV, Andersen PK: Does the risk of developing dementia increase with the number of episodes in patients with depressive disorder and in patients with bipolar disorder? J Neurol Neurosurg Psychiatry 75:1662–1666, 2004

Kessing LV, Andersen PK, Mortensen PB, et al: Recurrence in affective disorder, I: case register study. Br J Psychiatry 172:23–28, 1998

Ketter TA, Kimbrell TA, George MS, et al: Effects of mood and subtype on cerebral glucose metabolism in treatment-resistant bipolar disorder. Biol Psychiatry 49:97–109, 2001

Kim TS, Kim DJ, Yoon SJ, et al: Increased plasma brain-derived neurotrophic factor levels following unaided smoking cessation. Paper presented at the 160th annual meeting of the American Psychiatric Association, San Diego, CA, May 19–24, 2007

Korte M, Carroll P, Wolf E, et al: Hippocampal long-term potentiation is impaired in mice lacking brain-derived neurotrophic factor. Proc Natl Acad Sci U S A 92:8856–8860, 1995

Kowatch RA, Fristad M, Birmaher B, et al: Treatment guidelines for children and adolescents with bipolar disorder. J Am Acad Child Adolesc Psychiatry 44:213–235, 2005

Kraepelin E: Manic-Depressive Insanity and Paranoia. Edited by Robertson GM. Translated by Barclay RM. Edinburgh, Scotland, Livingstone, 1921

Kuma H, Miki T, Matsumoto Y, et al: Early maternal deprivation induces alterations in brain-derived neurotrophic factor expression in the developing rat hippocampus. Neurosci Lett 372:68–73, 2004

Kunzel HE, Binder EB, Nickel T, et al: Pharmacological and nonpharmacological factors influencing hypothalamic-pituitary-adrenocortical axis reactivity in acutely depressed psychiatric in-patients, measured by the Dex-CRH test. Neuropsychopharmacology 28:2169–2178, 2003

Kupka RW, Luckenbaugh DA, Post RM, et al: Comparison of rapid-cycling and non-rapid-cycling bipolar disorder based on prospective mood ratings in 539 outpatients. Am J Psychiatry 162:1273–1280, 2005

Lange KJ, McInnis MG: Studies of anticipation in bipolar affective disorder. CNS Spectr 7:196–202, 2002

Lapalme M, Hodgins S, LaRoche C: Children of parents with bipolar disorder: a metaanalysis of risk for mental disorders. Can J Psychiatry 42:623–631, 1997

Leibenluft E, Charney DS, Towbin KE, et al: Defining clinical phenotypes of juvenile mania. Am J Psychiatry 160:430–437, 2003

Leverich GS, Post RM: Life charting of affective disorders. CNS Spectr 3:21–37, 1998

Leverich GS, Suppes P, Denicoff KD, et al: Early trauma and bipolar disorder (34B), in Syllabus and Proceedings Summary, 154th Annual Meeting of the American Psychiatric Association, New Orleans, LA, May 5–10, 2001. Washington, DC, American Psychiatric Association, 2001

Leverich GS, Post RM, Keck PE Jr, et al: The poor prognosis of childhood-onset bipolar disorder. J Pediatr 150:485–490, 2007

Li R, el Mallakh RS: Triplet repeat gene sequences in neuropsychiatric diseases. Harv Rev Psychiatry 5:66–74, 1997

Lohoff FW, Sander T, Ferraro TN, et al: Confirmation of association between the Val66Met polymorphism in the brain-derived neurotrophic factor (BDNF) gene and bipolar I disorder. Am J Med Genet B Neuropsychiatr Genet 139:51–53, 2005

Machado-Vieira R, Dietrich MO, Leke R, et al: Decreased plasma brain derived neurotrophic factor levels in unmedicated bipolar patients during manic episode. Biol Psychiatry 61:142–144, 2007

MacLean PD: A triune concept of the brain and behavior, in The Clarence M. Hicks Memorial Lectures, 1969. Edited by Boag TJ, Campbell D. Toronto, ON, University of Toronto Press, 1973

Manji HK, Bersudsky Y, Chen G, et al: Modulation of protein kinase C isozymes and substrates by lithium: the role of myo-inositol. Neuropsychopharmacology 15:370–381, 1996

Manji HK, Quiroz JA, Sporn J, et al: Enhancing neuronal plasticity and cellular resilience to develop novel, improved therapeutics for difficult-to-treat depression. Biol Psychiatry 53:707–742, 2003

Marangell LB, George MS, Callahan AM, et al: Effects of intrathecal thyrotropin-releasing hormone (protirelin) in refractory depressed patients. Arch Gen Psychiatry 54:214–222, 1997

McMahon FJ, Hopkins PJ, Xu J, et al: Linkage of bipolar affective disorder to chromosome 18 markers in a new pedigree series. Am J Hum Genet 61:1397–1404, 1997

Mendlewicz J, Lindbald K, Souery D, et al: Expanded trinucleotide CAG repeats in families with bipolar affective disorder. Biol Psychiatry 42:1115–1122, 1997

Müller DJ, de Luca V, Sicard T: Brain-derived neurotrophic factor (BDNF) gene and rapid-cycling bipolar disorder: family-based association study. Br J Psychiatry 189:317–323, 2006

Neves-Pereira M, Mundo E, Muglia P, et al: The brain-derived neurotrophic factor gene confers susceptibility to bipolar disorder: evidence from a family-based association study. Am J Hum Genet 71:651–655, 2002

Nolen WA, Luckenbaugh DA, Altshuler LL, et al: Correlates of 1-year prospective outcome in bipolar disorder: results from the Stanley Foundation Bipolar Network. Am J Psychiatry 161:1447–1454, 2004

Pandey GN, Rizavi HS, Dwivedi Y, et al: Brain-derived neurotrophic factor gene expression in pediatric bipolar disorder: effects of treatment and clinical response. J Am Acad Child Adolesc Psychiatry 47:1077–1085, 2008

Papez JW: A proposed mechanism of emotion. Arch Neurol Psychiatry 38:725–743, 1937

Park SW, Lee SK, Kim JM, et al: Effects of quetiapine on the brain-derived neurotrophic factor expression in the hippocampus and neocortex of rats. Neurosci Lett 402:25–29, 2006

Pavuluri MN, Henry DB, Nadimpalli SS, et al: Biological risk factors in pediatric bipolar disorder. Biol Psychiatry 60:936–941, 2006

Pavuluri MN, O'Connor MM, Harral EM, et al: An fMRI study of the interface between affective and cognitive neural circuitry in pediatric bipolar disorder. Psychiatry Res 162:244–255, 2008

Perlis RH, Miyahara S, Marangell LB, et al: Long-term implications of early onset in bipolar disorder: data from the first 1000 participants in the Systematic Treatment Enhancement Program for Bipolar Disorder (STEP-BD). Biol Psychiatry 55:875–881, 2004

Pezawas L, Verchinski BA, Mattay VS, et al: The brain-derived neurotrophic factor val66met polymorphism and variation in human cortical morphology. J Neurosci 24:10099–10102, 2004

Post RM: Transduction of psychosocial stress into the neurobiology of recurrent affective disorder. Am J Psychiatry 149:999–1010, 1992

Post RM: Neural substrates of psychiatric syndromes, in Principles of Behavioral and Cognitive Neurology, 2nd Edition. Edited by Mesulam MM. New York, Oxford University Press, 2000, pp 406–438

Post RM: Preface and overview (to Bipolar Depression: The Stepchild). Clin Neurosci Res 2:122–126, 2002

Post RM: Kindling and sensitization as models for affective episode recurrence, cyclicity, and tolerance phenomena. Neurosci Biobehav Rev 31:858–873, 2007a

Post RM: Role of BDNF in bipolar and unipolar disorder: clinical and theoretical implications. J Psychiatr Res 41:979–990, 2007b

Post RM: Lithium and related mood stabilizers, in New Oxford Textbook of Psychiatry, 2nd Edition. Edited by Gelder MG, Lopez-Ibor JJ, Andreasen NC. Oxford, UK, Oxford University Press (in press)

Post RM, Altshuler LA: Mood disorders: somatic treatment (pharmacotherapy), in Kaplan & Sadock's Comprehensive Textbook of Psychiatry, 9th Edition. Edited by Sadock BJ, Sadock VA, Ruiz P. Philadelphia, PA, Lippincott Williams & Wilkins (in press)

Post RM, Kowatch RA: The heath care crisis of childhood onset bipolar illness: some recommendations for its amelioration. J Clin Psychiatry 67:115–125, 2006

Post RM, Leverich GS: The role of psychosocial stress in the onset and progression of bipolar disorder and its comorbidities: the need for earlier and alternative modes of therapeutic intervention. Dev Psychopathol 18:1181–1211, 2006

Post RM, Leverich GS: Treatment of Bipolar Illness: A Casebook for Clinicians and Patients. New York, WW Norton, 2008

Post RM, Weiss SR: Ziskind-Somerfeld Research Award 1992. Endogenous biochemical abnormalities in affective illness: therapeutic versus pathogenic. Biol Psychiatry 32:469–484, 1992

Post RM, Weiss SR: A speculative model of affective illness cyclicity based on patterns of drug tolerance observed in amygdala-kindled seizures. Mol Neurobiol 13:33–60, 1996

Post RM, Jimerson DC, Ballenger JC, et al: Cerebrospinal fluid norepinephrine and its metabolites in manic-depressive illness, in Neurobiology of Mood Disorders (Frontiers of Clinical Neuroscience). Baltimore, MD, Williams & Wilkins, 1984, pp 539–553

Post RM, Weiss SRB, Pert A: The role of context and conditioning in behavioral sensitization to cocaine. Psychopharmacol Bull 23:425–429, 1987

Post RM, Speer AM, Hough CJ, et al: Neurobiology of bipolar illness: implications for future study and therapeutics. Ann Clin Psychiatry 15:85–94, 2003

Post RM, Luckenbaugh DA, Leverich GS, et al: Incidence of childhood-onset bipolar illness in the USA and Europe. Br J Psychiatry 192:150–151, 2008

Prange AJ Jr, Lara PP, Wilson IC, et al: Effects of thyrotropin-releasing hormone in depression. Lancet 2:999–1002, 1972

Racine R: Kindling: the first decade. Neurosurgery 3:234–252, 1978

Rajkowska G: Postmortem studies in mood disorders indicate altered numbers of neurons and glial cells. Biol Psychiatry 48:766–777, 2000

Reichart CG, Nolen WA: Earlier onset of bipolar disorder in children by antidepressants or stimulants? An hypothesis. J Affect Disord 78:81–84, 2004

Rich BA, Fromm SJ, Berghorst LH, et al: Neural connectivity in children with bipolar disorder: impairment in the face emotion processing circuit. J Child Psychol Psychiatry 49:88–96, 2008

Roceri M, Hendriks W, Racagni G, et al: Early maternal deprivation reduces the expression of BDNF and NMDA receptor subunits in rat hippocampus. Mol Psychiatry 7:609–616, 2002

Roceri M, Cirulli F, Pessina C, et al: Postnatal repeated maternal deprivation produces age-dependent changes of brain-derived neurotrophic factor expression in selected rat brain regions. Biol Psychiatry 55:708–714, 2004

Rubinow DR, Post RM, Davis C, et al: Somatostatin and depression, in Somatostatin: Basic and Clinical Status. Edited by Reichlin S. New York, Plenum, 1987, pp 183–192

Sachar EJ, Hellman L, Roffwarg HP, et al: Disrupted 24-hour patterns of cortisol secretion in psychotic depression. Arch Gen Psychiatry 28:19–24, 1973

Sachs GS, Nierenberg AA, Calabrese JR, et al: Effectiveness of adjunctive antidepressant treatment for bipolar depression. N Engl J Med 356:1711–1722, 2007

Schildkraut JJ: The catecholamine hypothesis of affective disorders: a review of supporting evidence. Am J Psychiatry 122:509–522, 1965

Sheline YI, Barch DM, Donnelly JM, et al: Increased amygdala response to masked emotional faces in depressed subjects resolves with antidepressant treatment: an fMRI study. Biol Psychiatry 50:651–658, 2001

Sheline YI, Gado MH, Kraemer HC: Untreated depression and hippocampal volume loss. Am J Psychiatry 160:1516–1518, 2003

Shimizu E, Hashimoto K, Okamura N, et al: Alterations of serum levels of brain-derived neurotrophic factor (BDNF) in depression. Biol Psychiatry 54:70–75, 2003

Skibinska M, Hauser J, Czerski PM, et al: Association analysis of brain-derived neurotrophic factor (BDNF) gene Val66Met polymorphism in schizophrenia and bipolar affective disorder. World J Biol Psychiatry 5:215–220, 2004

Sklar P, Gabriel SB, McInnis MG, et al: Family-based association study of 76 candidate genes in bipolar disorder: BDNF is a potential risk locus. Brain-derived neutrophic factor. Mol Psychiatry 7:579–593, 2002

Stine OC, Xu J, Koskela R, et al: Evidence for linkage of bipolar disorder to chromosome 18 with a parent-of-origin effect. Am J Hum Genet 57:1384–1394, 1995

Szeszko PR, Lipsky R, Mentschel C, et al: Brain-derived neurotrophic factor val66met polymorphism and volume of the hippocampal formation. Mol Psychiatry 10:631–636, 2005

Tsankova NM, Berton O, Renthal W, et al: Sustained hippocampal chromatin regulation in a mouse model of depression and antidepressant action. Nat Neurosci 9:519–525, 2006

Weiss SR, Post RM: Caveats in the use of the kindling model of affective disorders. Toxicol Ind Health 10:421–447, 1994

Weissman MM, Klerman GL: Epidemiology of mental disorders: emerging trends in the United States. Arch Gen Psychiatry 35:705–712, 1978

Wilens TE, Biederman J, Kwon A, et al: Risk of substance use disorders in adolescents with bipolar disorder. J Am Acad Child Adolesc Psychiatry 43:1380–1386, 2004

Xing G, Russell S, Hough C, et al: Decreased prefrontal CaMKII alpha mRNA in bipolar illness. Neuroreport 13:501–505, 2002

Zarate CA Jr, Singh JB, Carlson PJ, et al: Efficacy of a protein kinase C inhibitor (tamoxifen) in the treatment of acute mania: a pilot study [published erratum appears in Bipolar Disord 9:932, 2007]. Bipolar Disord 9:561–570, 2007

6

Pharmacotherapy 1: Mood Stabilizers

Robert A. Kowatch, M.D., Ph.D.

Lithium was first used 36 years ago to treat "manic-depressive" illness in children (Annell 1969), and since that time, various mood stabilizers have been used to treat bipolar disorder in children and adolescents. The mood stabilizers can be divided into the traditional agents—lithium, valproate, and carbamazepine (see Table 6–1 for dosing and monitoring guidelines for these three agents)—and the newer, or "novel," agents. The novel mood stabilizers include lamotrigine, oxcarbazepine, topiramate, and gabapentin (Weisler et al. 2006). These novel agents, which were developed as antiepileptic agents, migrated from neurology to psychiatry after clinicians noticed their behavioral effects. All of these agents are used to treat children and adolescents with mood and behavior problems, and all of these agents, except lithium, are used to treat seizure disorders.

133

Table 6–1. Mood stabilizer dosing and monitoring in children and adolescents with bipolar disorder

Generic name	Trade name	How supplied (mg)	Starting dosage	Target dosage	Therapeutic serum level	Cautions
Carbamazepine	Tegretol	100, 200	Outpatients: 7 mg/kg/day given in 2–3 divided doses	Based on response and serum levels	8–11 mg/L	Monitor for P450 drug interactions
Carbamazepine XR	Tegretol XR Equetro	100, 200, 400				
Lithium carbonate	Lithobid	300 (and 150 generic)	Outpatients: 25 mg/kg/day given in 2–3 divided doses	Based on response and serum levels	0.8–1.2 mEq/L	Monitor for hyperthyroidism Avoid in pregnancy
	Eskalith	300 or 450 CR				
Lithium citrate	Cibalith-S	5 cc=300 mg				
Valproic acid	Depakene	250 250 mg/5 mL (syrup)	Outpatients: 15 mg/kg/day given in 2 divided doses	Based on response and serum levels	85–110 mg/L	Monitor liver function for pancreatitis and polycystic ovary syndrome in females Avoid in pregnancy
Divalproex sodium	Depakote DR Depakote ER	125, 250, 500 250, 500				

Note.   CR=controlled release; DR=delayed relase; ER=extended release; XR=extended release.

Lithium

Lithium carbonate (Li_2CO_3) is the most well-studied mood stabilizer in children and adolescents. It is the only mood stabilizer currently approved by the U.S. Food and Drug Administration (FDA) for the treatment of "manic episodes of manic-depressive illness" in patients age 12 years and older. Lithium carbonate is a naturally occurring salt that was discovered, in 1937 by the Australian urologist Joseph Cade (1949), to have mood-stabilizing properties. In addition, recent data suggest that lithium, along with valproate, may have neurotrophic effects via indirectly regulating several factors involved in cell survival pathways, including cyclic adenosine monophosphate response element–binding protein, brain-derived neurotrophic factor, Bcl-2, and mitogen-activated protein kinases (Manji and Zarate 2002). Lithium appears to be an effective agent for the treatment of both mania and bipolar depression in children and adolescents.

Efficacy

Lithium has been used for many years in children and adolescents to treat child- and adolescent-onset mania (Brumback and Weinberg 1977; Carlson et al. 1999; Hassanyeh 1980; Horowitz 1977; Strober et al. 1988; Varanka et al. 1988) and recently has been used for bipolar depression (Patel et al. 2006). There have been six older "controlled" trials of lithium in bipolar children and adolescents. Of these six studies, four (DeLong and Nieman 1983; Gram and Rafaelsen 1972; Lena 1979; McKnew et al. 1981) used a crossover design, which is not ideal for assessing outcome in a cyclical illness such as bipolar disorder. The average number of subjects in each of these older studies was 18, and response rates ranged from 33% to 80%, reflecting the heterogeneity of the samples and the differences among study designs. In general, several open-label studies suggested that approximately 40%–50% of manic children and adolescents with bipolar disorder will respond to lithium monotherapy (Findling et al. 2003; Kowatch et al. 2000; Youngerman and Canino 1978).

In the first prospective, placebo-controlled trial of lithium in children and adolescents with bipolar disorder and comorbid substance abuse, Geller et al. (1998a) reported that 25 subjects who received lithium or placebo for 6 weeks showed a significant improvement in global assessment of functioning (46% response rate in the lithium-treated group vs. 8% response rate in the placebo group). These patients had comorbid substance abuse, and there was a statistically significant decrease in positive urine toxicology screens following lithium treatment. However, this was a small study, not all of these subjects were bipolar, some were "bipolar with predictors," and no mania rating scales were used during the study. Kafantaris et al. (1992) reported the results of an open, prospective study of 100 adolescents, ages 12–18 years, who were being treated with lithium for an acute manic episode. Of these 100 participants, 63 met response criteria, and 26 achieved remission of manic symptoms at the week 4 assessment. Prominent depressive features, age at first mood episode, severity of mania, and co-morbidity with attention-deficit/hyperactivity disorder (ADHD) did *not* distinguish responders from nonresponders to lithium. Kafantaris et al. (2004) subsequently reported the results of a placebo-controlled, discontinuation study of lithium in 40 adolescents with mania (mean age=15 years). During the first part of this study, subjects received open treatment with lithium at therapeutic serum levels (mean=0.99 mEq/L) for at least 4 weeks. Responders to lithium then were randomly assigned to continue or discontinue lithium during a 2-week double-blind, placebo-controlled phase. Of these subjects, 58% experienced a clinically significant symptom exacerbation during the 2-week double-blind phase. However, the slightly lower exacerbation rate in the group maintained on lithium (53%) compared with the group switched to placebo (62%) did not reach statistical significance. This study does not appear to support a large effect for lithium continuation treatment of acute mania in adolescents, but with only a 2-week discontinuation period, it is difficult to make definitive conclusions about the efficacy of lithium in adolescents with mania. If the discontinuation period had been longer, a clear separation between the lithium and the placebo groups likely would have been observed.

Recently, Patel et al. (2006) evaluated the use of lithium in 27 adolescents (12–18 years old) to treat an episode of depression associated with bipolar I disorder. These patients received open-label lithium, which was adjusted to achieve a therapeutic serum level (1.0–1.2 mEq/L). The mean revised Childhood Depression Rating Scale scores in these patients decreased significantly from baseline to end point, resulting in a large effect size of 1.7. The findings of this study indicate that lithium appears effective for the treatment of an acute episode of depression in adolescents with bipolar disorder.

Lithium also may be useful for the prevention of mood episodes in children and adolescents with bipolar disorder. In an early study of maintenance treatment, Strober et al. (1990) prospectively evaluated 37 adolescents whose mood had been stabilized with lithium while the patients were hospitalized. After 18 months of follow-up, 35% of these patients discontinued lithium, and 92% of those who discontinued lithium subsequently relapsed as compared with 38% of those who were lithium compliant, supporting the potential utility of lithium for maintenance treatment of bipolar disorder in adolescents.

Safety

There is concern over the effect of long-term lithium use on renal function in children and adolescents. Long-term lithium use in adults is associated with a clinically significant reduction in the glomerular filtration rate and in the maximum urinary concentrating capacity (Bendz et al. 1994). In addition, because of its action on antidiuretic hormone in the distal tubules and collecting ducts, some rare cases of diabetes insipidus following treatment with lithium have been reported that were reversible after lithium was discontinued (Gelenberg et al. 1989). Focal glomerulosclerosis occasionally has been reported in children taking lithium, but in most cases, this condition remits once the lithium is discontinued (Sakarcan et al. 2002).

The use of lithium has been associated with the development of hypothyroidism, goiter, and thyroid autoantibodies in case reports of children and adolescents (Alessi et al. 1994). Gracious et al. (2004) found that in a group of children and adolescents taking lithium and valproate for a bipolar disorder, one-quarter of this group showed thyrotropin elevations of at least 10 mU/L within an average exposure to lithium of less than 3 months. The factors associated with elevation in thyrotropin in these lithium-treated subjects included a higher baseline thyrotropin level and a higher lithium level. Close monitoring of thyroid function in children and adolescents taking lithium is recommended. Adequate birth control measures must be followed in adolescent females taking lithium because lithium is associated with an increased rate of cardiac abnormalities in fetuses; lithium thus should not be used in pregnant females (Cohen et al. 1994).

Side Effects

Lithium is not easy to tolerate, and common side effects in children and adolescents include nausea, diarrhea, abdominal distress, sedation, tremor, polyuria, weight gain, and acne. Adherence to lithium is a major problem in adolescents who find the possibility of weight gain and acne a disincentive to continuing treatment. Children younger than 6 years are more prone to develop neurological side effects, especially during the initiation phase of lithium treatment (Hagino et al. 1998). With blood levels greater than 3.0 mEq/L, patients may develop more serious neurological symptoms, including seizures, coma, and death (Gelenberg et al. 1989). Lithium occasionally may affect cardiac conduction, causing first-degree atrioventricular block, irregular sinus rhythms, and increased premature ventricular contractions (Gelenberg et al. 1989). Reversible conduction abnormalities have been reported in children (Campbell et al. 1972, 1984). A baseline electrocardiogram (ECG) and another ECG once a therapeutic level has been reached are recommended.

Medications that increase lithium level include several antibiotics (e.g., ampicillin and tetracycline), nonsteroidal anti-inflammatory agents (e.g., ibuprofen), angiotensin-converting enzyme inhibitors, calcium channel blockers, antipsychotic agents, propranolol, and selective serotonin reuptake inhibitors (e.g., fluoxetine).

Baseline Assessments

Baseline studies prior to initiating treatment with lithium should include a general medical history and physical examination; serum electrolytes; creatinine, blood urea nitrogen, and serum calcium levels; thyroid function tests; an ECG; complete blood count with differential; and a pregnancy test for sexually active females (American Psychiatric Association 1994). Renal function should be tested every 2–3 months during the first 6 months of treatment with lithium carbonate, and thyroid function should be tested during the first 6 months of treatment. Thereafter, renal and thyroid functions should be checked every 6 months or when clinically indicated. Chronic treatment with lithium can potentially cause hypoparathyroidism, and serum calcium levels should be checked once a year (Bendz et al. 1996a, 1996b).

Dosing

Lithium is readily absorbed from the gastrointestinal system, with peak levels occurring 2–4 hours after each dose. Lithium is excreted by the kidneys, and the serum half-life in children and adolescents is estimated to be approximately 18 hours (Vitiello et al. 1988). Serum lithium levels in the range of 0.8–1.2 mEq/L are typically necessary for mood stabilization, although these levels are based on studies of adults with bipolar disorder. In general, lithium should be titrated to a total dose of 30 mg/kg/day given in two to three divided doses, which typically results in a therapeutic serum level of 0.8–1.2 mEq/L. Lithium should be administered cautiously and serum levels monitored carefully in patients with significant renal, cardiovascular, or thyroid disease or severe dehydration (Table 6–1).

Valproate

Valproate (divalproex sodium; 2-propylpentanoate) is a simple branched-chain fatty acid that was first introduced in the United States in 1978 as an antiseizure agent. It is currently approved by the FDA for the treatment of complex partial seizures, migraines, and manic episodes of bipolar illness in adults.

Efficacy

Valproate has been used to treat mania in adults for many years. A review of the five controlled studies of valproate for the acute treatment of mania in adults showed an average response rate of 54%, which indicated efficacy for valproate compared with placebo (McElroy and Keck 2000). In many of these studies, positive results were obtained, even though patients were selected from a population with symptoms previously refractory to lithium treatment and illness characterized by rapid cycling, mixed affective states, and irritability. Several case reports and open prospective trials have suggested the effectiveness of valproate for the treatment of bipolar disorders in children and adolescents (Deltito et al. 1998; Kastner and Friedman 1992; Kastner et al. 1990; Papatheodorou and Kutcher 1993; Papatheodorou et al. 1995; West et al. 1994, 1995; Whittier et al. 1995). Wagner and colleagues (2006) published the results of an open-label study of valproate in 40 children and adolescents (ages 7–19 years) with bipolar disorder. In the initial open-label phase of this study, subjects were given a starting dose of divalproex of 15 mg/kg/day. The mean final dosage was 17 mg/kg/day. Twenty-two subjects (55%) showed 50% or greater improvement in Mania Rating Scale scores during the open phase of treatment, suggesting that mania will respond to divalproex in approximately half of children and adolescents.

The results of a large randomized placebo-controlled, double-blind, multicenter study designed to evaluate the safety and efficacy of Depakote ER in the treatment of bipolar I disorder, manic or mixed episode, in children and adolescents ages 10–17 years have been released (Abbott Laboratories 2006), as presented at the annual meeting of the American Academy of Child and Adolescent Psychiatry, October 2007. During this trial, 150 subjects with a current clinical diagnosis of bipolar I disorder, manic or mixed episode, were enrolled at 20 study sites. Subjects were outpatients with a manic or mixed episode and a Young Mania Rating Scale (YMRS) score of 20 or greater at screening and baseline. Subjects were randomly assigned in a 1:1 ratio to receive active study medication (250- or 500-mg tablets of Depakote ER) or matching placebo tablets. The duration of the study was 6 weeks, including a screening period lasting 3–14 days, a 4-week treatment period, and an optional 1-week taper period. No statistically significant treatment difference was found between valproate and placebo on any of the efficacy variables, primary or secondary. This trial may have had negative results because the active treatment period of 4 weeks was not long enough or because the serum levels of divalproex were not high enough. The result of one possibly negative study of valproate in children and adolescents with bipolar disorder must be interpreted with caution, and child psychiatrists should not stop using valproate until there is a more in-depth examination of this trial and subsequent replications.

Kowatch et al. (2000) presented the results of a large National Institute of Mental Health–funded controlled trial of lithium versus divalproex versus placebo in subjects ages 7–17 years with bipolar I disorder. In this trial, 153 outpatients were randomly assigned in a double-blind fashion to treatment with lithium, divalproex, or placebo in a 2:2:1 ratio. Diagnoses were made with the Washington University Schedule for Affective Disorders and Schizophrenia for School-Aged Children (K-SADS) (Geller et al. 1998b), and the primary outcome measures were weekly YMRS and Clinical Global Impression (CGI)–Improvement scale ratings. The total trial length for each subject was 24 weeks. During the first 8 weeks, subjects received lithium, divalproex, or placebo in a double-blind fashion, and no other psychotropic medications were allowed other than as short-term "rescue" agents. The mean age of these subjects was 10.6±2.7 (range=7–17). Of these subjects, 86% were male. At the end of 8 weeks, divalproex showed efficacy on both a priori outcome measures but lithium did not. The response rates based on a CGI-Improvement score of "1 or 2" (much or very much improved) were divalproex, 54%; lithium, 42%; and placebo, 29%. There was a definite trend toward efficacy for lithium, but lithium did not clearly separate from placebo on the primary outcome measures.

Safety

Valproate is metabolized in the liver by cytochrome P450 enzymes and interacts with several medications that also are metabolized by this system. Medications that increase valproate levels include erythromycin, selective serotonin reuptake inhibitors, cimetidine, and salicylates. Valproate may increase the levels of phenobarbital, primidone, carbamazepine, phenytoin, tricyclics, and lamotrigine.

Polycystic ovary syndrome (PCOS) is an endocrine disorder characterized by ovulatory dysfunction and hyperandrogenism, affecting between 3% and 5% of women who are not taking psychotropic medications (Rasgon 2004). Common symptoms of PCOS include irregular or absent menstruation, lack of ovulation, weight gain, hirsutism, and acne. There are increasing concerns about the possible association between valproate and PCOS. The initial reports of the association between PCOS and divalproex exposure were in women with epilepsy. The association was particularly strong if their exposure was during adolescence (Isojärvi et al. 1993). In a recent report about adults with bipolar disorder, a sevenfold increased risk of new-onset oligomenorrhea with hyperandrogenism was found in women who were taking valproate (Joffe et al. 2006). All females who are taking valproate should have a baseline assessment of menstrual cycle patterns and continued monitoring for menstrual irregularities, weight gain, hirsutism, and acne that may develop during valproate treatment. If symptoms of PCOS develop, referral to an endocrinologist should be considered.

Side Effects

Common side effects of valproate in children and adolescents include nausea, increased appetite, weight gain, sedation, thrombocytopenia, transient hair loss, tremor, and vomiting. Rarely, pancreatitis (Sinclair et al. 2004; Werlin and Fish 2006) and liver failure (Ee et al. 2003; König et al. 1994; Treem

1994) also can occur in children taking valproate. Fetal exposure to valproate is associated with an increased rate of neural tube defects (Weisler et al. 2006).

Baseline Assessments

Baseline studies prior to initiating treatment with valproate in children and adolescents should include a general medical history and physical examination with height and weight measurements; liver function tests; a complete blood count with differential and platelets; and a pregnancy test for sexually active females. A complete blood count with differential, a platelet count, and liver function tests should be checked every 6 months or when clinically indicated.

Dosing

Valproate is readily absorbed from the gastrointestinal system, with peak levels occurring 2–4 hours after each dose. However, if valproate is given with meals to decrease nausea, peak levels may be reached in 5–6 hours. Valproate is highly protein bound, is metabolized in the liver, and has a serum half-life of 8–16 hours in children and young adolescents (Cloyd et al. 1993). A starting dose of divalproex sodium of 15 mg/kg/day in two to three divided doses in children and adolescents will produce serum valproate levels in the range of 50–60 μg/mL. Once this low serum level has been attained, the dose is usually titrated upward depending on the patient's tolerance and response, and it is optimal to measure serum valproate levels 12 hours after the last dose (see Table 6–1). Optimum serum levels for treating mania among adults are between 85 and 110 μg/mL, and the same is thought to be true for children and adolescents (Bowden et al. 1996). Valproate should be administered cautiously, and serum levels and liver function should be monitored carefully in patients with significant liver dysfunction (Asconape 2002) and in patients with inborn errors of ammonia metabolism (König et al. 1994; Treem 1994).

Carbamazepine

Carbamazepine is an anticonvulsant agent structurally similar to imipramine that was first introduced in the United States in 1968 for the treatment of seizures. Carbamazepine is metabolized by the cytochrome P450 hepatic system to an active metabolite: carbamazepine-10,11-epoxide. Carbamazepine induces its own metabolism, and this "autoinduction" is complete 3–5 weeks after a fixed dose is achieved. Initial carbamazepine serum half-life ranges from 25 to 65 hours and then decreases to 9–15 hours after autoinduction of the P450 enzymes (Wilder 1992).

Efficacy

Two recent controlled studies of a long-acting preparation of carbamazepine in adults with bipolar disorder demonstrated efficacy for carbamazepine as monotherapy for mania (Weisler et al. 2006). No controlled studies of carbamazepine for the treatment of bipolar disorder in children and adolescents have been done, and most reports in the literature concern its use in children and adolescents with ADHD or conduct disorder (Cueva et al. 1996; Evans et al. 1987; Kafantaris et al. 1992; Puente 1975). Pleak et al. (1988) reported worsening of behavior in 6 of 20 child and adolescent patients treated with carbamazepine for ADHD and conduct disorder. Thus, there is no strong evidence to support the use of carbamazepine as a first-line agent for bipolar children and adolescents, and this drug's numerous P450 drug interactions make its clinical use difficult.

Safety

Because of its stimulation of the hepatic P450 isoenzyme system, carbamazepine has many clinically significant drug interactions in children and adolescents. Carbamazepine decreases lithium clearance and increases the risk for lithium toxicity. Medications that increase carbamazepine levels include erythromycin, cimetidine, fluoxetine, verapamil, and valproate. Carbamazepine may increase the levels of the following medications: oral contraceptives, phenobarbital, primidone, phenytoin, tricyclics, and lamotrigine (Ciraulo et al. 1995). Carbamazepine decreases the serum levels of many of the atypical antipsychotics (Besag and Berry 2006), leading to symptomatic relapses in some patients.

Carbamazepine should not be used in patients with a history of bone marrow depression, hypersensitivity to the drug, or known sensitivity to any of the tricyclic compounds, such as amitriptyline or imipramine. Administration of carbamazepine and nefazodone may result in insufficient plasma concentrations of nefazodone and its active metabolite to achieve a therapeutic effect. Coadministration of carbamazepine with nefazodone is contraindicated. Carbamazepine can cause fetal harm and is therefore contraindicated during pregnancy.

Side Effects

Common side effects of carbamazepine in children and adolescents include sedation, ataxia, dizziness, blurred vision, nausea, and vomiting. Uncommon side effects of carbamazepine include aplastic anemia, hyponatremia, and Stevens-Johnson syndrome (Devi et al. 2005; Keating and Blahunka 1995).

Baseline Assessments

A complete pretreatment blood count, including platelets, should be obtained at baseline before treatment. A patient in the course of treatment who has low or decreased white blood cell or platelet counts should be monitored closely.

Dosing

A reasonable starting dose of carbamazepine is 100 mg twice daily for patients ages 6–12 years and 100 mg three times daily for patients age 12 and older. Carbamazepine serum levels between 8 and 11 µg/mL are necessary for seizure control, but the level for therapeutic effects in bipolar youths is unknown. The total daily dose of carbamazepine should not exceed 1,000 mg in children ages 6–12 years and 1,200 mg in patients age 13 years and older (see Table 6–1).

Lamotrigine

Lamotrigine is an antiseizure agent indicated as adjunctive therapy for partial seizures, the generalized seizures of Lennox-Gastaut syndrome, and primary generalized tonic-clonic seizures in adults and pediatric patients. Lamotrigine works by blocking voltage-sensitive sodium channels and secondarily inhibiting the release of excitatory neurotransmitters, particularly glutamate and aspartate (Ketter et al. 2003). Lamotrigine also inhibits serotonin reuptake, suggesting it might possess antidepressant properties. In 2003, the FDA approved lamotrigine for the "maintenance treatment" of bipolar I disorder in adults to delay the time to occurrence of mood episodes (depression, mania, hypomania, mixed episodes) in patients who receive standard therapy for acute mood episodes.

Efficacy

Several prospective studies in adults with bipolar disorder have suggested that lamotrigine may be beneficial for the treatment of mood (especially depressive) symptoms in bipolar disorder (Bowden et al. 2003; Calabrese et al. 1999). Only one study has examined the effectiveness of lamotrigine in adolescents with bipolar disorder. Chang et al. (2006) reported the results of an 8-week open-label trial of lamotrigine alone or as adjunctive therapy for the treatment of bipolar disorders in 20 adolescents ages 12–17 years (mean age = 15.8 years) who were experiencing a depressive or mixed episode. The mean final dosage was 131.6 mg/day, and 84% of these subjects were rated as much or very much improved on the CGI Scale. Larger placebo-controlled studies of lamotrigine in bipolar children and adolescents are needed.

Safety

Benign rashes develop in 12% of adult patients and typically within the first 8 weeks of lamotrigine therapy (Calabrese et al. 2002). Rarely, severe cutaneous reactions such as Stevens-Johnson syndrome and toxic epidermal necrolysis have been described. The risk of developing a serious rash is approximately three times greater in children and adolescents younger than 16 years compared with adults, and the FDA has issued a black-box warning in the *Physicians' Desk Reference* that states, "LAMICTAL® is not indicated for use in patients below the age of 16 years." The frequency of serious rash associated with lamotrigine (defined as rashes requiring hospitalization and discontinuation of treatment), including Stevens-Johnson syndrome, is approximately 1 in 100 children (1%) younger than 16 years and 3 in 1,000 adults (0.3%) ("Lamictal [Lamotrigine] Product Information" 2001).

Side Effects

The most common side effects of lamotrigine are dizziness, tremor, somnolence, nausea, asthenia, and headache. In case reports, side effects include lupus, leukopenia, agranulocytosis, hepatic failure, and multiorgan failure associated with lamotrigine treatment (reviewed in Sabers and Gram 2000).

However, lamotrigine has been well tolerated as long-term treatment in pediatric patients with epilepsy.

Lamotrigine is primarily eliminated by hepatic metabolism through glucuronidation processes (Sabers and Gram 2000). The glucuronidation of lamotrigine is inhibited by valproic acid and is induced by carbamazepine. The addition of carbamazepine to lamotrigine decreases lamotrigine blood levels by 50%. Concomitant treatment with valproate increases lamotrigine blood levels, and, therefore, it is advisable to use lower lamotrigine doses and proceed very cautiously when coadministering these medications. Additionally, when lamotrigine is coadministered with oral contraceptives, patients may require increased lamotrigine doses because estrogen induces the metabolism of lamotrigine. However, postpartum or following discontinuation of oral contraceptives, doses should be decreased because lamotrigine levels may double for a given dose (Reimers et al. 2005). Lamotrigine crosses the placenta and is excreted in breast milk.

Baseline Assessments

Before lamotrigine is started, a patient's complete blood count, differential, and platelet count and liver function tests should be assessed and monitored as often as clinically necessary.

Dosing

The starting dosage of lamotrigine for an adolescent not taking valproate is 25 mg/day for 2 weeks, with a gradual titration to 200–400 mg/day. If the patient is already taking valproate, the starting dose of lamotrigine is 25 mg every other day for 2 weeks. It is important to follow the revised dosing guidelines for lamotrigine to avoid serious rashes. For patients younger than 12 years, the dosing of lamotrigine is weight-based, and guidelines for dosing in this age group can be found at www.lamictal.com/epilepsy/hcp/dosing/pediatric_dosing.html.

Gabapentin

Gabapentin is an antiseizure agent approved for the treatment of partial seizures in patients older than 12 years with epilepsy and for postherpetic neuralgia in adults. It is structurally similar to γ-aminobutyric acid (GABA), increases GABA release from glia, and may modulate sodium channels. Gabapentin is eliminated from the systemic circulation by renal excretion as unchanged drug and is not appreciably metabolized in humans.

Efficacy

Adult double-blind, controlled studies of gabapentin as adjunctive therapy to lithium or valproate and as monotherapy suggest that it is no more effective than placebo for the treatment of mania (Pande et al. 2000); however, gabapentin may be useful in combination with other mood-stabilizing agents for the treatment of anxiety disorders in individuals with bipolar disorder (Keck et al. 2006). In children and adolescents, gabapentin may be useful as a second-line treatment for anxiety disorders comorbid with bipolar disorder. Gabapentin has been reported to cause behavioral disinhibition occasionally in younger children (Lee et al. 1996; Tallian et al. 1996).

Safety

No specific laboratory tests are necessary before gabapentin is started. Gabapentin is not metabolized or protein bound and does not alter hepatic enzymes or interact with other anticonvulsants. The half-life of gabapentin in children is, on average, 4.7 hours.

Side Effects

Gabapentin has a relatively benign side-effect profile. The most common side effects in studies involving bipolar patients are sedation, dizziness, tremor, headache, ataxia, fatigue, and weight gain.

Dosing

The effective dosage of gabapentin is 600–1,800 mg/day given in three divided doses, with a starting dosage of 50–100 mg three times a day. The bioavailability of gabapentin is decreased by 20% with concomitant use of aluminum or magnesium hydroxide antacids.

Topiramate

Topiramate is an antiseizure agent indicated as monotherapy in patients age 10 years and older with partial-onset or primary generalized tonic-clonic seizures and in adults for the prophylaxis of migraine headache. It has several potential mechanisms of action, including blockade of voltage-gated sodium channels, antagonism of the kainate/α-amino-3-hydroxy-5-methyl-4-isoxazolepropionic acid (AMPA) subtype of glutamate receptor, enhancement of GABA activity, and carbonic anhydrase inhibition. Pediatric patients have a 50% higher clearance of topiramate compared with adults, and consequently the elimination half-life is shorter in children and adolescents.

Efficacy

Topiramate has been shown to be moderately effective in causing weight loss in adult and adolescent patients with psychotropic-induced obesity (McElroy et al. 2007; Tramontina et al. 2007). It has not been shown to be an effective mood stabilizer.

Delbello et al. (2005) reported the results of an industry-funded double-blind, placebo-controlled study of topiramate monotherapy for acute mania in children and adolescents with bipolar disorder. This trial was discontinued early by the pharmaceutical company after several trials with topiramate for adult mania failed to show efficacy. During this pediatric trial, 56 children and adolescents (6–17 years) with a diagnosis of bipolar I disorder were randomly assigned in a double-blind fashion to topiramate (52%) or placebo (48%). The mean final dosage of topiramate was 278±121 mg/day. The reduction on the primary outcome variable, the mean YMRS score from baseline to final visit according to the last observation carried forward, was not statistically different between the topiramate group and the placebo group. This is considered a negative trial, with the caveat that the results are inconclusive because premature termination resulted in a limited sample size.

Safety

Topiramate is a weak inducer of cytochrome P450 enzymes and is, therefore, potentially associated with a risk of oral contraceptive failure (particularly, low-dose estrogen oral contraceptives). Topiramate decreases the serum levels of risperidone and valproate. Topiramate is associated with limb agenesis in rodents and should be used with caution in females of childbearing potential.

Side Effects

The side effects of topiramate include sedation, fatigue, impaired concentration (Thompson et al. 2000), and psychomotor slowing. A 1%–2% rate of nephrolithiasis due to carbonic anhydrase inhibition has been reported in patients with epilepsy. Word-finding difficulties have been reported in up to one-third of adult patients who received topiramate, and this also has been reported to occur in children.

Baseline Assessments

Measurement of baseline and periodic serum bicarbonate during topiramate treatment is recommended.

Dosing

Topiramate can be started at 25 mg twice daily, and the dosage can be titrated to 100–200 mg/day over 3–4 weeks. A lower starting dose and slower titration may decrease some of the side effects of topiramate.

Oxcarbazepine

Oxcarbazepine is indicated for use as monotherapy or adjunctive therapy in the treatment of partial seizures in adults and as monotherapy in the treatment of partial seizures in children. It is the 10-keto analogue of carbamazepine, which is biotransformed by hydroxylation to its active metabolite 10,11-dihydro-10-hydroxy-carbamazepine (monohydroxy derivative, MHD). MHD is the primary active metabolite and accounts for its antiseizure properties.

Wagner and colleagues (2006) reported the results of an industry-sponsored, multisite randomized double-blind, placebo-controlled study in children and adolescents with bipolar disorder. During this study, 116 youths with bipolar disorder (mean age=11.1±2.9 years) were randomly assigned to receive either oxcarbazepine or placebo. The difference in the primary outcome variable, change in YMRS mean scores, between the treatment groups was not statistically or clinically significant. This trial did not support the use of oxcarbazepine as monotherapy in the treatment of mania in children and adolescents. Whether this medication may be useful for the treatment of bipolar II disorder/hypomania, bipolar disorder not otherwise specified, or cyclothymia is unknown.

Conclusion

Both the traditional and the novel mood stabilizers may be effective in the treatment of bipolar disorder in children and adolescents. The evidence is strongest for lithium, somewhat strong for valproate, and weaker for the other agents. Also, emerging evidence indicates that the traditional mood stabilizers, lithium and valproate, may be "neuroprotective" in the central nervous system (Chuang 2004; Rowe and Chuang 2004). The mechanisms of these possible neuroprotective effects are complex but appear to cause changes at the level of the genome (Zhou et al. 2005). In clinical practice, the combination of a traditional mood stabilizer with an atypical antipsychotic is often very helpful for patients with bipolar I disorder.

References

Abbott Laboratories: Protocol No. M01-342: a double-blind, placebo-controlled trial to evaluate the safety and efficacy of Depakote ER for the treatment of mania associated with bipolar disorder in children and adolescents. 2006. Available at: www.clinicalstudyresults.org.

Alessi N, Naylor MW, Ghaziuddin M, et al: Update on lithium carbonate therapy in children and adolescents. J Am Acad Child Adolesc Psychiatry 33:291–304, 1994

American Psychiatric Association: Practice guideline for the treatment of patients with bipolar disorder. Am J Psychiatry 151 (12 suppl):1–36, 1994

Annell AL: Manic-depressive illness in children and effect of treatment with lithium carbonate. Acta Paedopsychiatr 36:292–301, 1969

Asconape JJ: Some common issues in the use of antiepileptic drugs. Semin Neurol 22:27–39, 2002

Bendz H, Aurell M, Balldin J, et al: Kidney damage in long-term lithium patients: a cross-sectional study of patients with 15 years or more on lithium. Nephrol Dial Transplant 9:1250–1254, 1994

Bendz H, Sjödin I, Aurell M: Renal function on and off lithium in patients treated with lithium for 15 years or more: a controlled, prospective lithium-withdrawal study. Nephrol Dial Transplant 11:457–460, 1996a

Bendz H, Sjödin I, Toss G, et al: Hyperparathyroidism and long-term lithium therapy—a cross-sectional study and the effect of lithium withdrawal. J Intern Med 240:357–365, 1996b

Besag FM, Berry D: Interactions between antiepileptic and antipsychotic drugs. Drug Saf 29:95–118, 2006

Bowden CL, Janicak PG, Orsulak O, et al: Relation of serum valproate concentration to response in mania. Am J Psychiatry 153:765–770, 1996

Bowden CL, Calabrese JR, Sachs G, et al: A placebo-controlled 18-month trial of lamotrigine and lithium maintenance treatment in recently manic or hypomanic patients with bipolar I disorder [published erratum appears in Arch Gen Psychiatry 61:680, 2004]. Arch Gen Psychiatry 60:392–400, 2003

Brumback RA, Weinberg WA: Mania in childhood, II: therapeutic trial of lithium carbonate and further description of manic-depressive illness in children. Am J Dis Child 131:1122–1126, 1977

Cade JF: Lithium salts in the treatment of psychotic excitement. Med J Aust 36:349–352, 1949

Calabrese JR, Bowden CL, Sachs GS, et al: A double-blind placebo-controlled study of lamotrigine monotherapy in outpatients with bipolar I depression. Lamictal 602 Study Group. J Clin Psychiatry 60:79–88, 1999

Calabrese JR, Sullivan JR, Bowden CL, et al: Rash in multicenter trials of lamotrigine in mood disorders: clinical relevance and management. J Clin Psychiatry 63:1012–1019, 2002

Campbell M, Fish B, Korein J, et al: Lithium and chlorpromazine: a controlled crossover study of hyperactive severely disturbed young children. J Autism Child Schizophr 2:234–263, 1972

Campbell M, Perry R, Green WH: Use of lithium in children and adolescents. Psychosomatics 252:95–101, 105–106, 1984

Carlson GA, Lavelle J, Bromet EJ: Medication treatment in adolescents vs. adults with psychotic mania. J Child Adolesc Psychopharmacol 9:221–231, 1999

Chang K, Saxena K, Howe M: An open-label study of lamotrigine adjunct or monotherapy for the treatment of adolescents with bipolar depression. J Am Acad Child Adolesc Psychiatry 45:298–304, 2006

Chuang DM: Neuroprotective and neurotrophic actions of the mood stabilizer lithium: can it be used to treat neurodegenerative diseases? Crit Rev Neurobiol 16:83–90, 2004

Ciraulo DA, Shader RJ, Greenblatt DJ, et al (eds): Drug Interactions in Psychiatry. Baltimore, MD, Williams & Wilkins, 1995

Cloyd JC, Fischer JH, Kriel RL, et al: Valproic acid pharmacokinetics in children, IV: effects of age and antiepileptic drugs on protein binding and intrinsic clearance. Clin Pharmacol Ther 53:22–29, 1993

Cohen LS, Friedman JM, Jefferson JW, et al: A reevaluation of risk of in utero exposure to lithium [published erratum appears in JAMA 271:1485, 1994]. JAMA 271:146–150, 1994

Cueva JE, Overall JE, Small AM, et al: Carbamazepine in aggressive children with conduct disorder: a double-blind and placebo-controlled study. J Am Acad Child Adolesc Psychiatry 35:480–490, 1996

Delbello MP, Findling RL, Kushner S, et al: A pilot controlled trial of topiramate for mania in children and adolescents with bipolar disorder. J Am Acad Child Adolesc Psychiatry 44:539–547, 2005

DeLong GR, Nieman MA: Lithium-induced behavior changes in children with symptoms suggesting manic-depressive illness. Psychopharmacol Bull 19:258–265, 1983

Deltito JA, Levitan J, Damore J, et al: Naturalistic experience with the use of divalproex sodium on an in-patient unit for adolescent psychiatric patients. Acta Psychiatr Scand 97:236–240, 1998

Devi K, George S, Criton S, et al: Carbamazepine—the commonest cause of toxic epidermal necrolysis and Stevens-Johnson syndrome: a study of 7 years. Indian J Dermatol Venereol Leprol 71:325–328, 2005

Ee LC, Shepherd RW, Cleghorn GJ, et al: Acute liver failure in children: a regional experience. J Paediatr Child Health 39:107–110, 2003

Evans RW, Clay TH, Gualtieri CT: Carbamazepine in pediatric psychiatry. J Am Acad Child Adolesc Psychiatry 26:2–8, 1987

Findling RL, McNamara NK, Gracious BL, et al: Combination lithium and divalproex sodium in pediatric bipolarity. J Am Acad Child Adolesc Psychiatry 42:895–901, 2003

Gelenberg AJ, Kane JM, Keller MB, et al: Comparison of standard and low serum levels of lithium for maintenance treatment of bipolar disorder. N Engl J Med 321:1489–1493, 1989

Geller B, Cooper TB, Sun K, et al: Double-blind and placebo-controlled study of lithium for adolescent bipolar disorders with secondary substance dependency. J Am Acad Child Adolesc Psychiatry 37:171–178, 1998a

Geller B, Warner K, Williams M, et al: Prepubertal and young adolescent bipolarity versus ADHD: assessment and validity using the WASH-U-KSADS, CBCL, and TRF. J Affect Disord 51:93–100, 1998

Gracious BL, Findling RL, Seman C, et al: Elevated thyrotropin in bipolar youths prescribed both lithium and divalproex sodium. J Am Acad Child Adolesc Psychiatry 43:215–220, 2004

Gram LF, Rafaelsen OJ: Lithium treatment of psychotic children and adolescents: a controlled clinical trial. Acta Psychiatr Scand 3:253–260, 1972

Hagino OR, Weller EB, Weller RA, et al: Comparison of lithium dosage methods for preschool- and early school-age children. J Am Acad Child Adolesc Psychiatry 37:60–65, 1998

Hassanyeh D: Bipolar affective psychosis with onset before age 16 years: report of 10 cases. Br J Psychiatry 137:530–539, 1980

Horowitz HA: Lithium and the treatment of adolescent manic depressive illness. Dis Nerv Syst 38:480–483, 1977

Isojärvi JI, Laatikainen TJ, Pakarinen AJ, et al: Polycystic ovaries and hyperandrogenism in women taking valproate for epilepsy. N Engl J Med 329:1383–1388, 1993

Joffe H, Cohen LS, Suppes T, et al: Valproate is associated with new-onset oligoamenorrhea with hyperandrogenism in women with bipolar disorder. Biol Psychiatry 59:1078–1086, 2006

Kafantaris V, Campbell M, Padron-Gayol MV, et al: Carbamazepine in hospitalized aggressive conduct disorder children: an open pilot study [published erratum appears in Psychopharmacol Bull 28:220, 1992]. Psychopharmacol Bull 28:193–199, 1992

Kafantaris V, Coletti DJ, Dicker R, et al: Lithium treatment of acute mania in adolescents: a placebo-controlled discontinuation study. J Am Acad Child Adolesc Psychiatry 43:984–993, 2004

Kastner T, Friedman DL: Verapamil and valproic acid treatment of prolonged mania. J Am Acad Child Adolesc Psychiatry 31:271–275, 1992

Kastner T, Friedman DL, Plummer AT, et al: Valproic acid for the treatment of children with mental retardation and mood symptomatology. Pediatrics 86:467–472, 1990

Keating A, Blahunka P: Carbamazepine-induced Stevens-Johnson syndrome in a child. Ann Pharmacother 29:538–539, 1995

Keck PE Jr, Strawn JR, McElroy SL: Pharmacologic treatment considerations in co-occurring bipolar and anxiety disorders. J Clin Psychiatry 67 (suppl 1):8–15, 2006

Ketter TA, Wang PW, Becker OV, et al: The diverse roles of anticonvulsants in bipolar disorders. Ann Clin Psychiatry 15:95–108, 2003

König SA, Siemes H, Bläker F, et al: Severe hepatotoxicity during valproate therapy: an update and report of eight new fatalities. Epilepsia 35:1005–1015, 1994

Kowatch RA, Suppes T, Carmody TJ, et al: Effect size of lithium, divalproex sodium and carbamazepine in children and adolescents with bipolar disorder. J Am Acad Child Adolesc Psychiatry 39:713–720, 2000

Lamictal (lamotrigine). Physicians' Desk Reference, 55th Edition. Research Triangle Park, NC, Thomson Healthcare, 2001

Lee DO, Steingard RJ, Cesena M, et al: Behavioral side effects of gabapentin in children. Epilepsia 37:87–90, 1996

Lena B: Lithium in child and adolescent psychiatry. Arch Gen Psychiatry 36 (8 spec no):854–855, 1979

Manji HK, Zarate CA: Molecular and cellular mechanisms underlying mood stabilization in bipolar disorder: implications for the development of improved therapeutics. Mol Psychiatry 7 (suppl 1):S1–S7, 2002

McElroy SL, Keck PE Jr: Pharmacologic agents for the treatment of acute bipolar mania. Biol Psychiatry 48:539–557, 2000

McElroy SL, Frye MA, Altshuler LL, et al: A 24-week, randomized, controlled trial of adjunctive sibutramine versus topiramate in the treatment of weight gain in overweight or obese patients with bipolar disorders. Bipolar Disord 9:426–434, 2007

McKnew DH, Cytryn L, Buchsbaum MS, et al: Lithium in children of lithium-responding parents. Psychiatry Res 4:171–180, 1981

Pande AC, Crockatt JG, Janney CA, et al: Gabapentin in bipolar disorder: a placebo-controlled trial of adjunctive therapy. Gabapentin Bipolar Disorder Study Group. Bipolar Disord 2 (3 pt 2):249–255, 2000

Papatheodorou G, Kutcher SP: Divalproex sodium treatment in late adolescent and young adult acute mania. Psychopharmacol Bull 29:213–219, 1993

Papatheodorou G, Kutcher SP, Katic M, et al: The efficacy and safety of divalproex sodium in the treatment of acute mania in adolescents and young adults: an open clinical trial. J Clin Psychopharmacol 15:110–116, 1995

Patel NC, DelBello MP, Bryan HS, et al: Open-label lithium for the treatment of adolescents with bipolar depression. J Am Acad Child Adolesc Psychiatry 45:289–297, 2006

Pleak RR, Birmaher B, Gavrilescu A, et al: Mania and neuropsychiatric excitation following carbamazepine. J Am Acad Child Adolesc Psychiatry 27:500–503, 1988

Puente RM: The use of carbamazepine in the treatment of behavioural disorders in children, in Epileptic Seizures—Behaviour—Pain. Edited by Birkmayer W. Baltimore, MD, University Park Press, 1975, pp 243–252

Rasgon N: The relationship between polycystic ovary syndrome and antiepileptic drugs: a review of the evidence. J Clin Psychopharmacol 24:322–334, 2004

Reimers A, Helde G, Brodtkorb E: Ethinyl estradiol, not progestogens, reduces lamotrigine serum concentrations. Epilepsia 46:1414–1417, 2005

Rowe MK, Chuang DM: Lithium neuroprotection: molecular mechanisms and clinical implications. Expert Rev Mol Med 6:1–18, 2004

Sabers A, Gram L: Newer anticonvulsants: comparative review of drug interactions and adverse effects. Drugs 60:23–33, 2000

Sakarcan A, Thomas DB, O'Reilly KP, et al: Lithium-induced nephrotic syndrome in a young pediatric patient. Pediatr Nephrol 17:290–292, 2002

Sinclair DB, Berg M, Breault R: Valproic acid-induced pancreatitis in childhood epilepsy: case series and review. J Child Neurol 19:498–502, 2004

Strober M, Morrell W, Burroughs J, et al: A family study of bipolar I disorder in adolescence: early onset of symptoms linked to increased familial loading and lithium resistance. J Affect Disord 15:255–268, 1988

Strober M, Morrell W, Lampert C, et al: Relapse following discontinuation of lithium maintenance therapy in adolescents with bipolar I illness: a naturalistic study. Am J Psychiatry 147:457–461, 1990

Tallian KB, Nahata MC, Lo W, et al: Gabapentin associated with aggressive behavior in pediatric patients with seizures. Epilepsia 37:501–502, 1996

Thompson PJ, Baxendale SA, Duncan JS, et al: Effects of topiramate on cognitive function. J Neurol Neurosurg Psychiatry 69:636–641, 2000

Tramontina S, Zeni CP, Pheula G, et al: Topiramate in adolescents with juvenile bipolar disorder presenting weight gain due to atypical antipsychotics or mood stabilizers: an open clinical trial. J Child Adolesc Psychopharmacol 17:129–134, 2007

Treem WR: Inherited and acquired syndromes of hyperammonemia and encephalopathy in children. Semin Liver Dis 14:236–258, 1994

Varanka TM, Weller RA, Weller EB, et al: Lithium treatment of manic episodes with psychotic features in prepubertal children. Am J Psychiatry 145:1557–1559, 1988

Vitiello B, Behar D, Malone R, et al: Pharmacokinetics of lithium carbonate in children. J Clin Psychopharmacol 8:355–359, 1988

Wagner KD, Kowatch RA, Emslier GJ, et al: A double-blind, randomized, placebo-controlled trial of oxcarbazepine in the treatment of bipolar disorder in children and adolescents [published erratum appears in Am J Psychiatry 163:1843, 2006]. Am J Psychiatry 163:1179–1186, 2006

Weisler RH, Cutler AJ, Ballenger JC, et al: The use of antiepileptic drugs in bipolar disorders: a review based on evidence from controlled trials. CNS Spectr 11:788–799, 2006

Werlin SL, Fish DL: The spectrum of valproic acid-associated pancreatitis. Pediatrics 118:1660–1663, 2006

West SA, Keck PE Jr, McElroy SL, et al: Open trial of valproate in the treatment of adolescent mania. J Child Adolesc Psychopharmacol 4:263–267, 1994

West SA, Keck PE Jr, McElroy SL: Oral loading doses in the valproate treatment of adolescents with mixed bipolar disorder. J Child Adolesc Psychopharmacol 5:225–231, 1995

Whittier MC, West SA, Galli VB, et al: Valproic acid for dysphoric mania in a mentally retarded adolescent. J Clin Psychiatry 56:590–591, 1995

Wilder BJ: Pharmacokinetics of valproate and carbamazepine. J Clin Psychopharmacol 12 (1 suppl):64S–68S, 1992

Youngerman J, Canino IA: Lithium carbonate use in children and adolescents: a survey of the literature. Arch Gen Psychiatry 35:216–224, 1978

Zhou R, Gray NA, Yuan P, et al: The anti-apoptotic, glucocorticoid receptor cochaperone protein BAG-1 is a long-term target for the actions of mood stabilizers. J Neurosci 25:4493–4502, 2005

7

Pharmacotherapy 2: Atypical Antipsychotics

Robert A. Kowatch, M.D., Ph.D.

The atypical antipsychotics are powerful psychotropic agents that are efficacious and effective for the treatment of mania in adults, adolescents, and children with bipolar disorder. These agents demonstrate both mood-stabilizing and antipsychotic properties with therapeutic effects on both depressive and manic symptoms. A recent meta-analysis of controlled clinical trials of the atypical antipsychotics concluded that all of the five newer atypical antipsychotics (aripiprazole, olanzapine, quetiapine, risperidone, and ziprasidone) were superior to placebo for the treatment of mania in adults with bipolar disorder (Perlis et al. 2006).

All of the atypical antipsychotics except clozapine have received U.S. Food and Drug Administration (FDA) approval for the treatment of mania associated with bipolar disorder in adults. Olanzapine, aripiprazole, and quetiapine have also received FDA approval as maintenance treatment for adults with bipolar disorder. Risperidone is indicated by the FDA for the short-term treatment of acute manic or mixed episodes associated with bipolar I disorder in children and adolescents ages 10–17 years. Aripiprazole is indicated for the acute and maintenance treatment of manic and mixed episodes associated with bipolar I disorder with or without psychotic features in pediatric patients 10–17 years of age. Olanzapine has a positive approval letter by the FDA for a bipolar indication in children and adolescents, and it is likely that quetiapine and ziprasidone will also be given an FDA indication in this population once the results of these industry-sponsored controlled studies are reviewed by the FDA. The atypical antipsychotics are better tolerated than the typical antipsychotics because they generally have a lower rate of extrapyramidal and other side effects (Stigler et al. 2001), and they are widely used in child psychiatry to treat autism, schizophrenia, conduct disorder, bipolar disorder, Tourette's syndrome, and posttraumatic stress disorder. Figure 7–1 compares the change in Young Mania Rating Scale (YMRS) scores across the five controlled studies of atypical antipsychotics in pediatric bipolar disorder versus scores from the Pediatric Bipolar Collaborative trial (Kowatch et al. 2007) for lithium and valproate discussed in Chapter 6 ("Pharmacotherapy 1: Mood Stabilizers") of this book. The figure shows the large changes in YMRS scores seen with the atypical antipsychotics versus the moderate changes seen with the mood stabilizers lithium and valproate.

Early Studies of Atypical Antipsychotics

There were several early reports suggesting that atypical antipsychotics, including clozapine (Kowatch et al. 1995), risperidone (Frazier et al. 1999), olanzapine (Chang and Ketter 2000; Soutullo et al. 1999), quetiapine (DelBello et al. 2002), and aripiprazole (Biederman et al. 2007), are effective for the treatment of mania in pediatric bipolar disorder. In a retrospective case series of children and adolescents who were severely ill (50% with bipolar disorder), Kowatch et al. (1995) found that Clinical Global Impression (CGI) severity ratings significantly improved from baseline to end point and that patients experienced minimal side effects following treatment with clozapine. However, the serious side effects of clozapine, including seizures, daytime sedation, and agranulocytosis, have limited clozapine's use in pediatric bipolar disorder.

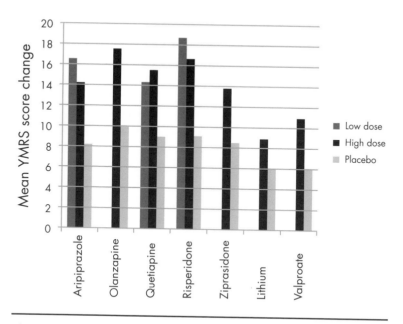

Figure 7–1.   Mean change in Young Mania Rating Scale (YMRS) scores from baseline across five controlled studies of atypical antipsychotics in pediatric bipolar disorder versus the scores from a controlled trial of lithium and valproate (Pediatric Bipolar Collaborative Study; Kowatch et al. 2007).

Risperidone

Risperidone is widely used in child psychiatry to treat irritability associated with pervasive developmental disorders (McCracken et al. 2002), aggressive behaviors associated with conduct disorder (Findling et al. 2000), psychotic disorders (Sikich et al. 2002), and bipolar disorder (Saxena et al. 2006). It is a very potent atypical antipsychotic that has been available in the U.S. market since 1993, making it the second-oldest atypical available in the United States after clozapine. In 2007 risperidone was given the first FDA indication for an atypical antipsychotic for the short-term treatment of acute manic or mixed episodes associated with bipolar I disorder in children and adolescents ages 10–17 years.

There were two early studies of risperidone for the treatment of youth with bipolar disorder. In the first, Frazier et al. (1999) performed a retrospective chart review evaluating risperidone as adjunctive treatment for pediatric mania ($N=28$). Subjects received risperidone at a mean dose of 1.7 ± 1.3 mg over an average period of 6.1 ± 8.5 months. The investigators found that response (defined as a CGI-Improvement score of ≤2) was achieved in 82% of youth with both manic and aggressive symptoms and 69% of youth with psychotic symptoms, but only 8% of youth with attention-deficit/hyperactivity disorder symptoms. In a more recent open-label prospective study, Biederman et al. (2005b) conducted an 8-week, open-label, prospective study of risperidone monotherapy (1.25 ± 1.5 mg/day) for 30 bipolar youths (manic, mixed, or hypomanic; 6–17 years of age) and reported that 70% responded positively, as defined by a CGI improvement score of ≤2. Weight increased significantly from baseline (2.1 ± 2.0 kg), and there was a fourfold increase in prolactin levels from baseline ($P<0.001$). Additionally, patients were permitted to continue their stimulant medications if needed during the course of this study. Side effects that are commonly reported with risperidone include extrapyramidal symptoms, weight gain, and prolactin elevation.

Risperidone's efficacy for short-term treatment of mania in children and adolescents was demonstrated in a 3-week, randomized, double-blind, placebo-controlled, multicenter study of 169 patients ages 10–17 who were experiencing a manic or mixed episode of bipolar I disorder (Pandina et al. 2007). Subjects in this trial were assigned to receive either low-dose risperidone, 0.5–2.5 mg/day, or high-dose risperidone, 3.0–6.0 mg/day. In both active medication groups, treatment with risperidone significantly decreased the total YMRS score, a measure of the severity of manic symptoms. No evidence of increased efficacy was observed at dosages higher than 2.5 mg/day. Adverse reactions in more than 5% of 169 pediatric patients during this trial included fatigue, dizziness, dystonia, parkinsonism, akathisia, abdominal pain, dyspepsia, nausea, vomiting, and diarrhea (Janssen Pharmaceuticals 2008). Subjects in the high-dose group had significantly more extrapyramidal symptoms than those in the low-dose group, 25% versus 5%.

The recommended dosage of risperidone in the *Physicians' Desk Reference* for children and adolescents with bipolar mania is initially 0.5 mg/day titrated in increments of 0.5–1 mg/day to a target dosage of 2.5 mg/day. Many patients can be adequately treated with 1–2 mg/day of risperidone. The half-lives of risperidone and its major active metabolite, 9-hydroxyrisperidone, in children are 3 ± 2.3 hours and 22 ± 46 hours, respectively (Aman et al. 2007). The pharmacological activity of 9-hydroxyrisperidone is similar to that of risperidone. The main metabolic pathway is through hydroxylation of risperidone to 9-hydroxyrisperidone by the hepatic enzyme cytochrome P450 (CYP) 2D6. Food does not affect the rate or extent of absorption. Risperidone is extensively metabolized in the liver by the CYP2D6 system (Aman et al. 2007). In long-term studies in children with autism, the most commonly reported adverse events associated with risperidone in children and adolescents have been rhinitis, abdominal pain, increased saliva, body pain, gynecomastia, and weight gain (Reyes et al. 2006).

Olanzapine

Several early case series and open-label prospective studies demonstrated that olanzapine was effective for the treatment of mania associated with pediatric bipolar disorder (Chang and Ketter 2000; Frazier et al. 2001; Khouzam and El-Gabalawi 2000; Soutullo et al. 1999). Recently, a large, industry-sponsored, double-blind, placebo-controlled study of olanzapine was completed (Tohen et al. 2007). This study included 159 children and adolescents (ages 10–17 years) with bipolar disorder who were randomly assigned to receive placebo or olanzapine (1:2 ratio) for 3 weeks. The modal daily dose of olanzapine was 9.7 ± 4.5 mg during this study. There was a statistically significant greater reduction in manic symptoms in the olanzapine group as compared with the placebo group. However, 42% of the children and adolescents gained $\geq 7\%$ of their baseline body weight. Other side effects of olanzapine included lipid profile abnormalities and elevated prolactin levels.

It is clear that bipolar disorder does not start at age 18 years and may actually manifest in preschoolers (Danielyan et al. 2007). Biederman et al. (2005a) compared 8 weeks of risperidone versus olanzapine monotherapy for the treatment of preschoolers with bipolar disorder. Risperidone was initiated at an open-label dosage of 0.25 mg/day, and the dosage was increased weekly according to response and tolerability to a maximum of 2.0 mg/day. Olanzapine was initiated at 1.25 mg/day, and the dosage was increased to no more than 10 mg/day. The authors reported decreases in YMRS scores of 18.3 ± 11.9 ($P < 0.001$) in risperidone-treated subjects and of 12.1 ± 10.4 ($P < 0.001$) in olanzapine-treated subjects that did not differ between groups (P=0.2). However, the small sample size of this trial limited the ability to detect statistically significant treatment group differences in response.

Quetiapine

There are two controlled studies that suggest the efficacy of quetiapine for adolescent mania (DelBello et al. 2002, 2006). In a double-blind, placebo-controlled study, DelBello et al. (2002) examined the efficacy, safety, and tolerability of quetiapine as an adjunct to divalproex for acute mania in adolescents with bipolar disorder. In this study, 30 adolescents with mania or with mixed bipolar I disorder (ages 12–18 years) received an initial divalproex dose of 20 mg/kg and were randomly assigned to 6 weeks of combination therapy with quetiapine, which was titrated to 450 mg/day (n=15), or placebo (n=15). Primary efficacy measures were change from baseline to end point in YMRS score and YMRS response rate. Safety and tolerability were assessed weekly. The divalproex and quetiapine group demonstrated a statistically significant greater reduction in manic symptoms than the divalproex and placebo group (P=0.03). Moreover, YMRS response rate was significantly greater in the divalproex and quetiapine group than in the divalproex and placebo group (87% vs. 53%, P=0.05). No significant group differences from baseline to end point in safety measures were noted. These data indicate that the combination of a mood stabilizer and an atypical antipsychotic agent may be more effective than a mood stabilizer alone for the treatment of mania in bipolar youths.

In a follow-up study, DelBello et al. (2006) randomly assigned 50 adolescents (ages 12–18 years) with bipolar I disorder, manic or mixed episode, to receive quetiapine (400–600 mg/day) or divalproex (serum level=80–120 µg/mL) for 28 days in a double-blind study. The patients receiving quetiapine had faster resolution of their manic symptoms and higher rates of remission than those treated with divalproex. Additionally, both medications were well tolerated.

In a large, industry-sponsored, controlled trial, 277 subjects with bipolar I disorder, manic episode, were assigned to receive quetiapine 400 mg/day, 600 mg/day, or placebo in a double-blind fashion for 3 weeks (DelBello et al. 2007). Quetiapine demonstrated efficacy at both dosages as compared with placebo. The most common adverse effects noted with quetiapine were somnolence, sedation, dizziness, and weight gain (+1.7 kg).

Aripiprazole

Two early retrospective case series reports of aripiprazole reported that approximately 70% of children and adolescents with bipolar disorders responded to aripiprazole (Barzman et al. 2004; Biederman et al. 2007). There also was a large, industry-supported, multisite clinical trial in which 296 subjects with bipolar I disorder, mixed or manic episode, were randomly assigned to receive aripiprazole or placebo for 4 weeks (Wagner et al. 2007). During this trial, subjects were randomly assigned to receive either 10 mg/day or 30 mg/day of aripiprazole or placebo in a 1:1:1 ratio. Aripiprazole demonstrated clinical and statistical superiority to placebo at both dosages, with 45% in the low-dose group versus 64% in the high-dose group demonstrating a ≥50% drop in their baseline YMRS scores. The most common adverse events reported during this trial were somnolence (23%), extrapyramidal disorder (18%), and fatigue (11%).

Ziprasidone

Ziprasidone has the advantage of being associated with the least amount of weight gain among the atypical antipsychotics in adults (Correll and Carlson 2006). In a recently completed dose-finding, 3-week, open-label study of ziprasidone for adolescents with psychosis ($N=63$; $n=46$ with bipolar disorder), patients were randomly assigned to receive 40 mg twice daily (low-dose group, $n=23$) or 80 mg twice daily (high-dose group, $n=40$) of ziprasidone, with the dose titrated over approximately 10 days. There was a mean ($\pm$SD) reduction in YMRS score of 17.2 ($\pm$8.2) for completers in the low-dose group and 13.1 ($\pm$8.9) for completers in the high-dose group (Versavel et al. 2005). The most common side effects in this study included sedation, nausea, headaches, and dizziness. QTc change over the course of the 3 weeks at the maximum serum concentration of ziprasidone was 1.3 msec for the low-dose group (80 mg/day) and 11.2 msec for the high-dose group (160 mg/day), indicating that ziprasidone in this trial had modest effects on the QTc interval.

Also, DelBello et al. (2008) recently completed a multisite, industry-sponsored study of ziprasidone, during which 238 subjects with bipolar I disorder, manic or mixed, were randomly assigned in a 2:1 ratio in a double-blind fashion to treatment with flexible-dose ziprasidone (80–160 mg/day) or placebo. In the intent-to-treat analysis, the estimated least squares mean changes from baseline to end point in the YMRS total score were −13.83 for ziprasidone and −8.61 for placebo ($P=0.0005$). Thus ziprasidone demonstrated an effect that was clinically and statistically significant in children and adolescents with bipolar I disorder. No significant changes in mean body mass index z scores or lipids, liver enzymes, or glucose levels were reported.

Management of Adverse Events With Atypical Antipsychotics

Although the atypical antipsychotics are very powerful psychotropics with demonstrated efficacy for pediatric mania, they also have significant adverse effects. Specific adverse effects of the use of atypical antipsychotics in children and adolescents that pose long-term concerns include tardive dyskinesia, weight gain, and increased serum prolactin levels.

Movement Disorders

In clinical trials that included 1,885 children and adolescents with autistic disorder or other psychiatric disorders treated with risperidone, 2 patients (0.1%) were reported to have tardive dyskinesia, which resolved when risperidone was discontinued (Janssen Pharmaceuticals 2008). The best way to monitor for the emergence of tardive dyskinesia is to use the Abnormal Involuntary Movement Scale at baseline and every 6 months for pediatric patients who are taking risperidone.

Weight Gain

In long-term, open-label trials, patients with autistic disorder or other psychiatric disorders treated with risperidone gained an average of 7.5 kg during 12 months of treatment; most of the weight gain occurred within the first 6 months (Croonenberghs et al. 2005). The expected normal weight gain in children is 3–3.5 kg per year adjusted for age, based on Centers for Disease Control and Prevention normative data.

It is good clinical practice to follow the American Diabetes Association et al. (2004) guidelines for monitoring antipsychotic treatment and intervene if clinically significant weight gain occurs. Klein et al. (2006) have demonstrated that metformin can aid in reversing the weight gain from atypical antipsychotics in children and adolescents. Potential side effects of metformin include hypoglycemia, diarrhea, nausea/vomiting, and, rarely, lactic acidosis. In this 16-week study, no adverse events were attributed to metformin.

Many agents used to treat children and adolescents with bipolar disorder are associated with weight gain. A series of general medical, metabolic problems may occur as a result of increases in weight. These include type 2 (noninsulindependent) diabetes mellitus, changes in lipid levels, and transaminase elevation (Clark and Burge 2003; Lebovitz 2003). Children who experience significant weight gain should be monitored especially closely for these possibilities and should be referred for exercise and nutritional counseling. Recently the American Diabetes Association, in collaboration with the American Psychiatric Association and other associations, published a monitoring protocol for all patients to be used before treatment with an atypical antipsychotic is initiated (American Diabetes Association et al. 2004). This protocol includes 1) inquiring about a personal and family history of obesity, diabetes, dyslipidemia, hypertension, or cardiovascular disease; 2) determining weight and height so that body mass index can be calculated; 3) measuring waist circumference (at the level of the umbilicus); 4) taking blood pressure; and 5) measuring fasting plasma glucose and a fasting lipid profile. This group recommended that the patient's weight be reassessed at 4, 8, and 12 weeks after initiation or changing of therapy with an atypical antipsychotic and quarterly thereafter at the time of routine visits. If a patient gains more than 5% of his or her initial weight at any time during therapy, the patient should be switched to an alternative agent.

Prolactin Elevation

All of the atypical antipsychotics except quetiapine elevate prolactin levels in children and adolescents as well as in adults. The long-term effects of this elevation on growth and sexual maturation have not been evaluated fully, but hyperprolactinemia may inhibit patients' reproductive function. All of the pediatric clinical trials for risperidone in autism (McCracken et al. 2002), disruptive behavior disorders with subaverage intelligence (Croonenberghs et al. 2005), schizophrenia (Janssen Pharmaceuticals 2008), and bipolar mania

Table 7–1. Dosing and monitoring guidelines for atypical antipsychotic use in youths with bipolar disorder

Generic name	Trade name	How supplied (po, mg)	Pediatric starting dosage (mg)	Target dose (mg/day)	Cautions
Aripiprazole	Abilify	2, 5, 10, 15, 20, 30	2.5–5 qhs	10–30	Monitor for P450 interactions (CYP3A4 and CYP2D6) Monitor for weight gain, lipids, and glucose
Clozapine	Clozaril	25, 100	25 bid	200–400	Monitor white blood count weekly for first 6 months, then every other week for 6 months, then every 4 weeks Seizures possible at higher doses Increased risk of myocarditis, hypercoagulable states, and arrhythmias Monitor for weight gain, lipids, and glucose
Olanzapine	Zyprexa Zydis	2.5, 5, 7.5, 10, 15, 20 5	2.5 bid	10–20	Monitor for CYP2D6 interactions Monitor for weight gain, lipids, and glucose
Quetiapine	Seroquel IR Seroquel XR	25, 50, 100, 200, 300, 400 200, 300, 400	50–100 qhs	400–1,200	Monitor for weight gain, lipids, and glucose

Table 7–1. Dosing and monitoring guidelines for atypical antipsychotic use in youths with bipolar disorder (*continued*)

Generic name	Trade name	How supplied (po, mg)	Pediatric starting dosage (mg)	Target dose (mg/day)	Cautions
Risperidone	Risperdal	0.25, 0.5, 1, 2, 3, 4	0.25 bid	1–2.5	Monitor for extrapyramidal symptoms and hyperprolactinemia (and associated sexual side effects, including galactorrhea) Monitor for weight gain, lipids, and glucose
Ziprasidone	Geodon	20, 40, 60, 80	20 bid	80–160	Check baseline electrocardiogram as dose increases or if reason for high level of concern Monitor for weight gain, lipids, and glucose

(Pandina et al. 2007) have demonstrated increased levels of serum prolactin from baseline (Janssen Pharmaceuticals 2008). Findling et al. (2003) analyzed data from five clinical trials (total $N=700$) during which children and adolescents ages 5–15 years with subaverage intelligence quotients and conduct or other disruptive behavior disorders received risperidone treatment for up to 55 weeks. They reported that the mean prolactin levels rose from 7.8 ng/mL at baseline to a peak of 29.4 ng/mL at weeks 4–7 of active treatment, then progressively decreased to 16.1 ng/mL at weeks 40–48 ($N=358$) and 13.0 ng/mL at weeks 52–55 ($N=42$). Females returned to a mean value within the normal range (≤ 30 ng/mL) by weeks 8–12, and males were close to normal values (≤ 18 ng/mL) by weeks 16–24. The authors concluded that serum prolactin levels tended to rise and peak within the first 1–2 months of treatment with risperidone and then steadily decline to values within or very close to the normal range by 3–5 months.

The biological significance of chronic, mild elevations of prolactin is unknown (Staller 2006). Both male and female adolescents entering puberty appear to be at the highest risk for elevated prolactin and clinical symptoms while being treated with risperidone (Holzer and Eap 2006). It is important to ask all adolescents treated with risperidone about increases in breast size and/ or galactorrhea. Patients who develop gynecomastia or galactorrhea should be switched to another atypical antipsychotic that does not increase serum prolactin levels.

Conclusion

Atypical antipsychotics are powerful psychotropics for the treatment of mania in children and adolescents. Table 7–1 summarizes dosing and safety information for these agents in children and adolescents. Additional studies are needed that evaluate the efficacy of atypical antipsychotics for depression associated with child and adolescent bipolar disorder and for long-term maintenance.

References

Aman MG, Vinks AA, Remmerie B, et al: Plasma pharmacokinetic characteristics of risperidone and their relationship to saliva concentrations in children with psychiatric or neurodevelopmental disorders. Clin Ther 29:1476–1486, 2007

American Diabetes Association, American Psychiatric Association, American Association of Clinical Endocrinologists, et al: Consensus development conference on antipsychotic drugs and obesity and diabetes. J Clin Psychiatry 65:267–272, 2004

Barzman DH, DelBello MP, Kowatch RA, et al: The effectiveness and tolerability of aripiprazole for pediatric bipolar disorders: a retrospective chart review. J Child Adolesc Psychopharmacol 14:593–600, 2004

Biederman J, Mick E, Hammerness P, et al: Open-label, 8-week trial of olanzapine and risperidone for the treatment of bipolar disorder in preschool-age children. Biol Psychiatry 58:589–594, 2005a

Biederman, J, Mick E, Wozniak J, et al: An open-label trial of risperidone in children and adolescents with bipolar disorder. J Child Adolesc Psychopharmacol 15:311–317, 2005b

Biederman J, Mick E, Spencer T, et al: An open-label trial of aripiprazole monotherapy in children and adolescents with bipolar disorder. CNS Spectr 12:683–689, 2007

Chang K, Ketter T: Mood stabilizer augmentation with olanzapine in acutely manic children. J Child Adolesc Psychopharmacol 10:45–49, 2000

Clark C, Burge MR: Diabetes mellitus associated with atypical anti-psychotic medications. Diabetes Technol Ther 5:669–683, 2003

Correll CU, Carlson HE: Endocrine and metabolic adverse effects of psychotropic medications in children and adolescents. J Am Acad Child Adolesc Psychiatry 45:771–791, 2006

Croonenberghs J, Fegert JM, Findling RL, et al: Risperidone in children with disruptive behavior disorders and subaverage intelligence: a 1-year, open-label study of 504 patients. J Am Acad Child Adolesc Psychiatry 44:64–72, 2005

Danielyan A, Pathak S, Kowatch RA, et al: Clinical characteristics of bipolar disorder in very young children. J Affect Disord 97:51–59, 2007

DelBello MP, Schwiers ML, Rosenberg HL, et al: A double-blind, randomized, placebo-controlled study of quetiapine as adjunctive treatment for adolescent mania. J Am Acad Child Adolesc Psychiatry 41:1216–1223, 2002

DelBello MP, Kowatch RA, Adler CM, et al: A double-blind randomized pilot study comparing quetiapine and divalproex for adolescent mania. J Am Acad Child Adolesc Psychiatry 45:305–313, 2006

DelBello M, Findling RL, Earley L, et al: Efficacy of quetiapine in children and adolescents with bipolar mania: a 3-week, double-blind, randomized, placebo-controlled trial. Paper presented at the 54th Annual Meeting of the American Academy of Child and Adolescent Psychiatry, Boston, MA, October 2007

DelBello M, Findling RL, Wang PP, et al: Safety and efficacy of ziprasidone in pediatric bipolar disorder (NR4-070), in 2008 New Research Program and Abstracts, American Psychiatric Association 161st Annual Meeting, Washington, DC, May 3–8, 2008. Washington, DC, American Psychiatric Association, 2008, pp 191–192

Findling R, McNamara N, Branicky LA, et al: A double-blind pilot study of risperidone in the treatment of conduct disorder. J Am Acad Child Adolesc Psychiatry 39:509–516, 2000

Findling RL, Kusumakar V, Daneman D, et al: Prolactin levels during long-term risperidone treatment in children and adolescents. J Clin Psychiatry 64:1362–1369, 2003

Frazier J, Meyer M, Biederman J, et al: Risperidone treatment for juvenile bipolar disorder: a retrospective chart review. J Am Acad Child Adolesc Psychiatry 38:960–965, 1999

Frazier JA, Biederman J, Tohen M, et al: A prospective open-label treatment trial of olanzapine monotherapy in children and adolescents with bipolar disorder. J Child Adolesc Psychopharmacol 11:239–250, 2001

Holzer L, Eap CB: Risperidone-induced symptomatic hyperprolactinaemia in adolescents. J Clin Psychopharmacol 26:167–171, 2006

Janssen Pharmaceuticals: Risperdal prescribing information. February 2008. Available at: http://www.risperdal.com/risperdal/shared/pi/risperdal.pdf. Accessed July 21, 2008.

Khouzam H, El-Gabalawi F: Treatment of bipolar I disorder in an adolescent with olanzapine. J Child Adolesc Psychopharmacol 10:147–151, 2000

Klein DJ, Cottingham EM, Sorter M, et al: A randomized, double-blind, placebo-controlled trial of metformin treatment of weight gain associated with initiation of atypical antipsychotic therapy in children and adolescents. Am J Psychiatry 163:2072–2079, 2006

Kowatch RA, Suppes T, Gilfillan SK, et al: Clozapine treatment of children and adolescents with bipolar disorder and schizophrenia: a clinical case series. J Child Adolesc Psychopharmacol 5:241–253, 1995

Kowatch RA, Suppes T, Carmody TJ, et al: Effect size of lithium, divalproex sodium and carbamazepine in children and adolescents with bipolar disorder. J Am Acad Child Adolesc Psychiatry 39:713–720, 2000

Lebovitz HE: Metabolic consequences of atypical antipsychotic drugs. Psychiatr Q 74:277–290, 2003

McCracken JT, McGough J, Shah B, et al: Risperidone in children with autism and serious behavioral problems. N Engl J Med 347:314–321, 2002

Pandina G, Delbello M, Kushner S, et al: Risperidone for the treatment of acute mania in bipolar youth. Presentation at the 54th Annual Meeting of the American Academy of Child and Adolescent Psychiatry. Boston, MA, October 2007

Perlis RH, Welge JA, Vornik LA, et al: Atypical antipsychotics in the treatment of mania: a meta-analysis of randomized, placebo-controlled trials. J Clin Psychiatry 67:509–516, 2006

Reyes M, Olah R, Csaba K, et al: Long-term safety and efficacy of risperidone in children with disruptive behaviour disorders: results of a 2-year extension study. Eur Child Adolesc Psychiatry 15:97–104, 2006

Saxena K, Chang K, Steiner H: Treatment of aggression with risperidone in children and adolescents with bipolar disorder: a case series. Bipolar Disord 8:405–410, 2006

Sikich L, Hamer R, Malekpour D, et al: Double-blind trial comparing risperidone, olanzapine, and haloperidol in the treatment of psychotic children and adolescents. Paper presented at the 57th Annual Meeting of the Society of Biological Psychiatry, Philadelphia, PA, May 2002

Soutullo C, Sorter M, Foster KD, et al: Olanzapine in the treatment of adolescent acute mania: a report of seven cases. J Affect Disord 53:279–283, 1999

Staller J: The effect of long-term antipsychotic treatment on prolactin. J Child Adolesc Psychopharmacol 16:317–326, 2006

Stigler KA, Potenza MN, McDougle CJ: Tolerability profile of atypical antipsychotics in children and adolescents. Paediatr Drugs 3:927–942, 2001

Tohen M, Kryzhanovskaya L, Carlson G, et al: Olanzapine versus placebo in the treatment of adolescents with bipolar mania. Am J Psychiatry 164:1547–1556, 2007

Versavel M, DelBello M, Ice K, et al: Ziprasidone dosing study in pediatric patients with bipolar disorder, schizophrenia, or schizoaffective disorder. Neuropsychopharmacology 30 (suppl 1):122, 2005

Wagner K, Nyilas M, Forbes R, et al: Acute efficacy of aripiprazole for the treatment of bipolar I disorder, mixed or manic, in pediatirc patients. Presentation at the American College of Neuropharmacology. Boca Raton, FL, December 2007

8

Pharmacotherapy 3: Medication Strategies and Tactics

Robert A. Kowatch, M.D., Ph.D.

The pharmacological treatment of a child or adolescent with bipolar disorder is often complicated because of the complex cycling pattern of the disorder, the presence of comorbid disorders, and the complex psychosocial matrix in which pediatric patients are immersed. Treatment guidelines often are helpful in treating patients with bipolar disorder because they summarize the current knowledge about the treatment of patients with bipolar disorder (Fountoulakis et al. 2005). There are multiple sets of guidelines developed to help clinicians manage adults with bipolar disorder (Bauer et al. 1999; Frances et al. 1998; "Practice Guideline for the Treatment of Patients With Bipolar Disorder" 1994; Sachs et al. 2000; Suppes et al. 2005), and two sets of guidelines have been developed specifically for children and adolescents with bipolar disorder: the Child and Adolescent Bipolar Foundation (CABF) guidelines and the American Academy of Child and Adolescent Psychiatry (AACAP) guidelines (Kowatch et al. 2005; McClellan et al. 2007). These two sets of pediatric guidelines are useful because they offer a concise review of the bipolar treatment literature and summarize reasonable options for initiating and maintaining treatment in the various clinical scenarios common to bipolar disorders. However, they are already outdated in light of the recent data about the efficacy of atypical antipsychotics for the treatment of mania in children and adolescents. The AACAP guidelines offer a thorough academic discussion of the phenomenological and diagnostic issues that surround pediatric bipolar disorder but little practical advice about how to treat pediatric patients with bipolar disorder. The CABF guidelines are more practical and offer specific treatment algorithms that are updated in this chapter.

Medication Strategies and Tactics

The paradigm of *strategies and tactics* was first used by A. J. Rush (1999) to describe the principles of maintenance phase treatment for adults with major depressive disorder. Rush defined strategies such as "what treatments to choose and in what order" and tactics such as "how to implement these strategies once chosen, in terms of dose and duration of treatment." This is a very useful way of conceptualizing treatment that we have adapted for the treatment of children and adolescents with bipolar disorders. For the purposes of this chapter, I have defined *strategies* as general good practice guidelines for assessing the patient, initiating treatment, and monitoring ongoing care, and *tactics* as the specific assessments and therapeutic agents used alone and in combination to achieve symptomatic remission and functional recovery with individual patients.

Strategy 1: Perform a Careful Assessment

Prior to initiation of pharmacological treatment, the following tactics are recommended: 1) confirming the diagnosis of bipolar disorder, 2) clarifying the DSM-IV-TR (American Psychiatric Association 2004) subtype of bipolar disorder, 3) assessing comorbid disorders, 4) assessing the patient's family history, 5) assessing the patient's medical and past treatment responses, and 6) identifying bipolar disorder target symptoms.

Tactic 1: Confirm the Diagnosis of Bipolar Disorder

The first tactic before initiating treatment is to verify that the patient you are considering for treatment of bipolar disorder is truly bipolar. Many children and adolescents are labeled "bipolar" without careful consideration of the diagnostic complexities and subtypes of this disorder. Other disorders that must be considered in the differential diagnosis of "mood swings" include generalized anxiety disorder, attention-deficit disorder; oppositional defiant disorder, obsessive-compulsive disorder, posttraumatic stress disorder, and fetal alcohol spectrum disorder. The symptoms of bipolarity in children and adolescents can be difficult to establish because of the effects of development on symptom expression, the variability of symptom expression depending on the context and phase of the illness, and other medications that the patient is currently taking. However, despite these differences in phenomenology, it is important to determine which subtype of bipolar disorder (per DSM-IV-TR) and episiode type the child or adolescent has—bipolar I disorder, bipolar II disorder, cyclothymia, or bipolar disorder not otherwise specified (NOS)—before initiating treatment.

Tactic 2: Verify the Subtype of Bipolar Disorder
It is important to verify the bipolar subtype and type of bipolar episode before starting treatment because this verification will determine which medications are used. The diagnostic classification system that DSM-IV-TR uses for bipolar disorders is complex, involving five types of episodes (manic, hypomanic, mixed, depressed, unspecified), four severity levels (mild, moderate, severe without psychosis, severe with psychosis), and three course specifiers (with or without interepisode recovery, seasonal pattern, rapid cycling). These DSM-IV-TR criteria were developed from data on adults with bipolar disorders, and none of these criteria take into account developmental differences between bipolar adults and bipolar children or adolescents. Pediatric bipolar patients often present with a mixed or "dysphoric" picture, characterized by frequent short periods of intense mood lability and irritability rather than classic euphoric mania. Clinicians who evaluate children with pediatric bipolar disorders often try to fit them into the DSM-IV-TR rapid-cycling subtype, but they find that this subtype does not fit bipolar children very well because these children often do not have clear episodes of mania. Rather, researchers report that bipolar children cycle far more frequently than four episodes per year, with Geller et al. (1995) reporting continuous cycling from mania or hypomania to euthymia or depression in 81% of well-defined samples of patients.

Tactic 3: Assess Comorbid Disorders
Children and adolescents with pediatric bipolar disorders often have comorbid disorders that complicate their treatment response. These comorbid dis-

orders most often include attention-deficit/hyperactivity disorder (ADHD), anxiety disorders, oppositional defiant disorder, and conduct disorder (Kovacs and Pollock 1995; West et al. 1995; Wozniak et al. 1995). ADHD is the most common comorbid disorder among pediatric bipolar patients, with leading research groups finding comorbid rates as high as 98% (Wozniak et al. 1995) and 97% (Geller et al. 1998). Pediatric bipolar disorder with comorbid ADHD can be difficult to treat because of the fear of exacerbating the patient's mood disorder while treating his or her ADHD with stimulants. However, in 1992 Carlson et al. reported a "synergistic rather than an antagonistic effect" of lithium and methylphenidate in seven hospitalized children with DSM-III-R bipolar disorder NOS and disruptive behavior disorders. Biederman et al. (1999) reported on a series of 38 pediatric patients who were diagnosed with DSM-III-R mania and ADHD and treated first with mood stabilizers and then stimulants. They noted that those patients who first had their mania treated with mood stabilizers responded very well to the addition of a stimulant medication (Biederman et al. 1999).

Tactic 4: Assess the Patient's Family History

The patient's family history may offer clues to the diagnosis of bipolar disorder because there is often a family history of bipolar disorder that may be helpful to ascertain before initiating treatment. If one of the child's first-degree relatives has bipolar disorder, then the child is four to five times more likely to also have a bipolar disorder (Youngstrom and Duax 2005). Although no one has ever determined if a parent's response to a specific agent predicts response in his or her child with bipolar disorder, it is often helpful to determine at what age the parent with bipolar disorder first became symptomatic, what his or her course has been, and to which agents he or she did or did not respond. Parents who have taken various psychotropic medications for their own bipolar illnesses are often in a better position to monitor for treatment and side effects.

Tactic 5: Assess the Patient's Past Treatment Responses

It is important as part of the patient's psychiatric workup to get a thorough history of what psychotropic medications the patient has been treated with in the past, including the dosages, duration of treatment, tolerance, and effect on bipolar symptoms. It is surprising how often children and adolescents with prominent bipolar symptoms have been treated with every psychotropic agent except a mood stabilizer. Specific selective serotonin reuptake inhibitors (SSRIs) and stimulant medications frequently may exacerbate bipolar symptoms, further clouding the picture of bipolar disorder. It is often extremely helpful to taper medications that may exacerbate bipolar disorder over a short period of time (e.g., 1 or 2 weeks) and then reevaluate the patient's bipolar disorder symptoms. If the patient's bipolar disorder symptoms are still present, then aggressive treatment is warranted.

Tactic 6: Identify Bipolar Disorder Target Symptoms

The symptoms of each patient with pediatric bipolar disorder are different depending on the patient, the phase of his or her illness, and the bipolar subtype. The treatment of a manic episode will differ markedly from that of a depressive episode, and it is important to differentiate the type of episode that the patient is currently experiencing and to identify the target symptoms of this episode to be resolved with treatment. Many patients experiencing a manic or mixed episode exhibit cardinal symptoms such as rapid daily mood swings, aggressive behavior, and irritability. During a depressive episode, symptoms may include decreased energy, social withdrawal, an increase in total sleep period, and a change in appetite.

Tactic 7: Perform a Medical Evaluation

Prior to treatment with any psychotropic agents, each patient should undergo a medical history, medical review of systems, physical examination, and appropriate laboratory examinations. There are also a number of medications and medical disorders that may exacerbate or mimic bipolar symptoms, and it is important to assess these potential confounds before initiating treatment. Potential medical disorders that cause mood cycling in children and adolescents should be considered before the diagnosis of a pediatric bipolar disorder is made (Table 8–1). Any concomitant medications that may increase mood cycling should be assessed and tapered and, if possible, stopped. Table 8–2 lists several medications that may increase mood cycling in children and adolescents.

The Schedule for Affective Disorders and Schizophrenia for School-Aged Children Mania Rating Scale (K-SADS-MRS) (see Appendix to this manual), developed by David Axelson and colleagues at Western Psychiatric Institute and

Table 8–1. Selected medical conditions that may mimic mania in children and adolescents

Hyperthyroidism

Closed or open head injury

Temporal lobe epilepsy

Multiple sclerosis

Systemic lupus erythematosus

Fetal alcohol spectrum disorder/alcohol-related neurodevelopmental disorder

Wilson's disease

Clinic in Pittsburgh, PA (Axelson et al. 2003), can be used by clinicians to assess manic symptoms in children and adolescents. This scale has excellent internal consistency and interrater reliability (Axelson et al. 2003). A score of 12 or higher on this scale differentiated bipolar patients who had clinically significant manic symptoms from those who did not, with a sensitivity of 87% and a specificity of 81%. The DSM-IV-TR criteria for mania and hypomania, as well as for psychotic symptoms, are assessed as part of the K-SADS-MRS, and clinicians easily can use the K-SADS-MRS during a diagnostic interview. The K-SADS-MRS is presented in the appendix to this manual.

Strategy 2: Using Specific Treatment Algorithms

Tactic 1: Treat Mania/Hypomania

The overall strategy when treating children and adolescents with bipolar disorder is to stabilize their mood first and then treat other comorbid disorders such as ADHD or anxiety disorders. The atypical antipsychotics, because of their effectiveness and ease of use, quickly are becoming first-line treatments for manic, mixed, and hypomanic episodes in children and adolescents. (This information is presented in Chapter 7, "Pharmacotherapy 2: Atypical Antipsychotics," of this manual.)

We have developed two general algorithms, one for the treatment of mania/hypomania (Figure 8–1) and one for bipolar depression (Figure 8–2), based on published adult guidelines, the emerging child and adolescent bipolar

Table 8–2. Medications that may increase mood cycling in children and adolescents

Antidepressants

    Tricyclic antidepressants

    Selective serotonin reuptake inhibitors

    Serotonin-norepinephrine reuptake inhibitors

Aminophylline

Oral or intravenous corticosteroids

Sympathomimetic amines (e.g., pseudoephedrine)

Antibiotics (e.g., clarithromycin, erythromycin, and amoxicillin)

treatment literature, and our own clinical experience. These algorithms recommend specific medications as tactics and may not be applicable to all patients. Together, the findings from the studies reviewed in Chapters 6 ("Pharmacotherapy 1: Mood Stabilizers") and 7 of this book suggest that atypical antipsychotics are more effective than lithium and/or valproate for the treatment of manic symptoms in children and adolescents. Because of their efficacy and lack of need for blood level monitoring, the atypical antipsychotics have become first-line treatments for mania/hypomania.

For a child or adolescent with mania/hypomania, stage 1A of this algorithm recommends monotherapy with the atypical antipsychotic quetiapine, ziprasidone, aripiprazole, or risperidone, in that order of preference. Quetiapine has the advantage of low risk of extrapyramidal symptoms (EPS) and tardive dyskinesia. Ziprasidone and aripiprazole have low weight-gain risk, with ziprasidone causing the least amount of weight gain. Risperidone, although very potent at low doses, increases prolactin levels; the long-term significance of this effect is unknown. Lithium and valproate were considered as second-line choices (stage 1B of this algorithm) because of their lower potency compared with atypical antipsychotics, and olanzapine, though very potent, causes significant weight gain and is also considered a stage 1B agent.

If a patient is not able to tolerate the first atypical agent chosen for monotherapy because of lack of response or intolerable side effects, then the next

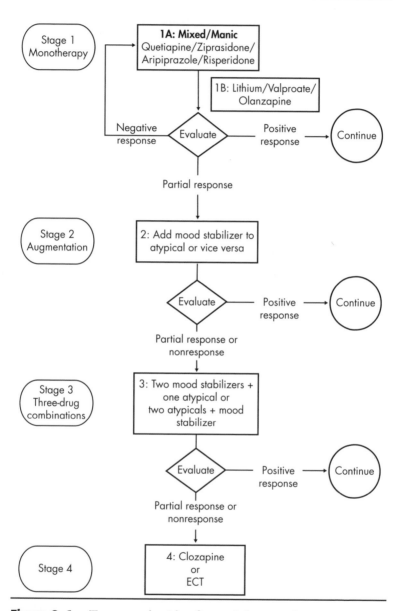

Figure 8–1. Treatment algorithm for mania/hypomania.

ECT = electroconvulsive therapy.

option is to cycle back up through an alternative agent from stage 1A or 1B. Stage 2 of this algorithm is for patients who show a "mild to moderately improved" response to monotherapy but who are not "much or very much improved."

Stage 3 of this algorithm recommends combination treatment with two mood stabilizers (e.g., lithium or valproate and an atypical antipsychotic). Alternatively, two atypical antipsychotics together or two atypical antipsychotics with a mood stabilizer are possible treatment combinations.

Stage 4, for patients with totally treatment-resistant mania/hypomania, involves a trial of either clozapine or electroconvulsive therapy. Monotherapy with clozapine can be used as a last resort, but is difficult to maintain in the long term because of the necessity for weekly blood draws and the large weight gain often seen with this agent.

Tactic 2: Treat Bipolar Depression

The treatment of bipolar depression especially can be problematic because antidepressants have a tendency to increase mood cycling, and there is limited evidence for other agents. There have been two recent prospective open-label studies assessing lamotrigine and lithium for bipolar depression in adolescents (Chang et al. 2006; Patel et al. 2006). Chang et al. (2006) conducted an 8-week, open-label trial of lamotrigine with 20 adolescents ages 12–17 years with diagnoses of bipolar I disorder, bipolar II disorder, or bipolar disorder NOS, with a current depressive episode. Lamotrigine was begun at 12.5–25 mg/day, and the mean final dosage was 131.6 mg/day. Sixteen subjects (84%) demonstrated a response, as defined by the primary response criteria, with 11 subjects (58%) considered in remission at week 8. Scores on the Young Mania Rating Scale and Overt Aggression Scale—Modified also decreased significantly during the trial. There was no significant weight change, rash, or other adverse effects during this trial. These preliminary results indicate that adolescents with bipolar depression appeared to respond to lamotrigine treatment, whether as adjunctive therapy or monotherapy, with decreases in depression, mania, and aggression, but larger, placebo-controlled studies of lamotrigine are needed in this population.

Patel et al. (2006) studied 27 adolescent inpatients (ages 12–18 years) with an episode of depression associated with bipolar I disorder. These subjects were treated openly with lithium 30 mg/kg per day, and the dosage was adjusted to achieve a therapeutic serum level (1.0–1.2 mEq/L). Response and remission rates were 48% and 30%, respectively. Side effects, which were generally mild to moderate in severity, included headache (74%), nausea/vomiting (67%), stomachache (30%), and abdominal cramps (19%). The findings of this study indicate that lithium appears effective and is relatively well tolerated for the treatment of an acute episode of depression in adolescents with bipolar disorder.

A retrospective study assessing treatment of depressed children and adolescents with bipolar disorder suggested that SSRIs may be effective for acute bipolar depression, but these agents may be associated with mood destabilization and exacerbation of manic symptoms (Biederman et al. 2000). In this study, depressive symptoms were 6.7 times more likely to improve when subjects received an SSRI. However, SSRIs were associated with a three times greater risk of relapse of manic symptomatology. In patients with active manic symptoms, the concomitant use of SSRIs with mood stabilizer treatment did not inhibit significantly the improvement of manic symptoms associated with mood stabilizer treatment (Biederman et al. 2000), suggesting that further studies of antidepressants in combination with mood stabilizers or atypical antipsychotics are needed. Antidepressant medications should be used with caution in children and adolescents with bipolar disorder because of the potential risk for increased mood instability and for the emergence of suicidal ideation.

On the basis of the previous studies, we developed the algorithm shown in Figure 8–2 for the treatment of depressive episodes during bipolar I or II disorder. This algorithm assumes that patients have already been treated for mania with an atypical antipsychotic or a mood stabilizer. Stage 1 of this algorithm recommends either starting lithium or increasing the current dose of lithium to achieve levels≥0.8 mEq/L. If the patient cannot tolerate lithium or does not have a full response to lithium, then stage 2 recommends a trial of lamotrigine. Stage 3 recommends a trial of either bupropion or an SSRI based on the patient's past treatment history.

Tactic 3: Consider Combination Therapy if Needed

The majority of children and adolescents with bipolar disorder will require combination pharmacotherapy for mood stabilization, but the data on combination treatment in children and adolescents are limited (Findling et al. 2003;

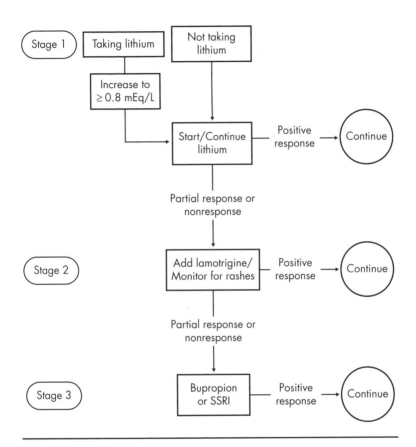

Figure 8–2. Bipolar depression algorithm.

ECT = electroconvulsive therapy; SSRI = selective serotonin reuptake inhibitor.

Kowatch et al. 2003). Kafantaris et al. (2001) evaluated acutely manic adolescents with psychotic features following treatment with lithium and an adjunctive antipsychotic to assess whether antipsychotics are necessary for psychotic mania in adolescents. Antipsychotics were gradually tapered and discontinued after 4 weeks of therapeutic lithium levels in patients whose psychotic symptoms resolved, and these patients were maintained with lithium monotherapy for up to 4 weeks. Significant improvement was seen in 64% of the sample with psychotic features after 4 weeks of combination treatment. However, 43% did not maintain their response after discontinuation of the antipsychotic medication, and this suggests that more than 4 weeks of antipsychotic treatment is required for some adolescents with psychotic mania. Variables associated with successful discontinuation of antipsychotic medication in this sample were first episode, shorter duration of psychosis, and the presence of thought disorder at baseline (Kafantaris et al. 2001).

In a double-blind, placebo-controlled study of an atypical antipsychotic for the treatment of bipolar adolescents, quetiapine in combination with divalproex resulted in a greater reduction of manic symptoms than divalproex monotherapy, suggesting that the combination of a mood stabilizer and an atypical antipsychotic is more effective than a mood stabilizer alone for the treatment of adolescent mania. In this study, quetiapine was titrated to a dosage of 450 mg/day in 7 days and was well tolerated (DelBello et al. 2006).

Findling et al. (2005) reported the results of a discontinuation trial of lithium and divalproex to determine whether divalproex was superior to lithium in the maintenance monotherapy of youths diagnosed with bipolar disorder who had been stabilized previously on the combination of lithium and divalproex. A total of 139 subjects with bipolar I or II disorder with a mean age of 10.8 years were treated initially with lithium and divalproex for a mean duration of 10.7 weeks. Patients meeting remission criteria for 4 consecutive weeks were then randomly assigned in a double-blind fashion to treatment with either lithium or divalproex for up to 76 weeks. Sixty youths were randomly assigned to receive monotherapy with either lithium ($n=30$) or divalproex ($n=30$). At the end of the study period, the lithium and divalproex treatment groups did not differ in survival time until emerging symptoms of relapse or survival time until discontinuation for any reason. The authors concluded that lithium was not found to be superior to divalproex as maintenance treatment in youths who had stabilized on combination lithium and divalproex pharmacotherapy, because the mean survival time in this trial for both agents was 113 days. This trial also demonstrated that monotherapy with either of these agents was not sufficient for maintenance treatment of children and adolescents with bipolar disorder.

The results of the three studies discussed previously support the use of combination therapy in children and adolescents with bipolar disorder. However, many more studies are needed that examine the various combinations of psychotropic agents that frequently are necessary to treat adequately patients with bipolar disorder and other comorbid disorders. For example, one of the treatment combinations that is being used frequently in clinical practice is two atypical antipsychotics used together (e.g., quetiapine with ziprasidone, low-dose risperidone with quetiapine). Although these atypical antipsychotic combinations fly in the face of theoretical psychopharmacology, in some cases these combinations are very effective.

Common Case Presentations

Complex-Cycling Bipolar Disorder

Complex-cycling bipolar disorder is the most common and complex type of pediatric bipolar disorder to diagnose and treat in prepubertal patients. The parents or guardians of patients with this disorder typically report four to six severe mood cycles per day, with almost constant minor mood swings and no clear episodes—the complex cycling pattern of pediatric bipolar disorder recently validated by Geller et al. and others in several large, well-controlled, longitudinal samples (Geller et al. 1995, 2000). These patients usually have been treated with every medication except a mood stabilizer or atypical antipsychotic and frequently have had negative reactions to stimulants or antidepressants. They often have comorbid ADHD or anxiety disorders, and parents report continuous cycling without clear episodes of mania or depression.

Case 1: Catherine With Mood Cycles

Catherine is a 9-year-old girl who, according to her mother, has extreme mood cycles, 5–10 times a day. Each of these mood cycles lasts 30 minutes to an hour and can occur with little or no provocation. On a typical day when Catherine wakes up, she will be in a "silly and hyper" mood that interferes with her getting ready for school almost every morning. When she returns home from school, her mood alternates between extreme anger and silliness. Catherine's energy level is usually very high, and it takes her several hours to fall asleep. She goes to bed about 9:30 P.M. but does not fall asleep until sometime around 11 P.M. or midnight. She is always up at 5 A.M.

Her mother reports that Catherine will go from 3–4 days of being "really hyper and silly" to 4–5 days of being very irritable and sad. During her down times Catherine's energy is low and she withdraws from the world. Her mother reports that there is no clear pattern to these episodes, but the down periods seem to last longer than the hyperactive periods. Her mother did recall a period last summer when Catherine was in a "hyper period" for several weeks and was only sleeping 3–4 hours per night and was hyperenergetic during the day: "We had to call her grandparents to come in and give us some relief. We thought we were going to have to commit her." Sometimes in school, Catherine gets in trouble for calling out in class and not paying attention when she is in a hyper period. During her down times she has a hard time completing assignments and will often want to stay home from school, saying that she does not feel well.

Her mother reports having had an episode of postpartum depression when she was 26 years old. Catherine's biological father suffers from alcoholism and has severe mood swings.

In the office, Catherine appears as a young prepubescent female who looks her stated age. She is alert and cooperative but rather intrusive: "Hey, doc, what you got in those cabinets? Any good books?" Her mood is mildly euphoric and her speech mildly pressured. When asked what she wants to be when she grows up, she replies, "Either president of the United States or a model." She denies visual or auditory hallucinations. She reports that during her good periods her thoughts sometimes "move as fast as a train and I can solve any math problem." Her insight into her mood swings is poor and her judgment impaired by her impulsivity. During her down periods she reports feeling "low and without any energy… my brain refuses to move." She denies suicidal or homicidal ideation.

Your evaluation of Catherine is that she is currently experiencing 3- to 4-day periods of hypomania with euphoria, irritability, grandiosity, racing thoughts, and poor sleep on a regular basis. She is currently being treated with 36 mg of methylphenidate, which she reports helps "a little" with her concentration in school. These episodes of hypomania are interspersed with short periods of depression. In the past she has met duration criteria for a manic episode. This is a very common cycling pattern for prepubertal children with bipolar I disorder.

You discuss Catherine's diagnosis of bipolar I disorder and possible treatment options with her and her mother together, and you decide that a trial of an atypical antipsychotic would be preferred over a mood stabilizer because of the less frequent need for blood draws. They decide to try quetiapine because of its safety profile. You also provide medication handouts, such as those from Mina K. Dulcan's (2007) book *Helping Parents, Youth, and Teachers Understand Medications for Behavioral and Emotional Problems: A Resource Book of Medication Information Handouts,* to help the patient and her mother understand the diagnosis and treatment of bipolar disorder.

The patient begins taking quetiapine 100 mg at bedtime, with an increase by 100 mg every other day until she is taking 300 mg at bedtime, and you see her for follow-up 1 week later. Her mother reports that Catherine's mood swings are somewhat improved. "Overall, she is 50% better but still is very manic when she gets home from school in the afternoon." You add another dose of quetiapine 100 mg after school, and at their next appointment 1 week later her mother reports that Catherine's mood is much more stable, she is sleeping 8–10 hours a night, and her silliness and irritability are almost gone. Catherine reports that she feels much calmer and is in control of her thoughts.

Treatment Strategy and Tactics for the Prepubertal Patient With Complex-Cycling Bipolar Disorder

The strategy with the prepubertal patient with complex cycling bipolar disorder is, first, to taper any medications that may be exacerbating his or her bipolar symptoms and initiate treatment with an atypical antipsychotic. This tapering usually can be done over a short period of time, usually 1–2 weeks. Most psychotropic medications can be tapered safely by halving the total daily dose every 3–5 days until the medication is discontinued, and then the patient's bipolar disorder symptoms can be more clearly evaluated. If the patient's manic symptoms continue after any manic medications are tapered, then algorithm stage 1A recommends monotherapy with quetiapine, ziprasidone, aripiprazole, or risperidone, in that order of preference. Stage 2 recommends combination therapy as discussed previously (see "Tactic 3: Consider Combination Therapy if Needed").

Bipolar II Disorder

In adolescents the first signs of a bipolar disorder may be the sudden appearance of a severe depressive episode with psychotic features or a manic or hypomanic episode precipitated by antidepressants (DelBello et al. 2007). However, differentiating an episode of major depression with psychotic features from a depressive episode of bipolar I or II disorder can be difficult. Wozniak et al. (2004) compared the clinical characteristics of depression, comorbidity, and family history in 109 children with unipolar depression and 43 with bipolar depression. They found that compared with children with unipolar depression, children with bipolar depression were more likely to have met criteria for depression caused by both "sad" and "mad" mood states and to have severe depression with suicidality, anhedonia, and hopelessness.

Case 2: Jason With Depression

You are asked to consult about a patient recently admitted to an adolescent psychiatry inpatient unit. Jason is a 14-year-old adolescent who was admitted to an inpatient unit following a 2-month history of severe depression and suicidal ideation. According to his biological mother, he became depressed in the fall of his freshman year of high school, when he suddenly became more withdrawn, his grades dropped, and he began staying up late and had trouble getting to school in the morning. His mood was extremely irritable and volatile, with periods of several hours a day when he reported feeling "dead inside." His appetite was very poor, and he lost approximately 20 lbs. He denied any substance abuse, and there were no unusual stressors in his life. He reported "thinking about suicide a lot" but not having the energy to do it. Prior to this episode he had done well in school, had never had any mood problems, and had several close friends. His biological father is estranged from the family and has a history of depression, mood swings, and treatment with lithium.

After 3 days of hospitalization, Jason was judged to have an episode of major depression, and citalopram 10 mg/day was initiated. Within 2 days, Jason's depressed mood improved, but he had difficulty sleeping and became "hyperactive," intrusive, and impulsive. He also reported hearing people calling his name when no one was around and was convinced that there were "ghosts on the unit" that only he could see at night. The citalopram was stopped, and Jason's mood and behavior stabilized after he received olanzapine 10 mg at bedtime for 2 nights. However, his treating psychiatrist was concerned that Jason might be bipolar and wanted a second opinion about his treatment.

Three days after the citalopram was stopped, you interview Jason. He appears as a thin adolescent male who is alert and cooperative. His mood is mildly euphoric and his speech pressured. He denies auditory or visual hallucinations, reporting that the "under-the-tongue medicine made the ghosts go away." His insight is poor.

You meet with the patient's mother and ask her to fill out the parent report version of the Mood Disorders Questionnaire (MDQ), a screening instrument for bipolar spectrum disorders (Figure 8–3). The original adult MDQ developed by Hirschfeld and colleagues (Hirschfeld 2003a, 2003b) is a self-report, single-page, paper-and-pencil inventory that can be scored quickly and easily by a clinician. The MDQ screens for a lifetime history of a manic or hypomanic syndrome by including 13 yes/no items derived from both DSM-IV-TR criteria and clinical experience. A yes/no question also asks whether several of any reported manic or hypomanic symptoms or behaviors were experienced during the same period of time. Although the MDQ was developed for and validated in adults, it can be used as a screening tool in older adolescents. Wagner et al. (2006) compared three versions of the Mood Disorder Questionnaire—Ado-

1. Has there ever been a time for a week or more when your adolescent was not his/her usual self and...   YES   NO

...felt too good or excited?   ☒   ☐
...was so irritable that he/she started fights or arguments with
  people?   ✗
...felt he/she could do anything?   ☐   ☒
...needed much less sleep?   ☒   ☐
...couldn't slow his/her mind down or thoughts raced through
  his/her head?   ☐   ☒
...was easily distracted by things?   ☒   ☐
...had much more energy than usual?   ☒   ☐
...was much more active or did more things than usual?   ☒   ☐
...had many boyfriends or girlfriends at the same time?   ☐   ☒
...was much more interested in sex than usual?   ☐   ☒
...did many things that were foolish or risky?   ☐   ☒
...spent too much money?   ☐   ☒
...used more alcohol or drugs?   ☐   ☒

**2. If you checked YES to more than one of the above, have
several of these ever happened to your adolescent during the
same period of time?**   ☒   ☐

**3. How much of a problem did any of these cause your adolescent—
like school problems, failing grades, problems with family and
friends, legal troubles? Please circle one response only.**

No Problem   Minor Problem   (Moderate Problem)   Serious Problem

Figure 8–3.   Parent report version of the Mood Disorders Questionnaire to gather information about the adolescent.

lescent Version: 1) self report of symptoms by the adolescent, 2) attributional report (how the adolescent believes teachers or friends would report his or her symptoms), and 3) a parent report of the adolescent's symptoms. They found that a score of 5 or more on the parent version yielded a sensitivity of 0.72 and specificity of 0.81, which was much better than the adolescent self-report and attributional versions. The adolescent self-report and attributional report are not useful for screening because adolescents with bipolar disorder generally have little insight into their moods and behaviors.

Treatment Strategy and Tactics for the Patient With Bipolar II Disorder

Review of the parent MDQ as rated by Jason's mother reveals a total score of ≥5, which is a positive screen for mania/hypomania and demonstrates that this patient has had episodes of hypomania in the past. The clinician decides that Jason meets criteria for bipolar II disorder based on his past history of hypomania and a current depressive episode. His current episode of mania appears to have been triggered by treatment with an SSRI and has not resolved 2 weeks after hospital discharge. Jason and his mother are not worried about weight gain, and Jason has responded well to olanzapine, so you begin a trial of olanzapine 5 mg at bedtime with appropriate metabolic monitoring.

Bipolar Depression

A depressive episode during the course of bipolar disorder can be very disabling in adults, adolescents, and children, with the probability of remaining ill for a year following an acute mood episode being 7% for manic bipolar disorder patients compared with 22% for depressed bipolar disorder patients (Keller et al. 1986). Moreover, bipolar disorder depression may be the most lethal phase of bipolar disorder, with marked rates of suicidality. Goldstein et al. (2005) reported that a third of child and adolescent patients with bipolar disorder had made a medically significant suicide attempt during the course of their illness. It is very important to recognize and treat aggressively depressive episodes during the course of bipolar disorder.

Case 3: Peggy With Depression

Peggy is a 16-year-old who has been treated for the last 2 years for bipolar I disorder following an episode of mania for which she was hospitalized. She was discharged on lithium, risperidone 1.0 mg/day and Adderall XR 20 mg/day for ADHD. She had been doing well at home and school up until last month, when her parents noticed increased irritability, poor appetite, difficulty getting out of bed in the morning, and increased isolation.

On mental status examination, Peggy appears as a mildly overweight, pubescent female. She is alert, oriented, and cooperative. Her mood is clearly depressed, but she denies suicidal ideation. She reports that "for the last month I have been feeling down for no good reason." She denies auditory or visual hallucinations but reports that her energy has been low, she is sleeping poorly, and she has lost her appetite. Her insight is good.

Treatment Strategy and Tactics for the Patient With Bipolar Depression
Peggy is diagnosed with bipolar I disorder, current episode depressed, with no psychotic features. Following stage 1 of the algorithm shown in Figure 8–2, her lithium level is checked. Her lithium level is 1.0 mEq/L, and she has been compliant with her other medications. The clinician suggests to the patient and her parents a course of cognitive therapy, but no therapist with cognitive-behavioral therapy training is available for at least 8 weeks. The clinician, in consultation with Peggy and her parents, then decides to begin lamotrigine 25 mg/day for 2 weeks, with a dosage increase to 50 mg/day in 2 weeks. When Peggy is seen in follow-up 2 weeks later, she reports feeling "somewhat better" with no side effects. The clinician encourages her to continue with the slow titration of the lamotrigine, and when the dosage reaches 150 mg/day, she reports that her depressive symptoms have remitted. She continues taking lithium, lamotrigine, and Adderall XR for the next year without any manic or depressive episodes.

Bipolar Disorder and ADHD

A significant proportion (40%–80%) of pediatric patients with bipolar disorder have comorbid ADHD and require treatment of comorbid ADHD for good functioning at home and school. The typical clinical presentation in this scenario is a prepubertal child who was diagnosed with ADHD at an early age and subsequently treated with stimulants around the age of 4–5 years for his or her "severe irritable hyperactivity." Then, usually at the age of 7–8 years, the child's bipolar symptoms emerge in full force. In the majority of such cases, even after the child's stimulant medications are discontinued, the child continues to manifest severe mood lability and other bipolar symptoms. Once a mood stabilizer is started, the child's mood improves, but he or she continues to manifest ADHD symptoms. Many times, the addition of a long-acting stimulant to the mood stabilizers improves the child's ADHD symptoms without exacerbating his or her mood disorder.

Our clinical and research experience, and the experience of others, suggest that if a pediatric bipolar patient with comorbid ADHD is first stabilized with either a mood stabilizer or an atypical antipsychotic, the addition of a stimulant is often very helpful in treating the comorbid ADHD (Biederman et al. 1999; Scheffer et al. 2005). The critical issue appears to be the sequence of treatment, with the patient's mania treated before stimulant medication is added or reintroduced.

Case 4: Kevin With ADHD

Kevin, a 12-year-old boy in the seventh grade, is brought to your office by his mother because he has had escalating behavior problems at home and school in the last several months. The middle school principal has called Kevin's parents about his recent "goofy" behavior with teachers and about other parents' complaints that he has made inappropriate comments to the girls he sits next to in class. As a result, Kevin is on the verge of being suspended for his inappropriate and disruptive behavior. His parents report that for the last month he has been staying up until 2:00–3:00 A.M., instant messaging his friends with his cell phone or watching television. They attribute his inappropriate sexual behavior to puberty and possibly Web sites he frequents on the Internet. They have tried blocking Kevin's access to these Web sites, but he was able to reinstall the operating system on their computer and erase the blocking software they had installed.

In taking his history, you learn that Kevin has not been sexually abused. It is important to inquire about such abuse, which could lead to a differential diagnosis in a child with a history of hypersexuality. Kevin was diagnosed with ADHD at age 6 years, and he took methylphenidate for about a year before it was discontinued because his parents were concerned about his decreased appetite. The family psychiatric history reveals that his mother has a past history of anxiety and depression and his father has a past history of alcoholism. Kevin scores 65 on the K-SADS-MRS, and you diagnose nonpsychotic bipolar I disorder with ADHD based on interviews with Kevin, his parents, school reports, and DSM-IV-TR criteria: significant elation and irritability lasting more than a week, increased goal-directed activity on the Internet, decreased need for sleep, hypersexual behavior, and distractibility.

Treatment Strategy and Tactics for the Patient With Bipolar Disorder and ADHD

The overall strategy in this scenario is to achieve a positive mood response (rated as much or very much improved) to a mood stabilizer or an atypical antipsychotic and then reassess the ADHD symptoms with an ADHD rating scale such as the Conners' abbreviated Parent-Teacher Questionnaire or the Vanderbilt ADHD Diagnostic Teacher Rating Scale (www.psychiatrictimes.com/clinical-scales/adhd/vadrs/).

Kevin's parents decide not to try an atypical antipsychotic because it is "an antipsychotic" and instead elect for a trial of valproate. Kevin weighs 120 lbs., and you prescribe divalproex 250 mg, one tablet in the morning and one in the evening, with an increase to two tablets in the evening after 5 days. One week later in the office, you see Kevin and his mother, who report that his moods and behaviors are unchanged. You check a predose valproate level and it is 55 mg/L, so you increase the divalproex to two tablets twice per day. Two weeks later, Kevin's mother reports that his moods are much improved and he is sleeping through the night, and his teachers have said that his inappropriate behaviors in school have ceased. A repeat valproate level check is 90 mg/L, and Kevin is tolerating the divalproex without any side effects.

On follow-up 1 month later, Kevin continues to have a positive mood response to the divalproex, but his teacher reports that he is very distractible in class, and a review of a Conners Teacher Questionnaire confirms the diagnosis of comorbid ADHD. Kevin is prescribed extended-release methylphenidate (Concerta) 36 mg, which helps with his attention and focusing in the classroom. In many cases of bipolar disorder and comorbid ADHD, if the patient is still manifesting significant ADHD symptoms despite a positive response to the mood stabilizer, it may be beneficial for the patient to begin taking a low dose of a long-acting stimulant medication. Many times, despite a negative mood response to stimulants in the past, the addition of a stimulant is beneficial for treating the patient's comorbid ADHD without exacerbating his or her bipolar disorder. Specific tactics include adding a long-acting stimulant such as extended-release methylphenidate (Concerta), controlled-delivery methylphenidate (Metadate CD), Adderall XR, or lisdexamfetamine (Vyvanse).

Clinical Pearls About Specific Medications

1. *Lithium.* Lithium is a good mood stabilizer with a moderate effect size. In some patients it may take as long as 6–8 weeks to get a full response to lithium. The side effects of weight gain, enuresis, and exacerbation of acne may limit lithium's use in some patients. There are still unanswered questions about lithium's long-term effect on renal function in children and adolescents.

2. *Valproate.* Valproate works faster than lithium and is generally well tolerated. All females treated with valproate should be monitored for signs of

polycystic ovary syndrome, which include hirsutism (abnormal hair growth), weight gain, and abnormal menses (Rasgon et al. 2005).

3. *Carbamazepine.* Carbamazepine remains a third-line mood stabilizer because of its strong cytochrome P450 interactions (Beasg and Berry 2006).

4. *Quetiapine.* It is very important to use adequate doses of quetiapine when treating mania in children and adolescents. For treatment of acute mania in inpatients, quetiapine can be dosed at "1–2–3–4"—100 mg at bedtime on day 1, then 200 mg on day 2, and so forth, until a dosage of 400 mg/day is reached. Sometimes 600–800 mg/day is required to achieve a full antimanic response. It is important to remember that quetiapine is more sedating at lower dosages (25–50 mg/day) than at higher dosages (300–400 mg/day).

5. *Olanzapine.* Olanzapine is a very effective antipsychotic and mood stabilizer. However, its powerful appetite-stimulating effects limit its use for many patients. The rapidly dissolving form of olanzapine, Zydis, is very effective in the emergency department or on inpatient units for the treatment of acute agitation.

6. *Aripiprazole.* Aripiprazole is indicated by the U.S. Food and Drug Administration (FDA) for acute and maintenance treatment of manic and mixed episodes associated with bipolar I disorder with or without psychotic features in adults and in pediatric patients 10–17 years of age. Aripiprazole can be used in a once-daily dose at bedtime in most patients. It is sedating and may cause significant EPS if started at too high a dose (e.g., 10 mg at bedtime). We usually start aripiprazole at 2.5–5 mg/day and titrate to a maintenance dosage of 10–20 mg/day.

7. *Ziprasidone.* Ziprasidone has the advantage of inducing very little weight gain, but patient responses to this atypical antipsychotic have been more erratic than to the other atypical antipsychotics. The intramuscular formulation of ziprasidone, a 10-mg dose, is very effective for the treatment of acute agitation.

8. *Risperidone.* Risperidone is indicated by the FDA as monotherapy in the short-term treatment of manic or mixed episodes of bipolar I disorder in children and adolescents ages 10–17 years. Risperidone remains one of the most potent atypical antipsychotics in child psychiatry and is currently the only atypical antipsychotic indicated to treat children and adolescents with autism, schizophrenia, or bipolar mania.

Important Treatment Issues

Duration of Treatment

A very important treatment issue is how long to continue treatment with mood stabilizers or atypical antipsychotics after treatment of an acute episode of mania or bipolar depression. There are now several studies in adolescents with bipolar disorder that provide guidance about the duration of treatment. Strober et al. (1990) followed a group of adolescents for 5 years who had been hospitalized for a manic episode, and demonstrated a threefold increase in relapse rates among adolescents with mania who discontinued lithium after hospital discharge. The lithium/valproate discontinuation trial discussed previously by Findling et al. (2005) had a duration of 76 weeks with either lithium or divalproex. There are two long-term continuation studies of atypical antipsychotics in children and adolescents with bipolar disorder. In the first, by Tohen et al. (2007), 146 adolescents who had been enrolled in a controlled trial of olanzapine versus placebo were treated openly with olanzapine for up to 26 weeks. These patients had significant symptom improvement during this open-label extension phase, but a large proportion of patients had increases in weight and prolactin and experienced changes in lipid parameters. In a second study, a 26-week open-label extension study with ziprasidone, 156 subjects ages 10–17 years with bipolar I disorder were treated openly with ziprasidone 40–80 mg twice daily. The most commonly reported treatment-emergent adverse events were sedation, headache, somnolence, dizziness, insomnia, nausea, and fatigue.

In treating a child or adolescent who has had a single manic episode, it is reasonable to maintain a mood-stabilizing agent or atypical antipsychotic for 12–18 months and then, if the patient is euthymic and in remission, to gradually reduce one medication over a 2- to 3-month period (Kowatch et al. 2005). If bipolar disorder symptoms recur, the mood-stabilizing agent should be reintroduced. Ultimately, the benefits of long-term treatment will have to be weighed against the risks of long-term maintenance treatment and a decision made by the patient and his or her guardians about how long to continue treatment. If a patient has had a manic or mixed episode that has necessitated hospitalization, the benefits of continued treatment with mood stabilizers outweigh the risks of long-term treatment.

Pregnancy and Sexually Transmitted Diseases

Many adolescents are sexually active, but adolescents with bipolar disorder can become hypersexual during a manic episode. This behavior during a manic episode is qualitatively different than the sexual behavior of a child or adolescent with posttraumatic stress disorder (PTSD). In a manic child or adolescent, his or her sexual behavior often is erotic and pleasure seeking as compared with the child or adolescent with PTSD, in whom this behavior is anxiety driven and more compulsive in nature. It is important to discuss the risk of impulsive and manic-driven sexual behavior with adolescents with bipolar disorder and their parents before it occurs. The risks of excessive involvement with erotic materials on the Internet and other sources should also be discussed with the patient. The dangers of sexually transmitted diseases and possible adverse effects of psychotropic medications on a fetus should also be discussed with female adolescents with bipolar disorder and their parents. A plan for reliable birth control should be implemented in consultation with the patient's pediatrician or gynecologist. Sexually active females with bipolar disorder can be started on low-dose progestogen birth control pills, which are less likely to affect their mood or interact with whatever psychotropic agents they are taking.

Insomnia

Many pediatric patients with bipolar disorder report having insomnia. A useful treatment strategy is to determine the cause of the patient's insomnia. If the insomnia is due to the patient's still having manic symptoms at the end of the evening that are causing initial insomnia, it may be helpful to shift whatever mood stabilizers he or she is taking to an hour before bedtime and ensure that these medications are maximized. If the insomnia is caused by anxiety, then adding either gabapentin or a low dose of an atypical antipsychotic agent to whatever mood stabilizer the patient is already taking may be helpful.

Weight Gain

Weight gain is a major side effect of mood stabilizers and most atypical antipsychotics. Important first strategies are to emphasize diet and exercise with restriction of high-carbohydrate foods and fast foods as much as possible. Another tactic for limiting weight gain is a trial of metformin, an agent indicated for type 2 diabetes. Metformin decreases hepatic glucose production, decreases intestinal absorption of glucose, and improves insulin sensitivity by increasing peripheral glucose uptake and utilization. Klein et al. (2006) studied 39 subjects with mood and psychotic disorders, ages 10–17, whose weight had increased by more than 10% during less than 1 year of olanzapine, risperidone, or quetiapine therapy. In this 16-week, double-blind, placebo-controlled trial, body weight, body mass index, and waist circumference were measured regularly, as were fasting insulin and glucose levels. Klein et al. reported that weight was stabilized in subjects receiving metformin, whereas those receiving placebo continued to gain weight (0.31 kg/week). Because the study was conducted with growing children, metformin treatment resulted in a reduction in z scores for both weight and body mass index. No serious adverse events resulted from metformin treatment. The investigators concluded that metformin therapy is safe and effective in reversing atypical antipsychotic–induced weight gain, decreased insulin sensitivity, and abnormal glucose metabolism resulting from treatment of children and adolescents with atypical antipsychotics.

The usual starting dosage of metformin is 500 mg twice per day, given with meals. Dosage increases should be made in increments of 500 mg weekly up to a maximum dosage of 2,000 mg/day, given in divided doses. Metformin comes in regular-release and extended-release formulations. Common side effects of metformin include diarrhea, nausea/vomiting, flatulence, asthenia, indigestion, abdominal discomfort, and headache.

Sedation

In many cases the teachers of a pediatric patient with bipolar disorder will notice that the child falls asleep in school, which seriously impairs his or her learning ability. One strategy for this common problem is to divide the doses of mood stabilizers and atypical antipsychotic agents into two or three smaller doses and avoid giving these medications all at bedtime. Treatment of excessive daytime somnolence with modafinil in patients with bipolar disorder is not recommended because it can cause mania (Frye et al. 2007; Vorspan et al. 2005).

Enuresis

Both nocturnal and daytime enuresis are common problems when lithium is prescribed, particularly when it is prescribed for young boys. The first step in these cases is to rule out any medical conditions that might be causing or exacerbating this problem, including genital-urinary deformations, renal impairment, and urinary tract infections. A specific tactic is the use of oral desmopressin 1–2 mg/day. Another tactic is to switch the patient from lithium to valproate, which does not typically cause enuresis.

Conclusion

The pharmacologic treatment of children and adolescents with bipolar disorder is complicated and best approached in a systematic manner. This chapter provides overall strategies and specific tactics for clinicians who treat these patients. The best treatment for these patients and their families usually requires medications and individual and family therapy.

References

American Psychiatric Association: Diagnostic and Statistical Manual of Mental Disorders, 4th Edition, Text Revision. Washington, DC, American Psychiatric Association, 2000

Axelson D, Birmaher B, Brent D, et al: A preliminary study of the Kiddie Schedule for Affective Disorders and Schizophrenia for School-Age Children Mania Rating Scale for children and adolescents. J Child Adolesc Psychopharmacol 13:463–470, 2003

Bauer MS, Callahan AM, Jampala C, et al: Clinical practice guidelines for bipolar disorder from the Department of Veterans Affairs. J Clin Psychiatry 60:9–21, 1999

Besag FM, Berry D: Interactions between antiepileptic and antipsychotic drugs. Drug Saf 292:95-118, 2006

Biederman J, Mick E, Prince J, et al: Systematic chart review of the pharmacologic treatment of comorbid attention deficit hyperactivity disorder in youth with bipolar disorder. J Child Adolesc Psychopharmacol 9:247–256, 1999

Biederman J, Mick E, Bostic JQ, et al: The naturalistic course of pharmacologic treatment of children with manic like symptoms: a systematic chart review. J Clin Psychiatry 59:628–637, 1998

Carlson GA, Rapport MD, Kelly KL, et al: The effects of methylphenidate and lithium on attention and activity level. J Am Acad Child Adolesc Psychiatry 31:262–270, 1992

Chang K, Saxena K, Howe M: An open-label study of lamotrigine adjunct or monotherapy for the treatment of adolescents with bipolar depression. J Am Acad Child Adolesc Psychiatry 45:298–304, 2006

DelBello MP, Kowatch RP, Adler CM, et al: A double-blind randomized pilot study comparing quetiapine and divalproex for adolescent mania. J Am Acad Child Adolesc Psychiatry 45:305-313, 2006

DelBello MP, Hanseman D, Adler CM, et al: Twelve-month outcome of adolescents with bipolar disorder following first hospitalization for a manic or mixed episode. Am J Psychiatry 164:582–590, 2007

Dulcan MK: Helping Parents, Youth, and Teachers Understand Medications for Behavioral and Emotional Problems: A Resource Book of Medication Information Handouts, 3rd Edition. Arlington, VA, American Psychiatric Publishing, 2007

Findling RL, McNamara NK, Gracious BL, et al: Combination lithium and divalproex sodium in pediatric bipolarity. J Am Acad Child Adolesc Psychiatry 42:895–901, 2003

Findling RL, McNamara NK, Youngstrom EA, et al: Double-blind 18-month trial of lithium versus divalproex maintenance treatment in pediatric bipolar disorder. J Am Acad Child Adolesc Psychiatry 44:409–417, 2005

Fountoulakis KN, Vieta E, Sanchez-Moreno J, et al: Treatment guidelines for bipolar disorder: a critical review. J Affect Disord 86:1–10, 2005

Frances AJ, Kahn DA, Carpenter D, et al: The Expert Consensus Guidelines for treating depression in bipolar disorder. J Clin Psychiatry 59 (suppl 4):73–79, 1998

Frye MA, Grunze H, Suppes T, et al: A placebo-controlled evaluation of adjunctive modafinil in the treatment of bipolar depression. Am J Psychiatry 164:1242–1249, 2007

Geller B, Sun K, Zimerman B, et al: Complex and rapid-cycling in bipolar children and adolescents: a preliminary study. J Affect Disord 34:259–268, 1995

Geller B, Cooper TB, Sun K, et al: Double-blind and placebo-controlled study of lithium for adolescent bipolar disorders with secondary substance dependency. J Am Acad Child Adolesc Psychiatry 37:171–178, 1998

Geller B, Zimerman B, Williams M, et al: Diagnostic characteristics of 93 cases of a prepubertal and early adolescent bipolar disorder phenotype by gender, puberty and comorbid attention deficit hyperactivity disorder. J Child Adolesc Psychopharmacol 10:157–164, 2000

Goldstein TR, Birmaher B, Axelson D, et al: History of suicide attempts in pediatric bipolar disorder: factors associated with increased risk. Bipolar Disord 7:525–535, 2005

Hirschfeld RM, Calabrese JR, Weissman MM, et al: Screening for bipolar disorder in the community. J Clin Psychiatry 64:53–59, 2003a

Hirschfeld RM, Holzer C, Calabrese JR, et al: Validity of the Mood Disorder Questionnaire: a general population study. Am J Psychiatry 160:178–180, 2003b

Kafantaris V, Coletti DJ, Dicker R, et al: Lithium treatment of acute mania in adolescents: a placebo-controlled discontinuation study. J Am Acad Child Adolesc Psychiatry 43:984–993, 2004

Keller MB, Lavori PW, Coryell W, et al: Differential outcome of pure manic, mixed/cycling, and pure depressive episodes in patients with bipolar illness. JAMA 255:3138–3142, 1986

Klein DJ, Cottingham EM, Sorter M, et al: Randomized, double-blind, placebo-controlled trial of metformin treatment of weight gain associated with initiation of atypical antipsychotic therapy in children and adolescents. Am J Psychiatry 163:2072-2079, 2006

Kovacs M, Pollock M: Bipolar disorder and comorbid conduct disorder in childhood and adolescence. J Am Acad Child Adolesc Psychiatry 34:715–723, 1995

Kowatch RA, Sethuraman G, Hume JH, et al: Combination pharmacotherapy in children and adolescents with bipolar disorder. Biol Psychiatry 53:978–984, 2003

Kowatch RA, Fristad MA, Birmaher B, et al: Treatment guidelines for children and adolescents with bipolar disorder. J Am Acad Child Adolesc Psychiatry 44:213–235, 2005

McClellan J, Kowatch RA, Findling RL; Work Group on Quality Issues: Practice parameter for the assessment and treatment of children and adolescents with bipolar disorder. J Am Acad Child Adolesc Psychiatry 46:107–125, 2007

Patel NC, DelBello MP, Bryan HS, et al: Open-label lithium for the treatment of adolescents with bipolar depression. J Am Acad Child Adolesc Psychiatry 45:289–297, 2006

Practice guideline for the treatment of patients with bipolar disorder. American Psychiatric Association. Am J Psychiatry 151 (12, suppl):1–36, 1994

Rasgon NL, Altshuler LL, Fairbanks L, et al: Reproductive function and risk for PCOS in women treated for bipolar disorder. Bipolar Disord 7:246–259, 2005

Rush AJ: Strategies and tactics in the management of maintenance treatment for depressed patients. J Clin Psychiatry 60 (suppl 14):21–26, 1999

Sachs GD, Printz D, Kahn DA, et al: The Expert Consensus Guideline Series: Medication Treatment of Bipolar Disorder 2000. Postgrad Med (spec no):1–104, 2000

Scheffer R, Kowatch R, Carmody T, et al: A randomized placebo-controlled trial of Adderall for symptoms of comorbid ADHD in pediatric bipolar disorder following mood stabilization with divalproex sodium. Am J Psychiatry 162:58–64, 2005

Strober M, Morrell C, Lampert C, et al: Relapse following discontinuation of lithium maintenance therapy in adolescents with bipolar I illness: a naturalistic study. Am J Psychiatry147:457–461, 1990

Suppes T, Dennehy EB, Hirschfeld RM, et al: The Texas Implementation of Medication algorithms: update to the algorithms for treatment of bipolar I disorder. J Clin Psychiatry 66:870–886, 2005

Tohen M, Kryzhanovskaya L, Carlson GA, et al: Olanzapine efficacy and tolerability in adolescents with bipolar mania: results from a 26-week, open-label extension study, in Abstracts of the 47th Annual Meeting of the New Clinical Drug Evaluation Unit, Boca Raton, FL, June 11–14, 2007, p 151

Wagner KD, Hirschfeld rm, Emslie gj, ET AL: Validation of the Mood Disorder Questionnaire for bipolar disorders in adolescents. J Clin Psychiatry 67:827–830, 2006

West SA, McElroy SL, Strakowski SM, et al: Attention deficit hyperactivity disorder in adolescent mania. Am J Psychiatry 152:271–273, 1995

Wozniak J, Biederman J, Kiely K, et al: Mania-like symptoms suggestive of childhood-onset bipolar disorder in clinically referred children. J Am Acad Child Adolesc Psychiatry 34:867–876, 1995

Youngstrom EA, Duax J: Evidence-based assessment of pediatric bipolar disorder, Part I: base rate and family history. J Am Acad Child Adolesc Psychiatry 44:712–717, 2005

9

Comorbidity

Robert L. Findling, M.D.

As a result of the variety of symptoms associated with diverse clinical manifestations, bipolar spectrum disorders are difficult to diagnose accurately in children and adolescents. Further complicating the diagnosis of bipolar disorders is the occurrence of high rates of psychiatric comorbidity in youths. In fact, one study of rates of syndromal and subsyndromal comorbid psychiatric diagnoses found that 97.9% (*n*=91) of children and adolescents with a bipolar spectrum disorder also had a comorbid psychiatric disorder (Tillman et al. 2003). Among the most common comorbid psychiatric conditions seen in young patients with bipolar disorders are attention-deficit/ hyperactivity disorder (ADHD), oppositional defiant disorder (ODD), and conduct disorder. Other comorbidities that frequently occur in children and adolescents with bipolar disorders are anxiety disorders and substance use disorders.

Comorbid Psychiatric Conditions: Findings From Selected Cohorts

Several groups of investigators have examined the rates of psychiatric comorbidity in populations of children and adolescents with bipolar illness. In what follows I discuss the most common comorbid psychiatric conditions in selected cohorts of patients with bipolar disorders. The findings for these cohorts are summarized in Table 9–1. It should be noted that these cohorts were selected because they included a sample size of greater than or equal to 50.

Attention-Deficit/Hyperactivity Disorder

ADHD is a very common comorbid diagnosis in children and adolescents with bipolar disorders. ADHD has been found to be a comorbid condition in approximately 37%–98% of youths with a bipolar disorder (Biederman et al. 2004; Geller et al. 1998; Masi et al. 2006; West et al. 1995; Wozniak et al. 1995a). It has been proposed that the high rates of comorbid ADHD are a result of symptoms common to both conditions: inattention, distractibility, impulsivity, psychomotor agitation, and sleep disturbances (Singh et al. 2006).

It is likely that earlier age at onset of a bipolar disorder is linked to a higher risk of comorbid ADHD. Several studies have found that the mean age at onset of bipolar disorders in bipolar patients with a history of childhood ADHD is significantly lower than in bipolar patients without a history of childhood ADHD (Sachs et al. 2000). In most cases, it appears that the onset of ADHD occurred before the onset of pediatric bipolar disorder. It has been suggested that hyperactivity is the first developmentally age-specific manifestation of early-onset bipolar disorder (Geller and Luby 1997). Additionally, ADHD may be a developmental marker of a very early-onset form of bipolar disorder (Biederman et al. 2005; Faraone et al. 1997b). Comorbid ADHD has been found to occur at rates as high as 98% in children with bipolar disorders; conversely, comorbid ADHD has generally been reported to occur at lower rates in adolescents with a bipolar disorder (West et al. 1995; Wozniak et al. 1995a). Some retrospective studies of adults with bipolar disorders have described higher rates of comorbid ADHD when bipolar onset occurred before the age of 19 (Sachs et al. 2000).

The presence of comorbid ADHD may complicate treatment strategies or may have a negative impact on clinical outcome. Furthermore, a comorbid diag-

Table 9–1.   Selected cohorts: comorbidity in pediatric bipolar illness

Investigators	N	Cohort demographics	Bipolar diagnosis	Comorbid diagnosis (%)				
				ADHD	ODD	CD	ADs	SUDs
Findling et al. 2001	90	Mean age[a]: 10.8±3.5 Males: 64 Females: 26	Bipolar I disorder	70.0	46.7	16.7	14.4	6.6
Tillman et al. 2003[b]	93	Mean age: 10.9±2.6 Males: 57 Females: 36	Bipolar I disorder	87.1	78.5	11.8	22.67	—
Faedda et al. 2004	82	Mean age: 10.6±3.6 Males: 54 Females: 28	Bipolar I disorder: 43 Bipolar II disorder: 33 Cyclothymia: 6	11.0	8.5[c]	—	50.0	3.7
Biederman et al. 2005[d]	299	Age: ≤18 Males: 222 Females: 77	Bipolar I disorder	84.3	85.3	41.8	49.5[e]	7.4
Axelson et al. 2006	438	Mean age: 12.7±3.2 Males: 233 Females: 205	Bipolar I disorder: 255 Bipolar II disorder: 30 Bipolar disorder not otherwise specified: 153	59.8	39.5	12.8	39.0	9.1

Note.   AD=anxiety disorder; ADHD=attention-deficit/hyperactivity disorder; CD=conduct disorder; ODD=oppositional defiant disorder; SUD= substance use disorder.
[a]Mean age is presented as age in years±standard deviation.
[b]Comorbid diagnosis rates for this study represent syndromal comorbidities only.
[c]Proportion of patients with comorbid ODD and/or comorbid CD were presented as one percentage.
[d]Data from two cohorts have been combined.
[e]Proportion represents only patients meeting criteria for multiple (≥2) anxiety disorders.

nosis of ADHD may also affect the clinical presentation of bipolarity. For instance, Masi et al. (2006) found that children and adolescents with both bipolar disorder and ADHD presented more often with irritability than elated mood in comparison to youths without a comorbid ADHD diagnosis. Additionally, the patients with a comorbid ADHD diagnosis appeared to be chronically ill rather than experiencing fluctuating episodes of illness (Masi et al. 2006).

High familial risk for comorbid ADHD and bipolar disorders has been reported. Data indicate that children of adults with ADHD and bipolar disorders are at an increased risk of developing a bipolar disorder; however, elevated risk for developing a bipolar disorder was not found in offspring of parents with ADHD only (Faraone et al. 1997a; Wozniak et al. 1995b). Furthermore, Chang et al. (2000) found that offspring of parents with bipolar illness commonly had ADHD (28%), major depression or dysthymia (15%), or bipolar disorder or cyclothymia (15%). Predictors of bipolarity in offspring of these parents with bipolarity included early parental symptom onset and parental history of childhood ADHD (Chang et al. 2000).

Disruptive Behavior Disorders

As a result of the behavioral disinhibition of bipolar illness, a large number of children and adolescents with bipolar disorders exhibit aggressive behavior and engage in antisocial acts (Wozniak et al. 2001). In fact, a substantial amount of symptom overlap exists between bipolar disorders and disruptive behavior disorders. For example, Tillman et al. (2003) found that 95.7% (n=89) of their sample of children and adolescents with bipolar disorder met criteria for syndromal (78.5%) or subsyndromal (17.2%) ODD. In addition, 25.8% (n= 24) of the youths with bipolar disorder also met diagnostic criteria for syndromal (11.8%) or subsyndromal (14.0%) conduct disorder.

Considerably high rates of conduct disorder have been reported in adolescents with bipolar disorder. Kovacs and Pollock (1995) reported a lifetime comorbidity rate of 69% and a 54% rate of episode comorbidity with conduct disorder in children and adolescents with bipolar disorder. The authors also suggested that comorbid conduct disorder may identify a subtype of very early-onset bipolar disorder (Kovacs and Pollock 1995; Reddy and Srinath 2000).

Common symptoms observed in children and adolescents referred for psychiatric evaluation are irritability and aggression. For instance, Danielyan et al. (2007) found that 84.6% (n=22) of a group of children with bipolar spectrum illnesses presented with irritability, and 88.5% ($n=23$) of the sample ($N=26$) presented with aggression. Both of these symptoms are observed in youths with a disruptive behavior disorder or those who are diagnosed with bipolar disorder. A posited delineation between conduct disorder and bipolar disorder aggression is that youths with conduct disorder without bipolarity present with predatory aggression. However, in children with bipolar disorder, the aggressive behaviors are less goal directed (Biederman et al. 1997).

In addition, children with bipolar disorders frequently meet diagnostic criteria for conduct disorder and vice versa (Wozniak et al. 2001). However, children with conduct disorder and bipolar illness may be misdiagnosed with conduct disorder only. The danger in such a misdiagnosis is that if the bipolar disorder remains undiagnosed, the affected child may not receive proper treatment (Biederman et al. 1997). On its own, conduct disorder is difficult to treat; however, once a comorbid disruptive behavior disorder in an individual with a bipolar disorder has been identified, there is a possibility the child will benefit from treatment for both disorders.

Also notable in children and adolescents with bipolar I disorder is the chronic irritability from which these youth suffer (Findling et al. 2001). These children are easily angered and annoyed, and they frequently lose their temper. Thus, children and adolescents with bipolar disorders are frequently diagnosed with comorbid ODD because they exhibit irritability and other symptoms of ODD during periods of euthymia (Findling et al. 2001).

Anxiety Disorders

Anxiety disorders—panic disorder, social anxiety disorder, obsessive-compulsive disorder (OCD), and posttraumatic stress disorder (PTSD)—are other relatively common comorbid conditions in children and adolescents with bipolar disorders. Extant adult data, specifically the Epidemiologic Catchment Area study that described phenomenology of persons with bipolar I and bipolar II disorders, indicate that 20.8% of adults with bipolar illness have a lifetime history of panic disorder and 21% have a lifetime history of OCD, compared with 0.8% and 2.5%, respectively, in the general population (reviewed by Freeman et al. 2002). The National Comorbidity Survey reported that 92.9% of individuals with bipolar I disorder also met criteria for an anxiety disorder, compared with 24.9% of the general population sample (Freeman et al. 2002). Additionally, data from the National Institute of Mental Health Systematic Treatment Enhancement Program for Bipolar Disorder (STEP-BD) indicate that very early age at onset of bipolar disorder (<13 years) is associated with a high rate of comorbid anxiety disorders (reviewed by Wagner 2006).

However, there is not yet a wealth of knowledge about anxiety disorder comorbidity in children and adolescents with bipolar disorders (Masi et al. 2001). What is known is that the presence of anxiety disorder symptoms during episodes of either depression or mania in children has been found to be associated with higher rates of rapid cycling, greater treatment resistance, poorer functional outcome, and higher risk for suicide (for a review, see Carlson and Meyer 2006).

In the literature, the rate of comorbid anxiety disorders has been reported to be as high as 77.4% in youths with bipolar disorders (Dickstein et al. 2005). Furthermore, in a literature review, Wagner (2006) noted the following rates of specific comorbid anxiety disorders in children and adolescents with bipolar disorder: OCD, 9.0%–48.9%; social phobia, 3.2%–39.5%; generalized anxiety disorder, 11.0%–33.3%; separation anxiety disorder, 13.3%–57.0%; panic disorder, 5.0%–52.0%; PTSD, 7.0%–27.0%; and multiple (more than one) anxiety disorders, 41.6%–53%.

Patients with comorbid anxiety symptoms may report that anxiety diagnoses and symptoms preceded the onset of the bipolar disorder, and therefore anxiety symptoms may be a marker of early-onset bipolar disorder (Carlson and Meyer 2006; Dickstein et al. 2005; Masi et al. 2001; Tillman et al. 2003; Wozniak et al. 2002). Similarly, it has been posited that children and adolescents with panic disorder are at higher risk for developing bipolar disorder and that panic disorder is likely an indicator of risk for bipolar disorder (Birmaher et al. 2002). Additionally, Dickstein et al. (2005) found that youths diagnosed with bipolar disorder and comorbid anxiety experienced greater functional impairment than youths without comorbid anxiety. It has also been found in adults that anxiety symptoms are often treatment resistant in patients with bipolar disorders, and consequently these patients appear to have a poorer prognosis than those who have bipolar disorder alone (Simon et al. 2004). The recent studies described above indicate that mood instability often exacerbates anxiety symptoms (Birmaher et al. 2002; Carlson and Meyer 2006; Dickstein et al. 2005; Masi et al. 2001; Simon et al. 2004; Tillman et al. 2003; Wozniak et al. 2002).

Substance Use

It is common for adults diagnosed with a bipolar disorder to have a comorbid substance use disorder (Grunebaum et al. 2006; Strakowski et al. 2000, 2007). Like other comorbid psychiatric conditions, substance use disorders complicate the course and treatment of bipolar disorder. With this in mind, it is imperative to assess regularly for a substance use disorder in adolescents with a bipolar disorder.

There is growing evidence that youths diagnosed with a bipolar disorder are at high risk for developing a substance use disorder. Specifically, substance use in youths with bipolar illness has been associated with earlier age at onset of bipolarity (Grunebaum et al. 2006) and a history of childhood hyperactivity (Strober et al. 2006). In the National Institutes of Health–funded Course and Outcome of Bipolar Illness in Youth study, 9.1% of the youths diagnosed with a bipolar disorder (mean age = 12.7 years) had a comorbid substance use disorder (Axelson et al. 2006). Wilens et al. (2004) found age at onset of bipolarity to be related to the risk of a substance use disorder. In that study, an age at onset of bipolar disorder of 13 years or older was a greater predictor of a substance use disorder than an age at onset of bipolar disorder prior to age 13 years. Additionally, comorbid conduct disorder is frequently present in children and adolescents with bipolar disorder and a substance use disorder (Wilens et al. 1999, 2004).

The substances generally most abused by patients with bipolar disorder are cigarettes, cannabis, and alcohol (Strakowski et al. 2000, 2005, 2007; Wilens et al. 2003). Wilens et al. (2003) found that there is a strong relationship between child-onset bipolar disorder and cigarette smoking and substance use disorder. Additionally, Strakowski et al. (2005) determined that patients between the ages of 12 to 45 years who had experienced the onset of bipolarity before the onset of alcohol use disorder exhibited symptoms of an alcohol use disorder more frequently than patients who experienced the onset of alcohol use disorder first. Furthermore, alcohol use increased during mixed episodes in patients who experienced bipolar onset before the onset of alcohol use disorder (Strakowski et al. 2005). Similarly, Strakowski et al. (2007) found that in patients who experienced the onset of bipolar disorder before the onset of a cannabis use disorder were more prone to cannabis abuse during periods of mania. The results of Strakowski et al. (2005, 2007) should be interpreted with caution when extrapolating this information to youths because despite the cohorts' inclusion of adolescents, the majority of both cohorts consisted of adults.

Some special considerations should be made in bipolar youths with a comorbid substance abuse. For instance, when considering treatment options for patients with bipolar disorder and comorbid substance abuse diagnoses, the clinician must assess the likelihood of medication misuse or abuse. In such patients, issues relating to treatment nonadherence also may be present.

Methodological Challenges

Notably, the rates of comorbid disorders vary according to the age of the child, sample selection (clinical versus community), and the methods used to ascertain the psychiatric symptomatology (Pavuluri et al. 2005). In addition, the high rates of reported comorbidity in youths with bipolar disorder may lead to a failure to diagnose a bipolar spectrum disorder. For example, early-onset bipolar disorders are commonly misdiagnosed as ADHD, major depressive disorder, anxiety disorders, ODD, and conduct disorders (Danielyan et al. 2007).

However, there is consensus that pediatric bipolar disorders are associated with high rates of comorbidity. Because more than one psychiatric syndrome frequently is present in children and adolescents with a bipolar disorder, once the diagnosis of bipolarity is made it is essential that the presence of a psychiatric comorbidity be determined. Identification of psychiatric comorbidities is imperative because effective treatment plans are dependent on the proper diagnosis of bipolar disorders and comorbid conditions.

Clinical Approach to Assessment

Many of the psychiatric disorders that occur as comorbidities in children and adolescents with bipolar disorders mistakenly can be perceived as manifestations of the bipolar illness itself. These misconceptions occur because the presentation of these other conditions can have a similar appearance to the symptoms of the affective illness. Specifically, restlessness and irritability are common symptoms across multiple diagnoses, and therefore it is important to ascertain symptom overlap before making a comorbid diagnosis. For example, many youngsters will appear obsessive or anxious during periods of mania or hypomania. Additionally, it is not uncommon for children with a bipolar disorder to be oppositional, surly, and defiant while either manic or depressed. These symptoms may "disappear" when the patient is experiencing neutral moods; however, frequently the symptoms do not ameliorate and are still present during periods of euthymia.

As mentioned earlier, optimal treatment of bipolar disorders requires treating both the affective illness and comorbid psychiatric conditions. Several methods exist for assigning the presence or absence of comorbid diagnoses. In the subtraction method, overlapping symptoms are not counted when making a diagnosis. As a result, the number of possible symptoms that can be considered is reduced significantly. To adjust for the reduction of symptoms in the subtraction method, the clinician can employ the proportion method. This method requires that the observed proportion of symptoms in the reduced set of symptoms obtained from the subtraction method be at least as large as the proportion of symptoms required by original diagnostic criteria (Milberger et al. 1995; see also Biederman et al. 2003). An additional way to assess for comorbidities is to use a "parsimonious" method, describing a patient's symptoms during his or her neutral moods or euthymic states (Findling et al. 2001). When symptoms persist during euthymic periods, a comorbid diagnosis can be inferred.

What follows is a case vignette that highlights the "parsimonious" method of diagnostic approaches to a youngster with bipolar disorder. This particular method is that which is employed in our center.

You are asked to evaluate a 12-year-old boy who has recently developed substantive difficulties with aggressive behavior and irritability.

The patient initially was brought to his pediatrician at age 8 because of long-standing difficulties with restlessness and overactivity. In addition, at that time, his teacher noted that this youth was distractible and frequently off task in school. As a result of these chronic difficulties, he was having marked problems with achievement and peer relationships. Besides these in-school issues, his family noted that at the time of his initial evaluation with his pediatrician, the patient had difficulties outside of school. His restlessness made it difficult to take him to religious services because he had a markedly more difficult time remaining seated than other children his own age. Because the patient had chronic, pervasive, and substantive difficulties with restlessness and distractibility, coupled with the observation that there were no particular external circumstances that could explain his symptoms, a diagnosis of ADHD was given. A behavior modification plan was implemented, and treatment with a psychostimulant was initiated. The youth responded well to treatment for the intervening 4 years.

Approximately 6 months before your evaluation, the patient developed new difficulties. Although there were no identifiable new stressors, and there were no changes in the patient's ADHD therapy, it appeared that the patient's ADHD "just got worse," and the "medication stopped working." During your evaluation, you learn that this youngster has become remarkably irritable, whereas he used to be pleasant and agreeable. Although he had made several good friends over the prior few years, he has started to get into physical altercations for the first time in his life. With further history, it is learned that the patient has had a change in sleep—he is now routinely sleeping 3 hours less per night than he used to. The family remarks that during the night, the patient will frequently rearrange furniture, compulsively work on new projects, and reorganize his baseball card collection again and again.

In addition, the patient has become much more talkative; in fact, there are periods of time when he will speak extremely rapidly and will be difficult to interrupt. There are also instances in which the patient will speak so rapidly that he is difficult to understand. The patient has also recently gotten into the habit of using curse words, not only at home but also at school.

Owing to concerns that the patient's psychostimulants were no longer of help, the patient's pediatrician discontinued his stimulant therapy 3 weeks before his evaluation with you. This change in pharmacotherapy yielded no change in the child's mood or behavior. Of note, there is a family history of a paternal aunt "who was on lithium" who completed suicide when she was in her 20s.

From this history, it appears that this youngster recently developed a bipolar spectrum disorder. In addition, because of the presence of a chronic history of dysfunctional/impairing restlessness and distractibility during periods of euthymia, this patient also appears to meet diagnostic criteria for ADHD. However, because this patient's compulsive behavior appears to occur only during periods of mania/hypomania, a diagnosis of obsessive-compulsive behavior might be deferred until the patient's mood disorder is treated effectively.

It is important that patients with a bipolar disorder and their families be aware of the likelihood of psychiatric comorbidity; if patients are otherwise unaware, then it may be difficult to describe symptoms during neutral moods. Once patients and their families are aware of the possibility of comorbidity, and once a patient's mood stabilizes, it is easier to assess for comorbid psychiatric disorders. Figure 9–1 summarizes possible approaches to evaluating and characterizing pediatric bipolarity. The assessment of psychiatric comorbidity in pediatric patients with bipolar illness is summarized in Figure 9–2.

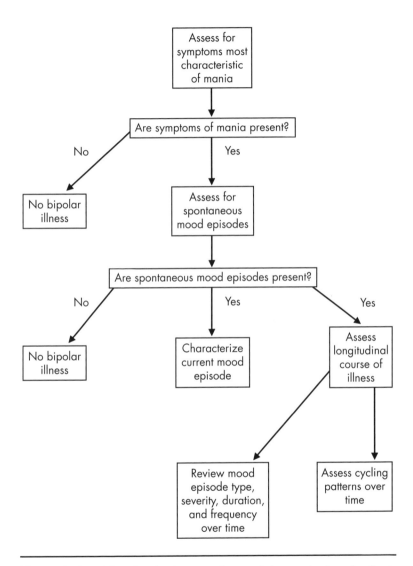

Figure 9–1. Selected evaluation procedures and characterization of pediatric bipolarity.

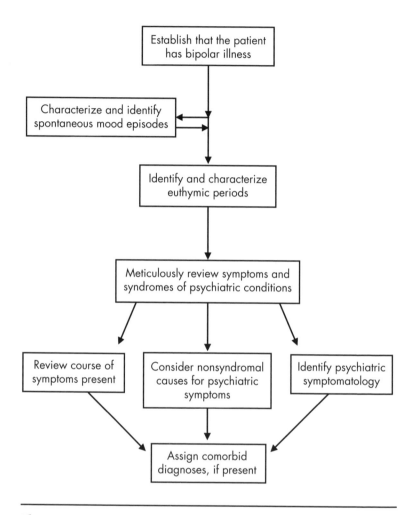

Figure 9–2. An approach to assessing comorbidity in pediatric bipolar illness.

Conclusion

The treatment of children and adolescents with bipolar disorder often is complicated by the presence of comorbid psychiatric diagnoses, the most common of which being ADHD, the disruptive behavior disorders, substance use disorders, and anxiety disorders. Careful assessment allows youth and their families to be provided with key information that will facilitate current and ongoing treatment planning. As a result, meticulous assessment and continued monitoring of comorbid disorders are necessary to ensure that the best treatment for a youth with a bipolar disorder is being given.

References

Axelson D, Birmaher B, Strober M, et al: Phenomenology of children and adolescents with bipolar spectrum disorders. Arch Gen Psychiatry 63:1139–1148, 2006

Biederman J, Faraone SV, Hatch M, et al: Conduct disorder with and without mania in a referred sample of ADHD children. J Affect Disord 44:177–188, 1997

Biederman J, Mick E, Faraone SV, et al: Current concepts in the validity, diagnosis and treatment of paediatric bipolar disorder. Int J Neuropsychopharmacol 6:293–300, 2003

Biederman J, Faraone SV, Wozniak J, et al: Further evidence of unique developmental phenotypic correlates of pediatric bipolar disorder: findings from a large sample of clinically referred preadolescent children assessed over the last 7 years. J Affect Disord 82 (suppl 1):S45–S58, 2004

Biederman J, Faraone SV, Wozniak J, et al: Clinical correlates of bipolar disorder in a large, referred sample of children and adolescents. J Psychiatr Res 39:611–622, 2005

Birmaher B, Kennah A, Brent D, et al: Is bipolar disorder specifically associated with panic disorder in youths? J Clin Psychiatry 63:414–419, 2002

Carlson GA, Meyer SE: Phenomenology and diagnosis of bipolar disorders in children, adolescents, and adults: complexities and developmental issues. Dev Psychopathol 18:939–969, 2006

Chang KD, Steiner H, Ketter TA: Psychiatric phenomenology of child and adolescent bipolar offspring. J Am Acad Child Adolesc Psychiatry 39:453–460, 2000

Danielyan A, Pathak S, Kowatch RA, et al: Clinical characteristics of bipolar disorder in very young children. J Affect Disord 97:51–59, 2007

Dickstein DP, Rich BA, Binstock AB, et al: Comorbid anxiety in phenotypes of pediatric bipolar disorder. J Child Adolesc Psychopharmacol 15:534–548, 2005

Faedda GL, Baldessarini RJ, Glovinsky IP, et al: Pediatric bipolar disorder: phenomenology and course of illness. Bipolar Disord 6:305–313, 2004

Faraone SV, Biederman J, Mennin D, et al: Attention-deficit hyperactivity disorder with bipolar disorder: a familial subtype? J Am Acad Child Adolesc Psychiatry 36:1378–1387, 1997a

Faraone SV, Biederman J, Wozniak J, et al: Is comorbidity with ADHD a marker for juvenile-onset mania? J Am Acad Child Adolesc Psychiatry 36:1046–1055, 1997b

Findling RL, Gracious BL, McNamara NK, et al: Rapid, continuous cycling and psychiatric co-morbidity in pediatric bipolar I disorder. Bipolar Disord 3:202–210, 2001

Freeman MP, Freeman SA, McElroy SL: The comorbidity of bipolar and anxiety disorders: prevalence, psychobiology, and treatment issues. J Affect Disord 68:1–23, 2002

Geller B, Luby J: Child and adolescent bipolar disorder: a review of the past 10 years. J Am Acad Child Adolesc Psychiatry 36:1168–1176, 1997

Geller B, Williams M, Zimerman B, et al: Prepubertal and early adolescent bipolarity differentiate from ADHD by manic symptoms, grandiose delusions, ultra-rapid or ultradian cycling. J Affect Disord 51:81–91, 1998

Grunebaum MF, Galfalvy HC, Nichols CM, et al: Aggression and substance abuse in bipolar disorder. Bipolar Disord 8:496–502, 2006

Kovacs M, Pollock M: Bipolar disorder and comorbid conduct disorder in childhood and adolescence. J Am Acad Child Adolesc Psychiatry 34:715–723, 1995

Masi G, Toni C, Perugi G, et al: Anxiety disorders in children and adolescents with bipolar disorder: a neglected comorbidity. Can J Psychiatry 46:797–802, 2001

Masi G, Perugi G, Toni C, et al: Attention-deficit hyperactivity disorder—bipolar comorbidity in children and adolescents. Bipolar Disord 8:373–381, 2006

Milberger S, Biederman J, Faraone SV, et al: Attention deficit hyperactivity disorder and comorbid disorders: issues of overlapping symptoms. Am J Psychiatry 152:1793–1799, 1995

Pavuluri MN, Birmaher B, Naylor MW: Pediatric bipolar disorder: a review of the past 10 years. J Am Acad Child Adolesc Psychiatry 44:846–871, 2005

Reddy YC, Srinath S: Juvenile bipolar disorder. Acta Psychiatr Scand 102:162–170, 2000

Sachs BS, Baldassano CF, Truman CJ, et al: Comorbidity of attention deficit hyperactivity disorder with early and late-onset bipolar disorder. Am J Psychiatry 157:466–468, 2000

Simon NM, Otto MW, Wisniewski SR, et al: Anxiety disorder comorbidity in bipolar disorder patients: data from the first 500 participants in the Systematic Treatment Enhancement Program for Bipolar Disorder (STEP-BD). Am J Psychiatry 161:2222–2229, 2004

Singh MK, DelBello MP, Kowatch RA, et al: Co-occurrence of bipolar and attention-deficit hyperactivity disorders in children. Bipolar Disord 8:710–720, 2006

Strakowski SM, DelBello MP, Fleck DE, et al: The impact of substance abuse on the course of bipolar disorder. Biol Psychiatry 48:477–485, 2000

Strakowski SM, DelBello MP, Fleck DE, et al: Effects of co-occurring alcohol abuse on the course of bipolar disorder following a first hospitalization for mania. Arch Gen Psychiatry 62:851–888, 2005

Strakowski SM, DelBello MP, Fleck DE, et al: Effects of co-occurring cannabis use disorders on the course of bipolar disorder after a first hospitalization for mania. Arch Gen Psychiatry 64:57–64, 2007

Strober M, Birmaher B, Ryan N, et al: Pediatric bipolar disease: current and future perspectives for study of its long-term course and treatment. Bipolar Disord 8:311–321, 2006

Tillman R, Geller B, Bolhofner K, et al: Ages of onset and rates of syndromal and subsyndromal comorbid DSM-IV diagnoses in a prepubertal and early adolescent bipolar disorder phenotype. J Am Acad Child Adolesc Psychiatry 42:1486–1493, 2003

Wagner KD: Bipolar disorder and comorbid anxiety disorders in children and adolescents. J Clin Psychiatry 67 (suppl 1):S16–S20, 2006

West SA, McElroy SL, Strakowski SM, et al: Attention deficit hyperactivity disorder in adolescent mania. Am J Psychiatry 152:271–273, 1995

Wilens TE, Biederman J, Millstein RB, et al: Risk for substance use disorders in youths with child- and adolescent-onset bipolar disorder. J Am Acad Child Adolesc Psychiatry 38:680–685, 1999

Wilens TE, Biederman J, Forkner P, et al: Patterns of comorbidity and dysfunction in clinically referred preschool and school-age children with bipolar disorder. J Child Adolesc Psychopharmacol 13:495–505, 2003

Wilens TE, Biederman J, Kwon A, et al: Risk of substance use disorders in adolescents with bipolar disorder. J Am Acad Child Adolesc Psychiatry 43:1380–1386, 2004

Wozniak J, Biederman J, Kiely K, et al: Mania-like symptoms suggestive of childhood-onset bipolar disorder in clinically referred children. J Am Acad Child Adolesc Psychiatry 34:867–876, 1995a

Wozniak J, Biederman J, Mundy E, et al: A pilot family study of childhood-onset mania. J Am Acad Child Adolesc Psychiatry 34:1577–1583, 1995b

Wozniak J, Biederman J, Faraone SV, et al: Heterogeneity of childhood conduct disorder: further evidence of a subtype of conduct disorder linked to bipolar disorder. J Affect Disord 64:121–131, 2001

Wozniak J, Biederman J, Monuteaux MC, et al: Parsing the comorbidity between bipolar disorder and anxiety disorders: a familial risk analysis. J Child Adolesc Psychopharmacol 12:101–111, 2002

10

Working With Patients and Their Families

Cardinal Symptom Monitoring and Mood Charting

Matthew E. Young, M.A.

Mary A. Fristad, Ph.D., A.B.P.P.

Psychosocial interventions, including group and individual psychotherapy, are an important component of comprehensive treatment for bipolar disorder in children and adolescents (Kowatch et al. 2005; McClellan et al. 2007). As adjuncts to medication, psychosocial treatments are intended to provide patients and their families with knowledge and skills. In this chapter we review a number of psychosocial therapy techniques used with children and adolescents with bipolar disorder. Psychoeducation to improve the family's understanding of bipolar disorder is a vital first step in therapy. Problem-solving and skills-training components are derived from cognitive-behavioral therapies and include skills for coping with negative emotions; modifying cognitions; maintaining healthy eating, sleeping, and exercise habits; and improving communication skills. Symptom monitoring is an important tool for children and their parents to learn, and aids the treatment team in monitoring response to medication and psychosocial treatments. Mood charting methods encourage patients and parents to take an active role in tracking treatment response and can increase insight into mood states.

A number of psychosocial interventions have been developed for use with children and adolescents with bipolar disorder. These treatments share several features in common, such as the use of psychoeducation and a focus on skill building, communication, and problem solving. Each has a foundation in cognitive-behavioral theory. However, limited data have been published to support the efficacy of these interventions. Published studies frequently have small sample sizes and lack random assignment or comparison groups. Table 10–1 describes the existing psychosocial treatments for bipolar disorder in children and adolescents and summarizes the available evidence regarding their efficacy. Large-scale randomized trials are necessary before any of these treatments can be considered an empirically supported treatment.

Psychoeducational Psychotherapy

Psychoeducation per se may be as simple as providing educational handouts in therapy. Significantly more extensive than psychoeducation is psychoeducational psychotherapy (PEP), an important component of all the treatments discussed in this chapter. It combines psychotherapy and education to improve an individual's ability to cope with an illness or problem by providing information and fostering skill building (Lukens and McFarlane 2004). In child and adolescent bipolar disorder, the patient and family are provided with information about the illness, its course and outcome, and methods of treatment. PEP may begin with several sessions devoted to increasing knowledge about the etiology, course, and prognosis of bipolar disorder; decreasing the stigma associated with bipolar disorder; and encouraging the patient and family to become active consumers of treatment (Fristad 2006).

An initial goal for parents is to learn about the illness and how they can improve treatment adherence and family functioning. Providing information

Table 10–1. Psychosocial treatments for bipolar disorder in children and adolescents

Treatment	Format	Target population, age range	Treatment components	Evidence
Multifamily psychoeducation groups (Fristad et al. 2002, 2003)	Concurrent child and parent groups	Bipolar disorder and depressive disorders, 8–12	Psychoeducation, communication training, problem-solving skills training, mood charting, medication compliance	Small-scale RCT ($N=35$): participants showed improvement in knowledge of mood disorders, family interaction, access to services, and social support, compared with wait-list control subjects. Participants continued TAU throughout the trial. Large-scale RCT ($N=165$): recently completed; results not yet published.
Individual family psychoeducation (IFP and IFP-24) (Fristad 2006)	Individual families (includes parent, parent-child, parent-child-sibling, and parent-child–school personnel sessions)	Bipolar disorder, 8–12	Psychoeducation, communication training, problem-solving skills training, mood charting, medication compliance, healthy habits (diet, exercise, and sleep); IFP-24 also includes sibling involvement and contact with the child's school	Small-scale RCT of IFP ($N=20$): significant improvement in family climate and positive family evaluations of treatment. Large effect size for mood symptoms, but small sample size limited power. Participants continued TAU throughout the trial. Seven families dropped out of treatment. Case series of IFP-24: recently completed; results not yet published.

Table 10–1. Psychosocial treatments for bipolar disorder in children and adolescents *(continued)*

Treatment	Format	Target population, age range	Treatment components	Evidence
Family-focused treatment (Miklowitz et al. 2004, 2006)	Individual family treatment	Bipolar disorder, 13–17	Psychoeducation, communication training, problem-solving skills training	Open trial (*N*=20): significant decrease in manic and depressive symptoms, as well as Child Behavior Checklist total problems *t*-score posttreatment. Improvements were maintained 1 year later. All participants were prescribed medication. No comparison group. RCT is under way.
Child- and family-focused cognitive-behavioral therapy (Pavuluri et al. 2004; West et al. 2007)	Individual (parent, child, parent-child, and parent-sibling sessions)	Bipolar disorder, 5–17	Psychoeducation, communication training, problem-solving skills training, sibling involvement, contact with child's school	Open trial (*N*=34): improvements in bipolar disorder and attention-deficit/hyperactivity disorder symptoms and global functioning, decreased aggression. Treatment gains maintained at 3-year follow-up with maintenance treatment sessions. All participants were prescribed medication. No comparison group.

Table 10–1.   Psychosocial treatments for bipolar disorder in children and adolescents *(continued)*

Treatment	Format	Target population, age range	Treatment components	Evidence
Cognitive-behavioral therapy (CBT) (Danielson et al. 2004; Feeny et al. 2006)	Individual (limited parent participation)	Bipolar disorder, 10–17	Psychoeducation, communication training, problem-solving skills training, mood charting, medication compliance, sleep regulation, identifying and modifying negative thoughts	Pilot study: CBT participants ($n=8$) did not differ from control group ($n=8$) on symptom measures. Large effect sizes were observed in most analyses, but small sample size limited power to detect statistically significant differences. Seven of 8 participants completed the 12-session protocol.
Dialectical behavior therapy (Goldstein et al. 2007)	Individual (alternating individual and family sessions; telephone skills coaching also incorporated)	Bipolar disorder, 12–18	Psychoeducation, mood charting, mood regulation skills training	Pilot study ($N=10$): 9 participants completed 1-year treatment; 90% of scheduled sessions were attended. Results indicate high consumer satisfaction and improvement in suicidality, mood dysregulation, and depressive symptoms. No significant improvements in manic symptoms or interpersonal functioning were observed.

Note.   RCT=randomized clinical trial; TAU=treatment as usual (i.e., receiving any additional treatment, including medication, the family felt was warranted).

about the biological etiology of bipolar disorder often decreases parents' feelings of blame or guilt about their child's illness. However, the therapist should also emphasize that the course of bipolar disorder is highly affected by psychosocial factors. This demonstrates to parents that their child's illness is not their fault but that management of bipolar disorder is their (along with their child's) responsibility. Therapists should also spend time debunking incorrect perceptions of mood disorders, such as the belief that they are a sign of weakness or that people can "just get over it" without intervention (Fristad et al. 1998). As comorbidity is common in child and adolescent bipolar disorder (Axelson et al. 2006; Lewinsohn et al. 1995), therapists should review this topic with parents. Psychoeducation regarding treatment for bipolar disorder should include a discussion of common medications, side-effect management, and strategies for maximizing adherence and tracking effectiveness (Fristad et al. 1998). Psychosocial treatments (e.g., individual, family, and group psychotherapy), school-based treatments, and other interventions (e.g., inpatient treatment, respite or out-of home placements, electroconvulsive therapy, herbal and nutritional supplementation) should be discussed. Providing parents with this information allows them to make educated decisions about the cost-benefit ratio of available interventions for their child.

PEP for children and adolescents with bipolar disorder requires adjustments for the patient's age, cognitive abilities, and level of symptoms. Acutely ill and unstable youth are poor candidates for psychosocial interventions, in general (Kowatch et al. 2005). However, as stabilization progresses, even young children often are able to participate in therapy and learn a great deal about their illness. Children should be provided with information about the symptoms of bipolar disorder, treatment methods, and their own role in managing the illness. One particularly useful exercise used in the Multifamily Psychoeducation Group (MFPG) study is called "Naming the Enemy" (Fristad et al. 1999). Once a child has been taught to recognize the symptoms that characterize his or her illness, this exercise allows the child to separate them from his or her "true self." Figure 10–1 is an example of this project. On the left, the child is asked to list positive attributes about himself or herself. On the right, the child is asked to describe symptoms of each of his or her diagnoses. By folding the right column over the left, the therapist can demonstrate how symptoms "cover up" the positive attributes of the individual. By folding the left column over the right, the therapist can demonstrate the goal of treat-

Name _____ Subject # _____

Session 2 Family Project - "Naming the Enemy"
The Symptom-Self Exercise

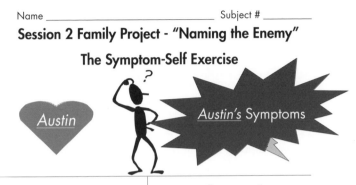

	Depression
Friendly	• Grouchy, sad
Likes to help with chores	• Crying a lot
	• Don't like myself
Great at spelling	• Not interested in playing
Creative	with friends
Kindhearted	Mania
Likes to draw	• "Super high" moods
Animal lover	• Talks too fast
	• Needs less sleep
Good at baseball	• Risky/unsafe behavior
Helps younger sibling	• Too much energy
	• Acting silly
Great smile	
Curious	ADHD
	• Attention problems
Good with computers	• Hyperactive
	• Gets out of seat in class
	• Forgetful

Figure 10–1.   "Naming the Enemy" exercise from Multifamily Psychoeducation Group.

ment: to reduce symptoms and allow the "true self" to show. This exercise allows the patient to demonstrate his or her newly acquired knowledge about bipolar disorder symptoms and assists in externalizing the illness (Fristad et al. 1999).

Skill Building and Problem Solving

Psychosocial interventions for bipolar disorder in children and adolescents contain therapeutic techniques that extend beyond the domain of psychoeducation. These techniques have been adapted from psychosocial treatments for adults with bipolar disorder or from treatments for other forms of child and adolescent psychopathology. Most often these methods are based on cognitive-behavioral and family systems theories. The goal of these treatments is to foster development of skills that allow the patient and family to cope better with bipolar disorder, anticipate and prevent relapse, and minimize the impairment caused by bipolar disorder in areas such as interpersonal relationships.

A variety of behaviors can be helpful for coping with mood symptoms. However, children and adolescents may have difficulty generating ideas for helpful behaviors in the midst of a mood episode. Therefore, the therapist can help the patient plan in advance for these stressful times by creating a list or "tool kit" of helpful coping skills. The tool kit technique has been used in psychotherapy for children with depression (Weisz et al. 1997) and is a component of MFPGs for children with bipolar disorder. In MFPGs, children are encouraged to generate a number of activities to help them cope with negative emotions from four domains: social, creative, physical, and rest and relaxation (R&R). For example, a child may list bike riding as a physical action, talking to a friend on the telephone as a social action, drawing as a creative action, and reading a book as an R&R behavior. Tool kit strategies can include enjoyable activities generated by the child and parents as well as techniques introduced by the therapist (e.g., deep breathing). Behaviors that can be used across a range of settings (e.g., at home during the day, at home at night when the child cannot make noise that will awaken family members, in school, riding in the car) should be included. When the patient experiences negative emotions, the tool kit serves as a menu of choices for coping with the situation. Younger children often enjoy making an actual tool kit rather than just writing a list of coping strategies. A small box, such as a shoebox, can be filled with small reminders of each social, creative, physical, and R&R activity (e.g., a picture of a basketball player to represent sports, one crayon as a reminder to try drawing). Children in the MFPG study frequently spent time alone or with their parents constructing and decorating their tool kits and then brought them to a subsequent session to share their coping strategies with therapists and peers.

Cognitive-behavioral techniques can also be used with children and adolescents with bipolar disorder to foster problem solving and the development of coping skills. The efficacy of cognitive-behavioral psychotherapy for children, adolescents, and families has been established for a number of disorders, including depression (Clarke et al. 1999; Lewinsohn et al. 1990; Weisz et al. 1997), anxiety (Albano and Kendall 2002; Flannery-Schroeder and Kendall 2000; Kendall 1994), and conduct disorder (Kazdin 1992). It is important to consider the client's developmental level when using cognitive-behavioral techniques. For example, younger children's reasoning and language abilities and the ability to understand the causal connection between cognitions and behaviors are less developed compared with those in adolescents and adults (Grave and Blissett 2004). Thinking-Feeling-Doing (TFD), an adaptation of cognitive-behavioral techniques for children, has been used with children with bipolar disorder in the MFPG study (Fristad et al. 2007).

TFD is used as an in-session exercise with children with bipolar disorder and their parents and is intended to "increase the child's and parents' 1) understanding of the connection between thoughts, feelings, and behavior; 2) awareness of their negative mood states and the negative thoughts and behaviors associated with that negative mood state; and 3) ability to generate alternative thoughts and behaviors that can lead to enhanced mood" (Fristad et al. 2007, p. 89). TFD utilizes a cartoon-like diagram (see Figure 10–2) to illustrate the connection between a patient's cognitions, emotions, and behavior. Arrows demonstrate how negative cognitions and behaviors can lead to negative emotions. The therapist leads the patient in a number of role-playing exercises to emphasize how changing one's cognitions and behaviors can result in improved emotions. In group therapy, patients are encouraged to help one another generate positive cognitions and behavior choices—a process that gives each patient additional practice with these skills. After these skills are practiced in the session, the TFD exercise is assigned as between-session homework to give patients an opportunity to generalize these skills to their daily environment. The patient chooses a real-life situation between sessions in which he or she can implement this technique and then shares results of the exercise in the next session.

Healthy Habits: Diet, Exercise, and Sleep

Healthy eating habits, physical exercise, and maintenance of a regular sleep schedule are important for children with bipolar disorder for a number of reasons. A number of medications commonly prescribed for children and adolescents are associated with weight gain. Physical activity and a healthy diet can minimize these effects, and exercise may help to alleviate symptoms of depression (Dunn 2005). Insomnia and decreased need for sleep are symptoms experienced by most children with bipolar disorder, and poorly regulated sleep patterns have the potential to trigger or maintain manic symptoms (Lofthouse et al. 2007, 2008). Therapists can work with the patient and family to identify which of these areas need improvement. The therapist may consider introducing the family to educational materials, such as the U.S. Department of Agriculture's food pyramid (MyPyramid available online at www.mypyramid. gov), as a guide for selecting healthy foods. A referral to a dietitian may be warranted for families with particularly poor eating habits. A number of options are available for physical exercise, ranging from simple behaviors (e.g., taking a daily walk with a pet or family members) to more involved activities such as martial arts or participation in team sports. Information about exercise for children, adolescents, and parents is available on the Internet at sites such as www.bam.gov, www.kidnetic.com, and www.verbnow.com. The therapist can work with families to improve sleep patterns by enforcing a set bedtime and removing items from the child's bedroom that interfere with sleep, such as televisions and video games.

Nonverbal Communication

Nonverbal communication training is an important component of psychosocial treatment for bipolar disorder in children and adolescents. Youth with bipolar disorder report more fear and perceive more hostility when viewing neutral faces, compared with control subjects (Rich et al. 2006). In adults with bipolar disorder, family-focused therapy is associated with an increase in positive nonverbal interactions between patients and family members (Simoneau et al. 1999). Nonverbal communication skills can be developed through

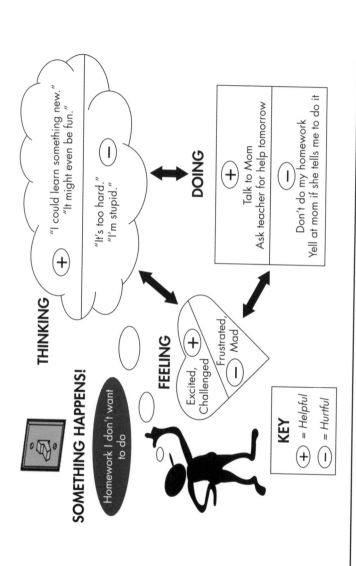

Figure 10–2. "Thinking-Feeling Doing" exercise from Multifamily Psychoeducation Group.

activities such as identifying and labeling pictures or photos that depict emotions. Role-play activities are particularly well suited for nonverbal communication skills training. In MFPGs, children practice nonverbal communication by playing "emotional charades" with their parents, taking turns acting out and identifying various emotional states without using words.

Verbal Communication

Verbal communication skills also are important to address in therapy. Younger children can be taught basic communication skills. For example, in the MFPG intervention, the therapist discusses the difference between verbal and nonverbal communication and "helpful" versus "hurtful" communication. Adolescents can address more advanced topics, such as assertiveness and active listening (Danielson et al. 2004). There is some evidence to suggest that certain types of communication and interaction among family members, including expressed emotion, can affect negatively the course of bipolar disorder (Simoneau et al. 1998). Therefore, parents and other family members should be involved in therapy whenever possible. Sessions with the parents alone can focus on identifying maladaptive family communication patterns. Family therapy sessions are particularly valuable because each individual has a chance to practice newly acquired communication skills. The therapist can facilitate this process by interrupting negative communication and ensuring that each family member is allowed to express his or her view in a constructive way. In MFPGs, children have an opportunity to practice verbal communication skills with their parents. Following the session on verbal communication, each child has an opportunity to suggest ways in which he or she thinks the family can improve communication. Parents are asked to practice active listening skills and refrain from interrupting or commenting while the child speaks. In the following session, parents have an opportunity to make similar suggestions, and children have an opportunity to practice active listening skills without commenting or objecting to parents' suggestions.

Symptom Monitoring

Because of the cyclical and fluctuating nature of bipolar disorder, mental health treatment providers, whether they are providing medication or psychosocial interventions, should monitor patients' symptoms. Information about symptom change and treatment response can help clinicians decide when to modify treatment. Symptoms of mania, depression, and any comorbid conditions should be assessed. Symptom monitoring, carried out with an unstructured interview, mood chart, or validated assessment measures, should be incorporated into each treatment session. Most self-report or parent-completed questionnaires regarding bipolar disorder are intended for initial screening and assessment (Youngstrom and Youngstrom 2005), and it is unclear whether these measures are useful for prospective symptom monitoring. More extensive data exist to support the use of mood symptom rating scales.

Mania Rating Scales

The most commonly used symptom rating scale for mania in research settings is the Young Mania Rating Scale (YMRS) (Young et al. 1978). This scale, which originally was developed for use with adults as an observation rating scale administered by psychiatric nurses in an inpatient setting, has been adapted for use with younger patients (Fristad et al. 1992, 1995). The YMRS is used in research with youth with bipolar disorder as a semistructured interview with the parent or child, as a parent questionnaire, and as an adolescent self-report questionnaire (Gracious et al. 2002; Youngstrom et al. 2003, 2004, 2005b). YMRS scores can be used to track response to pharmacological interventions (Patel et al. 2007). Administration is brief (approximately 20 minutes per informant as a semistructured interview), making the YMRS an attractive option for clinical settings. Despite its wide use, the YMRS has limitations. Some symptoms of mania are not included, other items do not correspond to DSM-IV-TR manic symptoms (American Psychiatric Association 2000), and irritability may be weighted too heavily in scoring (Hunt et al. 2005).

Another mania-specific symptom rating scale, the Kiddie Schedule for Affective Disorders and Schizophrenia Mania Rating Scale (K-SADS-MRS) (Axelson et al. 2003), is a semistructured interview that can be administered to the patient and/or parent to assess current symptom severity. The scale has high internal consistency and interrater reliability (Axelson et al. 2003). In an inpatient setting, parent K-SADS-MRS scores discriminated adolescents with bipolar disorder diagnoses from patients without bipolar disorder (Hunt et al. 2005). Similar to the YMRS, the K-SADS-MRS can be administered relatively quickly using the patient and/or parent as informants. A strength of the

K-SADS-MRS is that it allows the clinician to incorporate child and parent reports into a summary score for each symptom.

Depression Rating Scales

Symptoms of depression must also be monitored in children with bipolar disorder. This may be accomplished by the use of rating scales or interviews that focus on the symptoms of depression. The most commonly used self-report measure of depression symptoms for children and adolescents is the Children's Depression Inventory (Kovacs 1992). The Children's Depression Rating Scale—Revised (Poznanski et al. 1985) is a semistructured interview that assesses depression severity and can be administered to the patient or parent in a format similar to the YMRS. The K-SADS–Present Episode Version (K-SADS-P) depression rating scale, another semistructured interview, was adapted from the K-SADS-P diagnostic interview (Chambers et al. 1985). All of these measures are easily implemented in a clinical setting.

Symptom monitoring is essential for the treatment of patients with bipolar disorder. A number of measures are available for tracking mania and depression, and the patient and his or her parents can be used as informants. Clinicians should evaluate potential symptom severity measures based on their published psychometric properties and remember to track comorbid conditions in addition to mood symptoms to fully evaluate the patient's overall functioning.

Mood Charting

Daily or weekly mood charts, completed by a patient and/or the parents, can be an important component of psychosocial treatment. Mood charting methods provide the therapist with information about symptoms experienced between sessions, serving as a complement to symptom rating scales. Mood charting methods also allow patients and their families to practice monitoring moods at regular intervals. Goodwin and Jamison (2007) illustrate a number of ways that mood charting can be a beneficial component of psychotherapy for adults with bipolar disorder. Mood charting can provide the family and therapist with useful information about mood fluctuations associated with a variety of factors, including psychosocial stressors, physical health, seasonal patterns, and menstrual cycles. Mood chart data can also be used to monitor response to psychosocial and pharmacological interventions and provide the patient with a sense of control and collaboration (Goodwin and Jamison 2007).

Many of these benefits are experienced by children, adolescents, and their parents who utilize the mood charting method.

Mood charts can be relatively simple, with a place to record the child's overall mood for the day (see Figure 10–3). This type of chart is best used with children who are first learning to track their moods, with families who have difficulty completing more comprehensive charts, and for families who wish to have a simple method to chart on an ongoing basis. Mood charts for children are available at Web sites such as www.bpkids.org, the home page of the Child and Adolescent Bipolar Foundation, a parent support and advocacy group. Several charts are available at no cost for use by clinicians and families. Children and parents with greater insight into mood states and behavior can utilize more elaborate charts. These mood charts might include ratings of elevated, depressed, and irritable moods; sleep; medication use; compliance with psychotherapy assignments or strategies; and other relevant behaviors or emotions (e.g., anxiety, drug/alcohol use, diet, exercise). Figure 10–4 shows a detailed mood chart shared with families in the MFPG study. As cognitive abilities develop with age, and patients become skilled at monitoring their moods, a mood chart designed for adults with bipolar disorder may be appropriate. A comprehensive and commonly used adult mood chart is available from the Massachusetts General Hospital Bipolar Clinic and Research Program at www.manicdepressive.org/moodchart.html.

When making recommendations about mood charting to parents, clinicians must take into account family factors such as motivation, organization, and history of completing psychotherapy homework assignments. Comprehensive mood charts encourage in-depth monitoring of the child's mood, behavior, and treatment and provide the clinician and family with valuable information. However, they are more time-consuming and less likely to be completed than more simple mood charts. More impaired, disorganized, or chaotic families are often successful with basic mood charts. Clinicians should monitor the family's compliance with and response to mood charting and modify their recommendations to meet the family's needs. Consistent completion of a basic mood chart is preferable to sporadic completion of a complicated mood monitoring system. To maximize compliance with mood charting, clinicians can implement strategies that encourage psychotherapy homework completion. These include making assignments easy to complete (Conoley et al. 1994), letting the patient assist in formulating the assignment and

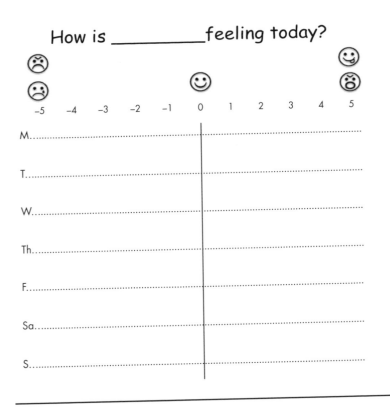

Figure 10–3.   Sample mood chart.

providing a written reminder (Burns and Auerbach 1992; Cox et al. 1988; Helbig and Fehm 2004), and reviewing the assignment during the next session (Garland and Scott 2002).

When clinicians ask children to track their own moods, the child's developmental level, cognitive abilities, and insight into his or her mood are the primary variables to consider. Children with mood disorders often have difficulty identifying their emotional states and may have difficulty rating their own mood. Therefore, a child's mood chart is usually not useful for monitoring treatment response. Despite this limitation, input from children is valuable in the assessment of bipolar disorder (Youngstrom et al. 2005a). Mood charting in children is useful as a strategy to increase the child's awareness and

Child's Name: _____ Treatment Provider/Program: _____

Medications (Type, Dose, Side Effects): _____

Month: _____

Date	Overall Rating (1=Great, 3=So-So, 5=Terrible)	Meds Taken?	Used Strategies (1=100%, 3=50%, 5=0%)	Weekly Comments (e.g., Life Event, Med Change, Med Side Effects, Sleep/Appetite Changes, Other)
1	1 2 3 4 5	Yes No	1 2 3 4 5	
2	1 2 3 4 5	Yes No	1 2 3 4 5	
3	1 2 3 4 5	Yes No	1 2 3 4 5	
4	1 2 3 4 5	Yes No	1 2 3 4 5	
5	1 2 3 4 5	Yes No	1 2 3 4 5	
6	1 2 3 4 5	Yes No	1 2 3 4 5	
7	1 2 3 4 5	Yes No	1 2 3 4 5	
8	1 2 3 4 5	Yes No	1 2 3 4 5	
9	1 2 3 4 5	Yes No	1 2 3 4 5	
10	1 2 3 4 5	Yes No	1 2 3 4 5	
11	1 2 3 4 5	Yes No	1 2 3 4 5	
12	1 2 3 4 5	Yes No	1 2 3 4 5	
13	1 2 3 4 5	Yes No	1 2 3 4 5	
14	1 2 3 4 5	Yes No	1 2 3 4 5	
15	1 2 3 4 5	Yes No	1 2 3 4 5	
16	1 2 3 4 5	Yes No	1 2 3 4 5	
17	1 2 3 4 5	Yes No	1 2 3 4 5	
18	1 2 3 4 5	Yes No	1 2 3 4 5	
19	1 2 3 4 5	Yes No	1 2 3 4 5	
20	1 2 3 4 5	Yes No	1 2 3 4 5	
21	1 2 3 4 5	Yes No	1 2 3 4 5	
22	1 2 3 4 5	Yes No	1 2 3 4 5	
23	1 2 3 4 5	Yes No	1 2 3 4 5	
24	1 2 3 4 5	Yes No	1 2 3 4 5	
25	1 2 3 4 5	Yes No	1 2 3 4 5	
26	1 2 3 4 5	Yes No	1 2 3 4 5	
27	1 2 3 4 5	Yes No	1 2 3 4 5	
28	1 2 3 4 5	Yes No	1 2 3 4 5	
29	1 2 3 4 5	Yes No	1 2 3 4 5	
30	1 2 3 4 5	Yes No	1 2 3 4 5	
31	1 2 3 4 5	Yes No	1 2 3 4 5	

Figure 10–4. Advanced mood chart.

monitoring of mood states. As patients progress into adolescence, greater insight into mood states can develop, and their mood charts become more useful in tracking treatment response and predicting relapse.

Ideally, mood charting should be an ongoing process that allows the patient and family to track mood symptoms over long periods of time. This approach also has the potential to reveal seasonal patterns of mood fluctuation. In reality, patients and families may not comply with mood charting indefinitely. Especially in times of mood stabilization, mood charting may not appear to be necessary to the family. At these times, the clinician might recommend a streamlined mood chart to provide the very basics of monitoring. However, therapists should emphasize the value of prospective mood charting to identify early signs of relapse. Mood charting is especially valuable during times of increased risk of relapse. In particular, events that involve goal attainment (Johnson 2005), stressful life events, and major life transitions can precipitate mood episodes. Mood charts are also particularly valuable when psychosocial and medication interventions are modified (e.g., dosage changes, addition of a new medication, transition from intensive psychotherapy to maintenance follow-up).

Conclusion

Psychosocial interventions are a valuable and necessary component of treatment for bipolar disorder. Psychosocial treatment is intended to augment medication and aims to foster skill development and coping strategies in patients and their families. Several psychosocial treatment programs have been developed for children and adolescents with bipolar disorder. Although research evidence is still developing to support the efficacy of these interventions, several common components are available for therapists to implement immediately with their patients. Psychoeducation is the foundation of all psychotherapy for bipolar disorder. By improving patients' and families' understanding of bipolar disorder and dispelling common misperceptions about this illness, the therapist helps families become better able to cope with bipolar disorder and act as active consumers of treatment. Skill building, based on cognitive-behavioral and family systems theories, allows patients and their families to modify problematic cognitive and communication patterns and take an active role in improving outcome. Symptom monitoring measures, completed by therapists in session, and mood charting, completed by patients and their parents between sessions, allow for improved monitoring of treatment response and early identification of relapse. These methods allow therapists to build a collaborative alliance with patients and families to minimize the psychosocial impairment bipolar disorder causes.

References

Albano AM, Kendall PC: Cognitive behavioural therapy for children and adolescents with anxiety disorders: clinical research advances. Int Rev Psychiatry 14:129–134, 2002

American Psychiatric Association: Diagnostic and Statistical Manual of Mental Disorders, 4th Edition, Text Revision. Washington, DC, American Psychiatric Association, 2000

Axelson D, Birmaher B, Brent D, et al: A preliminary study of the Kiddie Schedule for Affective Disorders and Schizophrenia for School-Age Children Mania Rating Scale for children and adolescents. J Child Adolesc Psychopharmacol 13:463–470, 2003

Axelson D, Birmaher B, Strober M, et al: Phenomenology of children and adolescents with bipolar spectrum disorders. Arch Gen Psychiatry 63:1139–1148, 2006

Burns DD, Auerbach AH: Does homework compliance enhance recovery from depression? Psychiatr Ann 22:464–469, 1992

Chambers WJ, Puig-Antich J, Hirsch M, et al: The assessment of affective disorders in children and adolescents by semistructured interview: test–retest reliability of the Schedule for Affective Disorders and Schizophrenia for School-Age Children, Present Episode Version. Arch Gen Psychiatry 42:696–702, 1985

Clarke GN, Rohde P, Lewinsohn PM, et al: Cognitive-behavioral treatment of adolescent depression: efficacy of acute group treatment and booster sessions. J Am Acad Child Adolesc Psychiatry 38:272–279, 1999

Conoley CW, Padula MA, Payton DS, et al: Predictors of client implementation of counselor recommendations: match with problem, difficulty level, and building on client strengths. J Couns Psychol 41:3–7, 1994

Cox DJ, Tisdelle DA, Culbert JP: Increasing adherence to behavioral homework assignments. J Behav Med 11:519–522, 1988

Danielson CK, Feeny NC, Findling RL, et al: Psychosocial treatment of bipolar disorders in adolescents: a proposed cognitive-behavioral intervention. Cogn Behav Pract 11:283–297, 2004

Dunn AL: Exercise treatment for depression: efficacy and dose response. Am J Prev Med 28:1–8, 2005

Feeny NC, Danielson CK, Schwartz L, et al: Cognitive-behavioral therapy for bipolar disorders in adolescents: a pilot study. Bipolar Disord 8:508–515, 2006

Flannery-Schroeder EC, Kendall PC: Group and individual cognitive-behavioral treatments for youth with anxiety disorders: a randomized clinical trial. Cognit Ther Res 24:251–278, 2000

Fristad MA: Psychoeducational treatment for school-aged children with bipolar disorder. Dev Psychopathol 18:1289–1306, 2006

Fristad MA, Weller EB, Weller RA: The Mania Rating Scale: can it be used in children? A preliminary report. J Am Acad Child Adolesc Psychiatry 31:252–257, 1992

Fristad MA, Weller RA, Weller EB: The Mania Rating Scale (MRS): further reliability and validity studies with children. Ann Clin Psychiatry 7:127–132, 1995

Fristad MA, Gavazzi SM, Soldano KW: Multi-family psychoeducation groups for childhood mood disorders: a program description and preliminary efficacy data. Contemporary Family Therapy: An International Journal 20:385–402, 1998

Fristad MA, Gavazzi SM, Soldano KW: Naming the enemy: learning to differentiate mood disorder "symptoms" from the "self" that experiences them. J Fam Psychother 10:81–88, 1999

Fristad MA, Goldberg-Arnold JS, Gavazzi SM: Multifamily psychoeducation groups (MFPG) for families of children with bipolar disorder. Bipolar Disord 4:254–262, 2002

Fristad MA, Goldberg-Arnold JS, Gavazzi SM: Multi-family psychoeducation groups in the treatment of children with mood disorders. J Marital Fam Ther 29:491–504, 2003

Fristad MA, Davidson KH, Leffler JM: Thinking-Feeling-Doing: a therapeutic technique for children with bipolar disorder and their parents. J Fam Psychother 18:81–104, 2007

Garland A, Scott J: Using homework in therapy for depression. J Clin Psychol 58:489–498, 2002

Goldstein TR, Axelson DA, Birmaher B, et al: Dialectical behavior therapy for adolescents with bipolar disorder: a 1-year open trial. J Am Acad Child Adolesc Psychiatry 46:820–830, 2007

Goodwin FK, Jamison KR: Manic-Depressive Illness: Bipolar Disorders and Recurrent Depression, 2nd Edition. New York, Oxford University Press, 2007

Gracious BL, Youngstrom EA, Findling RL, et al: Discriminative validity of a parent version of the Young Mania Rating Scale. J Am Acad Child Adolesc Psychiatry 41:1350–1359, 2002

Grave J, Blissett J: Is cognitive behavior therapy developmentally appropriate for young children? A critical review of the evidence. Clin Psychol Rev 24:399–420, 2004

Helbig S, Fehm L: Problems with homework in CBT: rare exception or rather frequent? Behavioural and Cognitive Psychotherapy 32:291–301, 2004

Hunt JI, Dyl J, Armstrong L, et al: Frequency of manic symptoms and bipolar disorder in psychiatrically hospitalized adolescents using the K-SADS Mania Rating Scale. J Child Adolesc Psychopharmacol 15:918–930, 2005

Johnson SL: Mania and dysregulation in goal pursuit: a review. Clin Psychol Rev 25:241–262, 2005

Kazdin AE: Cognitive problem-solving skills training and parent management training in the treatment of antisocial behavior in children. J Consult Clin Psychol 60:733–747, 1992

Kendall PC: Treating anxiety disorders in children: results of a randomized clinical trial. J Consult Clin Psychol 62:100–110, 1994

Kovacs M: The Children's Depression Inventory (CDI) Manual. Toronto, ON, Canada, Multi-Health Systems, 1992

Kowatch RA, Fristad MA, Birmaher B, et al; Child Psychiatric Workgroup on Bipolar Disorder: Treatment guidelines for children and adolescents with bipolar disorder. J Am Acad Child Adolesc Psychiatry 44:213–239, 2005

Lewinsohn PM, Clarke GN, Hops H, et al: Cognitive-behavioral treatment for depressed adolescents. Behav Ther 21:385–401, 1990

Lewinsohn PM, Klein DN, Seeley JR: Bipolar disorders in a community sample of older adolescents: prevalence, phenomenology, comorbidity, and course. J Am Acad Child Adolesc Psychiatry 34:454–463, 1995

Lofthouse N, Fristad MA, Splaingard M, et al: Parent and child reports of sleep problems associated with early onset bipolar spectrum disorders. J Fam Psychol 21:114–123, 2007

Lofthouse N, Fristad MA, Splaingard M, et al: Web survey of sleep problems associated with early-onset bipolar spectrum disorders. J Pediatr Psychol 33:349–357, 2008 (Epub ahead of print)

Lukens EP, McFarlane WR: Psychoeducation as evidence-based practice: considerations for practice, research, and policy. Brief Treatment and Crisis Intervention 4:205–225, 2004

McClellan J, Kowatch R, Findling RL: Practice parameter for the assessment and treatment of children and adolescents with bipolar disorder. J Am Acad Child Adolesc Psychiatry 46:107–125, 2007

Miklowitz DJ, George EL, Axelson DA, et al: Family focused treatment for adolescents with bipolar disorder. J Affect Disord 82 (suppl 1):S113–S128, 2004

Miklowitz DJ, Biuckians A, Richards JA: Early onset bipolar disorder: a family treatment perspective. Dev Psychopathol 18:1247–1265, 2006

Patel NC, Patrick DM, Youngstrom EA, et al: Response and remission in adolescent mania: signal detection analyses of the Young Mania Rating Scale. J Am Acad Child Adolesc Psychiatry 46:628–635, 2007

Pavuluri MN, Graczyk PA, Henry DB, et al: Child- and family-focused cognitive-behavioral therapy for pediatric bipolar disorder: development and preliminary results. J Am Acad Child Adolesc Psychiatry 43:528–537, 2004

Poznanski EO, Freeman LN, Mokros HB: Children's Depression Rating Scale—Revised. Psychopharmacol Bull 21:979–989, 1985

Rich BA, Vinton DT, Roberson-Nay R, et al: Limbic hyperactivation during processing of neutral facial expressions in children with bipolar disorder. Proc Natl Acad Sci U S A 103:8900–8905, 2006

Simoneau TL, Miklowitz DJ, Richards JA, et al: Expressed emotion and interactional patterns in the families of bipolar patients. J Abnorm Psychol 107:497–507, 1998

Simoneau TL, Miklowitz DJ, Richards JA, et al: Bipolar disorder and family communication: effects of a psychoeducational treatment program. J Abnorm Psychol 108:588–597, 1999

Weisz JR, Thurber CA, Sweeney L, et al: Brief treatment of mild-to-moderate child depression using primary and secondary control enhancement training. J Consult Clin Psychol 65:703–707, 1997

West AE, Henry DB, Pavuluri MN: Maintenance model of integrated psychosocial treatment in pediatric bipolar disorder: a pilot feasibility study. J Am Acad Child Adolesc Psychiatry 46:205–212, 2007

Young RC, Biggs JT, Ziegler VE, et al: A rating scale for mania: reliability, validity and sensitivity. Br J Psychiatry 133:429–435, 1978

Youngstrom EA, Youngstrom JK: Evidence-based assessment of pediatric bipolar disorder, part II: incorporating information from behavior checklists. J Am Acad Child Adolesc Psychiatry 44:823–828, 2005

Youngstrom EA, Gracious BL, Danielson CK, et al: Toward an integration of parent and clinician report on the Young Mania Rating Scale. J Affect Disord 77:179–190, 2003

Youngstrom EA, Findling RL, Calabrese JR, et al: Comparing the diagnostic accuracy of six potential screening instruments for bipolar disorder in youths aged 5 to 17 years. J Am Acad Child Adolesc Psychiatry 43:847–858, 2004

Youngstrom EA, Findling RL, Youngstrom JK, et al: Toward an evidence-based assessment of pediatric bipolar disorder. J Clin Child Adolesc Psychol 34:433–448, 2005a

Youngstrom EA, Meyers O, Demeter C, et al: Comparing diagnostic checklists for pediatric bipolar disorder in academic and community mental health settings. Bipolar Disord 7:507–517, 2005b

Pavuluri MN, Graczyk PA, Henry DB, et al: Child- and family-focused cognitive-behavioral therapy for pediatric bipolar disorder: development and preliminary results. J Am Acad Child Adolesc Psychiatry 43:528–537, 2004

Poznanski EO, Freeman LN, Mokros HB: Children's Depression Rating Scale—Revised. Psychopharmacol Bull 21:979–989, 1985

Rich BA, Vinton DT, Roberson-Nay R, et al: Limbic hyperactivation during processing of neutral facial expressions in children with bipolar disorder. Proc Natl Acad Sci U S A 103:8900–8905, 2006

Simoneau TL, Miklowitz DJ, Richards JA, et al: Expressed emotion and interactional patterns in the families of bipolar patients. J Abnorm Psychol 107:497–507, 1998

Simoneau TL, Miklowitz DJ, Richards JA, et al: Bipolar disorder and family communication: effects of a psychoeducational treatment program. J Abnorm Psychol 108:588–597, 1999

Weisz JR, Thurber CA, Sweeney L, et al: Brief treatment of mild-to-moderate child depression using primary and secondary control enhancement training. J Consult Clin Psychol 65:703–707, 1997

West AE, Henry DB, Pavuluri MN: Maintenance model of integrated psychosocial treatment in pediatric bipolar disorder: a pilot feasibility study. J Am Acad Child Adolesc Psychiatry 46:205–212, 2007

Young RC, Biggs JT, Ziegler VE, et al: A rating scale for mania: reliability, validity and sensitivity. Br J Psychiatry 133:429–435, 1978

Youngstrom EA, Youngstrom JK: Evidence-based assessment of pediatric bipolar disorder, part II: incorporating information from behavior checklists. J Am Acad Child Adolesc Psychiatry 44:823–828, 2005

Youngstrom EA, Gracious BL, Danielson CK, et al: Toward an integration of parent and clinician report on the Young Mania Rating Scale. J Affect Disord 77:179–190, 2003

Youngstrom EA, Findling RL, Calabrese JR, et al: Comparing the diagnostic accuracy of six potential screening instruments for bipolar disorder in youths aged 5 to 17 years. J Am Acad Child Adolesc Psychiatry 43:847–858, 2004

Youngstrom EA, Findling RL, Youngstrom JK, et al: Toward an evidence-based assessment of pediatric bipolar disorder. J Clin Child Adolesc Psychol 34:433–448, 2005a

Youngstrom EA, Meyers O, Demeter C, et al: Comparing diagnostic checklists for pediatric bipolar disorder in academic and community mental health settings. Bipolar Disord 7:507–517, 2005b

completed by therapists in session, and mood charting, completed by patients and their parents between sessions, allow for improved monitoring of treatment response and early identification of relapse. These methods allow therapists to build a collaborative alliance with patients and families to minimize the psychosocial impairment bipolar disorder causes.

References

Albano AM, Kendall PC: Cognitive behavioural therapy for children and adolescents with anxiety disorders: clinical research advances. Int Rev Psychiatry 14:129–134, 2002

American Psychiatric Association: Diagnostic and Statistical Manual of Mental Disorders, 4th Edition, Text Revision. Washington, DC, American Psychiatric Association, 2000

Axelson D, Birmaher B, Brent D, et al: A preliminary study of the Kiddie Schedule for Affective Disorders and Schizophrenia for School-Age Children Mania Rating Scale for children and adolescents. J Child Adolesc Psychopharmacol 13:463–470, 2003

Axelson D, Birmaher B, Strober M, et al: Phenomenology of children and adolescents with bipolar spectrum disorders. Arch Gen Psychiatry 63:1139–1148, 2006

Burns DD, Auerbach AH: Does homework compliance enhance recovery from depression? Psychiatr Ann 22:464–469, 1992

Chambers WJ, Puig-Antich J, Hirsch M, et al: The assessment of affective disorders in children and adolescents by semistructured interview: test–retest reliability of the Schedule for Affective Disorders and Schizophrenia for School-Age Children, Present Episode Version. Arch Gen Psychiatry 42:696–702, 1985

Clarke GN, Rohde P, Lewinsohn PM, et al: Cognitive-behavioral treatment of adolescent depression: efficacy of acute group treatment and booster sessions. J Am Acad Child Adolesc Psychiatry 38:272–279, 1999

Conoley CW, Padula MA, Payton DS, et al: Predictors of client implementation of counselor recommendations: match with problem, difficulty level, and building on client strengths. J Couns Psychol 41:3–7, 1994

Cox DJ, Tisdelle DA, Culbert JP: Increasing adherence to behavioral homework assignments. J Behav Med 11:519–522, 1988

Danielson CK, Feeny NC, Findling RL, et al: Psychosocial treatment of bipolar disorders in adolescents: a proposed cognitive-behavioral intervention. Cogn Behav Pract 11:283–297, 2004

Dunn AL: Exercise treatment for depression: efficacy and dose response. Am J Prev Med 28:1–8, 2005

Feeny NC, Danielson CK, Schwartz L, et al: Cognitive-behavioral therapy for bipolar disorders in adolescents: a pilot study. Bipolar Disord 8:508–515, 2006

Flannery-Schroeder EC, Kendall PC: Group and individual cognitive-behavioral treatments for youth with anxiety disorders: a randomized clinical trial. Cognit Ther Res 24:251–278, 2000

Fristad MA: Psychoeducational treatment for school-aged children with bipolar disorder. Dev Psychopathol 18:1289–1306, 2006

Fristad MA, Weller EB, Weller RA: The Mania Rating Scale: can it be used in children? A preliminary report. J Am Acad Child Adolesc Psychiatry 31:252–257, 1992

Fristad MA, Weller RA, Weller EB: The Mania Rating Scale (MRS): further reliability and validity studies with children. Ann Clin Psychiatry 7:127–132, 1995

Fristad MA, Gavazzi SM, Soldano KW: Multi-family psychoeducation groups for childhood mood disorders: a program description and preliminary efficacy data. Contemporary Family Therapy: An International Journal 20:385–402, 1998

Fristad MA, Gavazzi SM, Soldano KW: Naming the enemy: learning to differentiate mood disorder "symptoms" from the "self" that experiences them. J Fam Psychother 10:81–88, 1999

Fristad MA, Goldberg-Arnold JS, Gavazzi SM: Multifamily psychoeducation groups (MFPG) for families of children with bipolar disorder. Bipolar Disord 4:254–262, 2002

Fristad MA, Goldberg-Arnold JS, Gavazzi SM: Multi-family psychoeducation groups in the treatment of children with mood disorders. J Marital Fam Ther 29:491–504, 2003

Fristad MA, Davidson KH, Leffler JM: Thinking-Feeling-Doing: a therapeutic technique for children with bipolar disorder and their parents. J Fam Psychother 18:81–104, 2007

Garland A, Scott J: Using homework in therapy for depression. J Clin Psychol 58:489–498, 2002

Goldstein TR, Axelson DA, Birmaher B, et al: Dialectical behavior therapy for adolescents with bipolar disorder: a 1-year open trial. J Am Acad Child Adolesc Psychiatry 46:820–830, 2007

Goodwin FK, Jamison KR: Manic-Depressive Illness: Bipolar Disorders and Recurrent Depression, 2nd Edition. New York, Oxford University Press, 2007

Gracious BL, Youngstrom EA, Findling RL, et al: Discriminative validity of a parent version of the Young Mania Rating Scale. J Am Acad Child Adolesc Psychiatry 41:1350–1359, 2002

Grave J, Blissett J: Is cognitive behavior therapy developmentally appropriate for young children? A critical review of the evidence. Clin Psychol Rev 24:399–420, 2004

Helbig S, Fehm L: Problems with homework in CBT: rare exception or rather frequent? Behavioural and Cognitive Psychotherapy 32:291–301, 2004

Hunt JI, Dyl J, Armstrong L, et al: Frequency of manic symptoms and bipolar di in psychiatrically hospitalized adolescents using the K-SADS Mania Rating J Child Adolesc Psychopharmacol 15:918–930, 2005

Johnson SL: Mania and dysregulation in goal pursuit: a review. Clin Psych 25:241–262, 2005

Kazdin AE: Cognitive problem-solving skills training and parent management ing in the treatment of antisocial behavior in children. J Consult Clin P 60:733–747, 1992

Kendall PC: Treating anxiety disorders in children: results of a randomized trial. J Consult Clin Psychol 62:100–110, 1994

Kovacs M: The Children's Depression Inventory (CDI) Manual. Toronto, ON ada, Multi-Health Systems, 1992

Kowatch RA, Fristad MA, Birmaher B, et al; Child Psychiatric Workgroup on Disorder: Treatment guidelines for children and adolescents with bipolar di J Am Acad Child Adolesc Psychiatry 44:213–239, 2005

Lewinsohn PM, Clarke GN, Hops H, et al: Cognitive-behavioral treatment pressed adolescents. Behav Ther 21:385–401, 1990

Lewinsohn PM, Klein DN, Seeley JR: Bipolar disorders in a community san older adolescents: prevalence, phenomenology, comorbidity, and course Acad Child Adolesc Psychiatry 34:454–463, 1995

Lofthouse N, Fristad MA, Splaingard M, et al: Parent and child reports o problems associated with early onset bipolar spectrum disorders. J Fam 21:114–123, 2007

Lofthouse N, Fristad MA, Splaingard M, et al: Web survey of sleep problem ciated with early-onset bipolar spectrum disorders. J Pediatr Psychol 33:34 2008 (Epub ahead of print)

Lukens EP, McFarlane WR: Psychoeducation as evidence-based practice: co ations for practice, research, and policy. Brief Treatment and Crisis Interv 4:205–225, 2004

McClellan J, Kowatch R, Findling RL: Practice parameter for the assessment an ment of children and adolescents with bipolar disorder. J Am Acad Child Psychiatry 46:107–125, 2007

Miklowitz DJ, George EL, Axelson DA, et al: Family focused treatment for adol with bipolar disorder. J Affect Disord 82 (suppl 1):S113–S128, 2004

Miklowitz DJ, Biuckians A, Richards JA: Early onset bipolar disorder: a family ment perspective. Dev Psychopathol 18:1247–1265, 2006

Patel NC, Patrick DM, Youngstrom EA, et al: Response and remission in ado mania: signal detection analyses of the Young Mania Rating Scale. J Am Child Adolesc Psychiatry 46:628–635, 2007

11

The Bipolar Child and the Educational System

Working With Schools

Benjamin W. Fields, M.A., M.Ed.

Mary A. Fristad, Ph.D., A.B.P.P.

Children and adolescents spend more time in school than in any other setting outside of the home, with time spent at school accounting for more than 12,000 hours over the course of the primary and secondary school years (Clarizio 1994). Thus, it is no wonder that school adjustment is of crucial importance to every child. This is no less true, of course, for students with pediatric bipolar disorder—a group, unfortunately, that research suggests exhibits considerable school impairment. The high prevalence of academic dysfunction in these children and adolescents "highlight[s] the need for clinicians caring for patients with [pediatric bipolar disorder] to carefully attend to school performance as a potential domain where the illness might be causing functional impairment" (Pavuluri et al. 2006a, p. 955).

Academic Problems in Pediatric Bipolar Disorder

The extent and nature of academic impairment in children and adolescents with bipolar disorder are significant and varied, encompassing problems in reading, writing, math, and behavior. In Wozniak et al.'s (1995) cohort of 43 children with bipolar disorder, 42% experienced reading and writing difficulties, whereas 30% evidenced difficulty in math. These students also had lower arithmetic and reading scores than either children with attention-deficit/hyperactivity disorder (ADHD) or children with no disorder. Likewise, Pavuluri et al. (2006a) reported reading and writing difficulties in 46% and math difficulties in 29% of their sample of 55 children and adolescents with bipolar disorder.

Geller et al. (2002a) found that 79% of their sample of children with bipolar disorder had behavior problems at school. Additionally, 44% had low grades, 14% had a learning disability, 11% were in a remedial class, and 8% had repeated a grade. In Faedda et al.'s (2004) cohort of 82 pediatric bipolar patients, 16% had a comorbid learning disorder.

Lagace et al. (2003) reported that adolescents in remission from bipolar I disorder had significantly lower mathematics achievement than adolescents in remission from major depressive disorder or with no psychiatric history.

What is behind this academic dysfunction? Pavuluri et al. (2006a) suggest that neuropsychological deficits associated with pediatric bipolar disorder, as opposed to purely behavioral factors, play a significant role; in fact, a growing body of evidence supports this explanation.

Memory deficits have been noted frequently in recent studies of pediatric bipolar disorder. Pavuluri et al. (2006b), for example, found impairment in working memory in patients with pediatric bipolar disorder. Interestingly, this impairment was present regardless of whether the subjects were acutely symptomatic or euthymic, or medicated or unmedicated. The authors offer this as evidence that neuropsychological deficits are "trait-like characteristics of pediatric bipolar disorder" (p. 286).

Glahn et al. (2005) also found evidence of memory impairment in children and adolescents, but only in those diagnosed with bipolar I disorder and not in those with bipolar II disorder or bipolar disorder not otherwise specified; however, mood severity was not related to memory in this sample. This finding fits with Bearden et al.'s (2006) report that adult outpatients with bipolar disorder experienced impaired memory and that this deficit was not secondary to their clinical state, leading the authors to suggest bipolar disorder is associated with "an underlying pathophysiology" (p. 139).

Other neuropsychological deficits observed in patients with pediatric bipolar disorder include lowered verbal and performance IQ and impairment in motor inhibition, attention, response flexibility, and processing speed (Doyle et al. 2005; Leibenluft et al. 2007; McCarthy et al. 2004; McClure et al. 2005; Pavuluri et al. 2006b; Wozniak et al. 1995).

What is striking is the common finding that neuropsychological deficits often persist, even when subjects are euthymic and not actively manic or depressed (Deckersbach et al. 2005). Thus, as noted by Malhi et al. (2007), "an absence of symptoms does not necessarily equate to 'recovery'" (p. 114). This point is especially relevant when addressing the academic needs of students with bipolar disorder, because even when these children are between periods of acute illness, they may still require accommodation and specialized instruction.

The school impairment seen in children and adolescents with bipolar disorder may be even more troubling to parents, teachers, and, indeed, the children themselves, because these children may have achieved at high levels before the onset of the disorder. Quackenbush et al. (1996) and Kutcher et al. (1998), for example, assessed the premorbid functioning of individuals with adolescent-onset bipolar I disorder and found them to "[demonstrate] good to excellent peer and academic functioning prior to illness onset." Likewise, Cannon et al.'s (1997) examination of premorbid functioning in childhood and adolescence of individuals with bipolar disorder revealed that whereas patients with bipolar disorder evidenced more social impairment than healthy control subjects, they functioned well in school. These findings, however, are inconsistent with Pavuluri et al.'s (2006a) report of learning difficulties in young children with bipolar disorder. This discrepancy is potentially indicative of a cognitive picture of childhood-onset bipolar disorder that may differ from the impairment associated with adolescent-onset bipolar disorder.

Identifying the cognitive dysfunction that appears to be at least partially responsible for academic difficulties seen in children and adolescents with bipolar disorder is, as stated by Pavuluri et al. (2006a), "the first step toward educational remediation. Intervention strategies can then be targeted to reduce neurocognitive dysfunctions or circumvent them by teaching compensatory strategies, thereby enhancing the learning potential of individuals with [pediatric bipolar disorder] during their years of formal education" (p. 951).

Impairment Caused by Manic Symptoms

Many symptoms of mania may be particularly or uniquely impairing in the school context. Indeed, if one examines the phenomenology of the disorder, as elucidated by Kowatch et al.'s (2005b) meta-analysis, all of the most common manic symptoms seen in children and adolescents—increased energy, distractibility, pressured speech, irritability, grandiosity, elated mood, decreased need for sleep, and racing thoughts—have the potential to create havoc in a young person's academic environment, and that of fellow students, teachers, and other school personnel.

Outside of a very few select circumstances encountered during the school day, the increased energy so typical of children in manic or hypomanic episodes is rarely adaptive. Instead, this intense physical activation tends to be disruptive to students experiencing the symptoms and to those around them, because these children may have problems remaining seated or appropriately still when in their seats. They may also have trouble remaining quiet or channeling their increased energy into fine motor activities emphasized in the classroom. Physical education classes may provide the one school environment in which increased energy might be more productively focused; unfortunately, legislation such as No Child Left Behind places little emphasis on physical education, and this perhaps explains why very few schools meet even the Centers for Disease Control and Prevention's minimal recommendations for weekly physical education time (Burgeson et al. 2001; Centers for Disease Control and Prevention 2007; Murnan et al. 2006). Even when opportunities for physical activity are present, the activities tend to require relatively focused and controlled energy, unlike that often seen in manic episodes, which has been described as "[involving] an energy level that would leave an adult, trying to imitate [the episode], exhausted" (DuVal 2005, p. 40).

Manic distractibility also can be impairing to students with bipolar disorder, although this may be less salient for the educational environment of other students. For the student experiencing distractibility, however, this symptom may be as detrimental as any associated with bipolar disorder, because not being able to concentrate on material presented in the classroom puts these children at risk of falling behind academically. Pavuluri et al. (2006a) found that disturbance in attention in children and adolescents with bipolar disorder, in fact, predicted difficulties in reading, writing, and math, even after controlling for the presence of comorbid ADHD.

Pressured speech, although perhaps not as academically deleterious in and of itself as some other manic symptoms, is certainly noticeable and negatively differentiates a student in a manic episode from his or her classmates. In addition, because such speech may reflect underlying racing thoughts, it may be difficult to follow, impairing communication. Racing thoughts may make it difficult to attend to and process information presented in class and may lead to frequent disciplinary action for talking to peers during class and talking out of turn (Fristad and Goldberg-Arnold 2004; Kowatch and Fristad 2006).

Irritability has been considered a controversial indicator of bipolar status because of its association with so many other disorders. Manic irritability, in fact, may be attributed mistakenly to a host of other disorders, including ADHD and oppositional defiant disorder, or even to just "another exchange in an ongoing power struggle" (Weckerly 2002, p. 49). Kowatch et al. (2005b) compared irritability to fever or pain, in that it "provides a sensitive indicator that something is wrong, but it is not specific to any particular condition" (p. 493). Nonetheless, irritability is ubiquitous in the symptomatic presentation of pediatric bipolar disorder (Axelson et al. 2006; Faedda et al. 2004; Geller et al. 1998, 2000, 2002a, 2002b; Weller et al. 2003; Wozniak et al. 1995). At the more mild end of the spectrum, manic irritability may manifest as uncooperative or oppositional behavior at school; at a severe level, however, it may manifest in aggressive or even dangerous behavior, which can easily lead to suspension or expulsion, especially if the behavior is not identified as the product of a serious mental illness (Kim and Miklowitz 2002, p. 217).

Elated mood, the first of two cardinal symptoms of mania, has been described in the school context by Geller et al. (2002c). They describe a child with bipolar disorder who could not stop giggling in class and who was subsequently sent to the principal's office and suspended. Again, this may be especially problematic when school personnel are not aware of the child's bipolar diagnosis. For example, when a child experiencing manic elation is referred to a school administrator for discipline, only to continue laughing in the face of punishment, his or her inappropriate affect may be misinterpreted as disrespect or an unwillingness to accept responsibility for his or her actions.

The second cardinal symptom of mania, *grandiosity*, can also be disruptive, as seen in Geller and Luby's (1997) description of children with bipolar disorder as commonly harassing teachers about how best to teach the class, or even "fail[ing] subjects intentionally because they believe the courses are taught incorrectly" (p. 1169). Adolescents are described as often believing they will achieve professional success, despite their failing school grades. This grandiosity is impairing, not only because it may undermine a teacher's authority and classroom management but also because it may make it more difficult to motivate the student to master subject material he or she considers unimportant.

Decreased need for sleep is yet another manic symptom that can interfere with a child or adolescent's school performance. Although a child in a manic episode may not have any problems staying awake in class (unlike a child in a depressive episode), learning, memory, and attention all appear to be adversely impacted by lack of sleep, regardless of whether the child appears to be alert or not (Crick and Mitchison 1983; Karni et al. 1994). Additionally, sleep may aid in the process of unlearning unnecessary or even maladaptive information (Crick and Mitchison 1983).

Impairment Caused by Depressive Symptoms

Symptoms characteristic of the depressive side of bipolar disorder, including irritability, sadness, impaired concentration, decreased productivity, loss of interest, negative self-image, fatigue, insomnia or hypersomnia, and psychomotor agitation or retardation, can also pose challenges for affected students and result in academic underperformance and school disruption (Evans et al. 2002; Hammen et al. 1999; Kumpulainen et al. 1999; Reynolds and Johnston 1994; Waslick et al. 2002).

Much like the irritability seen in manic episodes, depressive irritability may manifest as oppositional or disruptive behavior in school, which can lead to conflict with both teachers and peers. This conflict, however, is less likely to be aggressive or potentially violent than that seen in the context of a manic episode and thus, perhaps, is less likely to come to the attention of school administrators responsible for disciplinary action. Anecdotally, depressive irritability is described as being more "Oscar the Grouch" than "Tasmanian Devil," and whereas most teachers would probably express a preference for a grumpy student over a destructive one, neither helps to foster a cooperative, pleasant classroom environment.

The sadness associated with depression may often be overshadowed in the classroom by externalizing behaviors, which may be "more readily expressed than…internal, subjective suffering" (Hammen and Rudolph 2002, p. 233). However, the "unresponsiveness [that sadness] may cause" (Puura et al. 1998, p. 583) frequently is noticed by teachers, who often find it a struggle to motivate students suffering from depressive symptoms of bipolar disorder.

Motivation may also be affected by the loss of interest that often accompanies depressive phases of bipolar disorder. Fristad and Goldberg-Arnold (2004) note that students who were once driven to succeed academically may find themselves unable to "muster the energy or interest" to engage in learning (p. 189) and that resulting poor grades can then lead to a lowered opinion of oneself. This negative self-image often appears in stark contrast to the grandiosity that may accompany mania. Feelings of worthlessness, inferiority, and incapability may further undermine a student's willingness to put forth effort in the classroom, because of the belief that he or she will be unable to succeed.

Insomnia, hypersomnia, and the fatigue associated with each are perhaps some of the most academically debilitating of all the depressive symptoms of bipolar disorder. A student who cannot stay awake in class is benefiting from his or her education no more than one who is not in the building at all. Because of a lack or poor quality of sleep, children and adolescents with depressive insomnia often find it hard to function at school, especially during the early part of the day. A hypersomnolent student may face additional difficulties upon returning home from school, because long naps may interfere with the completion of homework or participation in after-school activities. Further, these long naps may have the unintended consequence of making it more difficult for the student to fall asleep at bedtime, thus maintaining a vicious cycle of sleeplessness at night and fatigue and sleepiness during the day.

Much like irritability, psychomotor agitation and retardation may be more evident in the school setting than, for example, depressed mood, because of these symptoms' externalizing nature. As noted by Abikoff et al. (1993), however, psychomotor agitation in depressed students is often identified by teachers as a symptom of ADHD. On the other hand, psychomotor retardation may be the antithesis of the proverbial "squeaky wheel"—that is, easily overlooked or discounted because it does not tend to disrupt other students or classroom activities. The psychomotor retardation that may be indicative of a depressive episode, especially in a student with a history of manic and disruptive behavior, unfortunately may come as a relief to teachers and fellow students alike.

Peer Relations in School

The association between pediatric bipolar disorder and academic underperformance is well established. Of course, the school experience, as described by Feshbach and Feshbach (1987), is composed of more than just academic tasks and in fact encompasses a number of factors, ranging from the acquisition of subject matter to the essential development of social skills and personality attributes. Each of these domains is apt to be affected negatively by pediatric bipolar disorder.

Peer relationships in particular may suffer as a result of bipolar symptomatology, with common social skills difficulties including misinterpretation of jokes, shyness, bullying, and being bullied (Lofthouse et al. 2004). Further, other children may be disturbed by the sometimes bizarre presentation of a classmate in a manic or hypomanic episode, and even after symptoms have subsided, the affected student may not be easily accepted (Chandler 2006). Not surprisingly, Quackenbush et al. (1996) found "marked deterioration" in peer relationships and extracurricular involvement in adolescents after the onset of bipolar disorder (p. 16). Besides the obvious negative social impact of bipolar features such as irritability, grandiosity, and negative self-image, children and adolescents with bipolar disorder also may lack the social cognition necessary for effective peer engagement. McClure et al. (2005), for example, found that patients with pediatric bipolar disorder performed more poorly on measures of facial expression recognition and pragmatic judgment of language. Goldstein (2003) found that although adolescents with bipolar disorder had age-appropriate knowledge of social skills during periods of symptom remission, they nonetheless displayed impaired social skills performance. Further, Rich et al. (2006) reported that older children and adolescents with bipolar disorder were more apt to perceive hostility in neutral faces and report more fear when viewing these faces.

With these deficits in interpreting and utilizing social cues, it is no wonder that these students often struggle within what even psychiatrically healthy youths can find to be a treacherous social environment.

Dealing With Medication Side Effects in School

Lofthouse et al. (2004) assert that psychopharmacological intervention is "the foundation of effective treatment for early onset [bipolar disorder]" and that "most children require multiple medications to alleviate symptoms of mania, depression, and co-occurring conditions" (p. S5-14). This sentiment was echoed in Kowatch et al.'s (2005a) treatment guidelines for bipolar disorder in children and adolescents.

These medications, however, can produce a number of side effects that may present additional challenges at school for children with bipolar disorder. Table 11–1 contains a list of medications frequently used to treat pediatric bipolar disorder and common comorbid conditions such as ADHD, along with side effects that may warrant attention when planning accommodations and modifications.

Special Education and Bipolar Disorder

As Doyle et al. (2005) have observed, "The need for special educational placement may not be obvious to those interacting with these youths in the school setting, where poor academic performance may be attributed purely to behavioral difficulties" (p. 546). Nonetheless, evidence from several studies indicates that a large proportion of children with bipolar disorder do receive special education services, with reports ranging from one-fifth to nearly two-thirds (Faedda et al. 2004; Findling et al. 2001; Pavuluri et al. 2006a). However, because of the high comorbidity of learning disabilities and ADHD with bipolar disorder, it is not clear whether high rates of special education class placement are due to these co-occurring disorders, to bipolar disorder, or to some combination thereof. Although a child's bipolar diagnosis (or any diagnosis, for that matter) does not automatically qualify him or her for special education services, it may, even in the absence of comorbid conditions, still merit and result in such a placement.

Table 11–1. Most common side effects of medications used in the treatment of pediatric bipolar disorder, organized by medication class

Antidepressants

Bupropion: agitation, headache, dry mouth, nausea, vomiting, tremor

Citalopram: apathy, confusion, drowsiness, insomnia, weakness, abdominal pain, diarrhea, dry mouth, indigestion, flatulence, nausea, sweating, tremor

Escitalopram: insomnia, diarrhea, nausea

Fluoxetine: anxiety, drowsiness, headache, insomnia, nervousness, diarrhea, sweating, tremor, itching

Fluvoxamine: dizziness, drowsiness, headache, insomnia, nervousness, weakness, constipation, diarrhea, dry mouth, indigestion, nausea

Mirtazapine: drowsiness, constipation, dry mouth, increased appetite, weight gain

Nefazodone: dizziness, insomnia, sleepiness, constipation, dry mouth, nausea

Sertraline: dizziness, drowsiness, fatigue, headache, insomnia, diarrhea, dry mouth, nausea, sweating, tremor

Antihypertensives

Clonidine: drowsiness, dry mouth

Guanfacine: drowsiness, weakness, constipation, dry mouth

Antipsychotics

Aripiprazole: constipation

Clozapine: dizziness, sedation, constipation

Olanzapine: agitation, dizziness, headache, restlessness, sedation, weakness, constipation, dry mouth, weight gain, tremor

Quetiapine: dizziness, weight gain

Risperidone: aggressive behavior, dizziness, headache, insomnia, sedation, visual disturbance, cough, constipation, diarrhea, dry mouth, nausea, itching, weight gain

Ziprasidone: dizziness, drowsiness, restlessness, constipation, diarrhea, nausea

Table 11–1. Most common side effects of medications used in the treatment of pediatric bipolar disorder, organized by medication class *(continued)*

Mood stabilizers

Carbamazepine: loss of coordination, drowsiness

Divalproex: nausea, vomiting, indigestion

Lamotrigine: loss of coordination, dizziness, headache, nausea, vomiting, photosensitivity, rash

Lithium: fatigue, headache, impaired memory, abdominal pain, diarrhea, nausea, muscle weakness, dehydration, tremor

Oxcarbazepine: dizziness, vertigo, drowsiness, fatigue, headache, abnormal vision, abdominal pain, nausea, vomiting, loss of coordination, tremor

Tiagabine: dizziness, drowsiness, nervousness, weakness

Topiramate: dizziness, drowsiness, fatigue, impaired concentration and memory, nervousness, psychomotor retardation, speech problems, abnormal vision, nausea, weight loss, loss of coordination

Psychostimulants

Adderall: hyperactivity, insomnia, restlessness, tremor, loss of appetite

Dextroamphetamine: hyperactivity, insomnia, restlessness, tremor, loss of appetite

Dexmethylphenidate: abdominal pain

Methylphenidate: hyperactivity, insomnia, restlessness, tremor, loss of appetite

Nonstimulant

Atomoxetine: dizziness, fatigue, mood swings, insomnia, nausea, vomiting, dry mouth, constipation, decreased appetite

Source. Adapted from Deglin and Vallerand 2006.

Ideally, every child in need of special education services would be identified quickly by school personnel, and modifications and accommodations would be created to help the child reach his or her academic potential. Unfortunately, schools face budgetary restrictions and handle such large numbers of students that it often falls to parents to advocate for their children to ensure they are receiving the free appropriate public education (FAPE) mandated by federal law (Papalos et al. 2002a).

Warner et al. (2003) noted that because pediatric bipolar disorder is unfamiliar to many people, including school personnel, "schools often provide inadequate support and educational accommodations to affected students and their families…and handle these manifestations as disciplinary issues rather than symptoms of a complex mental health condition."

Clinicians should be aware of the challenges parents may face in securing specialized educational services for children with bipolar disorder, both to offer guidance in navigating what can be a confusing and intimidating process and because clinicians may be called on to participate in the process of securing appropriate accommodations and modifications for these children (Warner et al. 2003). A list of possible accommodations and modifications for children with bipolar disorder and comorbid conditions, including learning disorders and behavioral disorders such as ADHD, is provided in Table 11–2. It is not expected that all of these modifications would be used for any single child. For ease of use, the table is organized by types of impairment that may be common in children with bipolar disorder.

Information regarding the biological nature of bipolar disorder may be important to present to school personnel when requesting services for a child with the disorder, because an illness presumed to be biologically based may make it easier to secure special education services (Harris 2005).

When a parent decides to pursue special education services for his or her child with bipolar disorder (or when a school decides to initiate such a process independently), the child may qualify under two different statutes: the Individuals with Disabilities Education Act (IDEA) or Section 504 of the Rehabilitation Act, each of which has its own eligibility criteria and provides for its own level of services (National Alliance for the Mentally Ill 2004). Eligibility for either IDEA or Section 504 is determined by a school-provided multifactor evaluation, in which several aspects of the child's functioning are assessed to avoid basing eligibility on only one area or on the results of only one measure or assessment. All suspected areas of disability are to be assayed in such an evaluation.

A child qualifies for IDEA by falling under 1 of 13 different categories of disability. Children with bipolar disorder typically qualify under the auspices of 1 of 3 of these categories: emotional disturbance, specific learning disabil-

Table 11–2. Possible educational modifications and accommodations for students with bipolar disorder, organized by type of impairment

Cognitive impairment (including attentional difficulty/distractibility and comorbid learning disorders)

Reduced course load

Fewer advanced courses

Course audits to gauge academic readiness

Enrichment in areas of particular interest or strength (e.g., music and art)

Smaller class size

Frequent scheduled breaks

Clear but discreet visual or auditory cues from teacher to aid student in focusing or staying on task

Preferential seating closer to teacher to aid in focus

Reduction in homework or allowances for late work without penalty

Extended time to complete in-class assignments, tests, and homework

Testing in area separate from classmates, away from distractions and with trusted staff member

Use of simplified instructions on tests/assignments

Instructions read aloud and clarified if necessary

Availability of readers for tests

Word banks or multiple-choice format on tests instead of open-ended questions

Reduced options on multiple-choice format tests

Allowing student with problems related to written expression to dictate responses

Information provided in bulleted format

Allowing composition of essays in bulleted format

No penalties for reversal of letters or numbers, spelling errors, or handwriting

Assistance and training in breaking down assignments, especially larger, more complex ones, into manageable steps, and checks to see that assignments are progressing on schedule

Teaching student to accurately estimate time needed for tasks/assignments

Table 11–2.   Possible educational modifications and accommodations for students with bipolar disorder, organized by type of impairment *(continued)*

Cognitive impairment (including attentional difficulty/distractibility and comorbid learning disorders) *(continued)*

Availability of a resource room late in school day for a student whose concentration wanes as day progresses or who needs assistance to remember and organize materials to take home

Use of student planner, checked daily for completeness

Daily/weekly communication to parents regarding assignment completion, upcoming assignments, and grade status

Providing student with (or helping student to create) daily list at end of each day regarding what assignments need to be completed at home and materials needed for each

Frequent opportunities to clean out locker, desk, or book bag

Color-coded materials for different classes (e.g., all notebooks and textbooks for science labeled in yellow)

Visually oriented curricular materials

Copies of notes and board work

Extra set of textbooks for home use—two sets for students splitting time between divorced parents

Use of large-print materials

Textbooks with important information already highlighted (or, conversely, allow student to highlight directly in textbook)

Use of condensed or simplified version of text

Books on tape

Use of tape recorder in class

Use of calculator

Graph paper to aid student in keeping numbers in appropriate columns

In-class use of keyboard to take notes and complete assignments

Use of reading software that scans text and repeats text aloud (e.g., Kurzweil)

Use of writing software that repeats what student has typed (e.g., Co:Writer, Kurzweil)

Use of voice recognition software to aid in composition of written assignments (e.g., Microsoft Word)

Table 11–2.   Possible educational modifications and accommodations for students with bipolar disorder, organized by type of impairment *(continued)*

Decreased motivation/loss of interest

Scheduling of classes that take advantage of student's particular strengths and interests, especially during time of day when student is least motivated

Dispersal of classes of interest throughout school day

Alternating of assignments that emphasize student's unique interests and talents (e.g., art, music)

Fatigue/somnolence

Delayed start time or shortened school day

Scheduling of classes of particular interest early in day, when student is less alert

Scheduling of the most demanding classes for time of day when student is most alert and awake

Availability of a resource room during first period for student with trouble waking, or late in day to allow student to catch up on material missed earlier in day

Scheduling of testing at time of day when student is functioning best

Reduction in homework or extending of deadlines for students who fall asleep soon after arriving home from school

Copies of notes from classes missed

Allowing student to move around classroom or go for brief walk

Seating in brightest area in room, preferably near natural light

Providing area for brief nap (e.g., nurse's office)

Increased absences (e.g., because of medication changes, doctor's appointments, illness relapse, hospitalization)

Estimated grades, based on already completed work, when work cannot be completed due to absence

Tutoring during extended absences

Assignments regularly communicated to parents and students via telephone, fax, email, or school Web site

Virtual learning academies (Internet schooling)

Home instruction or therapeutic day school/boarding school may be warranted if absences become too frequent or disruptive to student's academic progress

Table 11–2.　Possible educational modifications and accommodations for students with bipolar disorder, organized by type of impairment *(continued)*

Irritability/aggression

Access to safe place where student can go when feeling overwhelmed or "ready to blow"

Allowing student to go for walk or providing opportunities for physical activity to dissipate stress and defuse volatile situations

Preferential seating close to teacher if educator is skilled in recognizing and defusing student's irritability—close to door if student needs to remove himself or herself from classroom

Seating that allows for buffer space

Preferential seating near calm, model students

Providing a resource room closer to end of day if student struggles to maintain control after long school day

Meetings with school-based mental health professional (e.g., school psychologist, social worker) to develop anger management techniques and self-calming strategies

Speech-language services to help student develop improved communication skills that may allow him or her to effectively communicate frustration with words before situation escalates to physical aggression

Advance preparation and warning before transitions or disruptions in classroom routine

Extra time to transition between classes or activities, avoiding crowded or boisterous hallways

Opportunities for less competitive physical education activities such as yoga or strength training

Staff supervision in hallways, cafeteria, and bus (for especially explosive students)

Medication side effects

Allowing students with hand tremors to dictate answers

Allowing water bottle at all times for medication-induced thirst

Allowing healthy, low-calorie snacks in class for students with increased hunger

Table 11–2.   Possible educational modifications and accommodations for students with bipolar disorder, organized by type of impairment *(continued)*

Medication side effects *(continued)*

Permanent bathroom pass for students with gastrointestinal distress and those with medication-induced thirst

For students with visual blurring, provision of reader, books on tape, or scribe; reduction in assigned reading and writing; allowing student to tape-record answers to assignments/tests

Access to plenty of fluids and rest during recess or physical education classes, where dehydration and overheating may occur

Seating close to door to allow student to exit classroom discreetly to visit restroom, nurse

Psychomotor agitation/increased energy

Allowing student to go for walk or providing opportunities for physical activity to dissipate increased energy

Scheduling routine breaks from class work

Visual or auditory cue for student to indicate need for break

Psychomotor retardation

Extra travel time between classes

Credit for attendance rather than participation in physical education classes

Social difficulties/impaired peer relationships

Peer assistant or buddy to help student adjust to school routines (e.g., class transitions, lunch)

Social skills training

Use of social stories to prepare child for novel or difficult situations

Peer education regarding diversity, including learning differences (maintaining appropriate levels of confidentiality is critical, however)

Source.   Adapted from Child and Adolescent Bipolar Foundation 2002, 2007; Packer 2002a, 2002b; Papolos et al. 2002b, 2002b; Quackenbush et al. 1996; Warner et al. 2003.

ity, or other health impairment. To qualify for special education services under IDEA, however, it must be demonstrated that the student's disability has an adverse impact on his or her school performance and that he or she requires special education services (National Alliance for the Mentally Ill 2004). Once he or she is qualified under IDEA, the student is able to receive services that are funded, in part, by the state and federal government but that must follow established guidelines regarding how the student is to be evaluated, supported, and monitored. These services are carefully outlined in the child's individualized education plan.

There has been debate as to which category of disability delineated by IDEA is most appropriate or advantageous for a child with bipolar disorder. The prevailing wisdom suggests that an "other health impairment" classification is most appropriate, because the "other health impairment" criteria stipulate that the child must have a chronic or acute health problem that negatively affects school performance (Gilcher et al. 2004; Papolos and Papolos 2006). Using this classification acknowledges the biologically based, medical nature of bipolar disorder.

On the other hand, it has been suggested that a classification of emotional disturbance may be preferable to that of "other health impairment" because of the perception that an emotional disturbance classification may provide more opportunities for extensive accommodations (e.g., a residential treatment facility) should the need arise (Papolos and Papolos 2006). IDEA, however, stipulates that accommodations and modifications not be based on category of disability but rather on the needs of the particular student (Gilcher et al. 2004). Thus, although a concern over available services may be justified because of misapplication or misinterpretation of IDEA classifications on the part of school districts, the law, itself, does not tie the provision of particular services to any one classification.

In addition, there are potential drawbacks associated with an emotional disturbance classification. For example, there is some concern children labeled as such may be relegated to classrooms in which the prevailing focus is on behavior and discipline rather than on academic subject matter and related skills (Gilcher et al. 2004).

In contrast to IDEA, a child does not qualify for Section 504 under any specific category of disability. Rather, Section 504 provides for coverage for any physical or mental disability. Also unlike in IDEA, a child may qualify for Section 504 if his or her impairment limits a "major life activity." Though academic performance may, in fact, be considered a major life activity, it is not the only domain liable to be affected by a disability, and, thus, Section 504 allows students to qualify with impairment in functioning in any number of areas. Finally, Section 504 does not provide funding for services; as such, it also does not involve as many requirements that the school must follow in its implementation, often making this a more attractive option to school districts that may be wary of being "locked in" to providing potentially expensive services to a child with a disability like bipolar disorder. Neither IDEA nor Section 504, however, allows the cost of the intervention to determine whether services are provided to the student.

Figure 11–1 presents a flow chart illustrating the general process needed to qualify any child, including one with bipolar disorder, for an individualized education plan or Section 504 plan. Specific details, such as the time allotted for schools to complete evaluations, are not included because these vary from state to state. A clinician involved in the treatment of children with bipolar disorder, or any psychological disorder for that matter, should be familiar with the particular educational guidelines established by the state in which he or she practices; such information should be readily available through the state's department of education and should be available online. Web links to each state's department of education, including offices dealing with special education, can be found on the U.S. Department of Education's Web site, www.ed.gov. Additionally, Table 11–3 provides a list of common abbreviations and terms related to special education.

Conclusion

Regardless of whether parents wish to pursue school-based services for a child with bipolar disorder, establishing open communication between parents, mental health clinician(s), and school personnel is essential. Although bipolar disorder has gained increasing acceptance as a legitimate diagnosis for children and adolescents, its relatively low base rate makes it unlikely that school personnel will have substantial experience in dealing with the needs of a child with this disorder. Thus, educating school personnel about pediatric bipolar disorder may be of paramount importance.

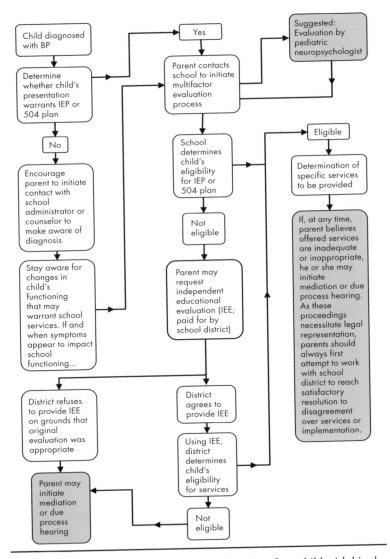

Figure 11–1.   Process of obtaining school services for a child with bipolar disorder.

Shaded boxes represent steps that may entail substantial expense to parents and that may not necessarily be reimbursed by school district. BP = bipolar disorder; IEP = individualized education plan.

Table 11–3. Common educational terms (with abbreviations and acronyms)

Assistive technology device	Any item, product, or equipment used to increase, maintain, or improve the functional capabilities of a child with a disability, the use and provision of which may be stipulated in an IEP. The term does not include surgically implanted medical devices (e.g., cochlear implants) or replacement of such devices.
Behavior intervention plan (BIP)	Plan devised by an IEP team outlining behavioral intervention strategies, modifications, and additional services that may be necessary to address the problem behavior of a child with a disability. This plan is meant to address the findings of a functional behavior assessment.
Emotional disturbance (ED)	Category of disability specified under IDEA, defined as having significant emotional dysregulation that negatively affects educational performance and that cannot be explained by intellectual, sensory, or health factors.
Free appropriate public education (FAPE)	Special education and related services provided at public expense and under public supervision that meet established state standards. This includes an appropriate preschool, elementary school, and secondary school education that conforms to the child's IEP.
Functional behavior assessment (FBA)	Process by which an IEP team attempts to determine the function of a child's problem behavior. Ideally, this process leads to interventions that assist the child in replacing problem behaviors with more appropriate behaviors. Under certain circumstances (e.g., after child's disability is found to be substantially related to serious disciplinary infractions, or after such a child has been suspended more than 10 days in a school year), an FBA is required.

Table 11–3.   Common educational terms (with abbreviations and acronyms) *(continued)*

Term	Definition
Inclusion	The placement of children with disabilities in the regular classroom. This assumes the child will benefit from being in the class and not necessarily that the child will achieve at the same level as students without disabilities. A special education teacher may coteach the class with a regular education teacher or may simply coordinate services and consult with the regular teacher.
Independent educational evaluation (IEE)	Assessment conducted by a qualified professional not employed by the school district responsible for a child's education. Parents may request that an IEE be conducted, at the school district's expense, if they disagree with the district's findings regarding a child's educational needs. This provides parents an opportunity to participate more fully in development of a child's IEP. A school district may also initiate an IEE if the district lacks the personnel to conduct an appropriate evaluation.
Individualized education plan (IEP)	A written statement, periodically reviewed and revised, for a child with a disability detailing how the disability affects the child's involvement and progress in the general education curriculum; special education and related services to be provided to the child; measurable annual goals, both academic and functional; accommodations needed to measure the child's performance on state- and district-wide achievement tests; and transition services needed to assist the child in reaching goals related to training, education, employment, and independent living skills.
Individuals with Disabilities Education Act (IDEA)	Law ensuring educational services to children with disabilities.

Table 11–3. Common educational terms (with abbreviations and acronyms) *(continued)*

Individuals with Disabilities Education Improvement Act (IDEIA)	Law reauthorizing and updating IDEA.
Least restrictive environment (LRE)	Term in law that stipulates that children with disabilities be educated in the "least restrictive environment" possible (i.e., educated, to the maximum extent appropriate, with children who are not disabled in the regular classroom).
Multifactor evaluation (MFE)	School-provided evaluation performed by a multidisciplinary team to determine eligibility for either IDEA or Section 504 of the Rehabilitation Act. Several aspects of the child's functioning are assessed to avoid basing eligibility on only one area or the results of only one measure or assessment.
No Child Left Behind Act (NCLB)	Federal law including requirements regarding highly qualified teachers, research-based instructional methods, supplemental educational services, school district report cards, annual testing, and parental involvement. For children with disabilities, NCLB is perhaps most often salient regarding the qualifications of special education teachers, the determination of how fully to include these children in state-wide achievement testing, and keeping parents involved and informed.
Other health impairment (OHI)	Category of disability specified under IDEA, defined as having limited strength, vitality, or alertness because of a chronic or acute health problem and that negatively affects a child's educational performance.
Resource room	Substitute for a core academic class, in which a small number of children with disabilities are taught at their own instructional levels by a special education teacher.

Table 11–3.   Common educational terms (with abbreviations and acronyms) *(continued)*

Severe behavioral handicap (SBH)	Term used by some state departments of education to denote a child with an emotional disturbance, despite the fact that children with emotional and behavioral difficulties may have very different needs. Because SBH is not a category of disability defined by law, it is important for clinicians and parents to investigate exactly what such a label means if applied to a child.
Section 504 of the Rehabilitation Act (504 plan)	Civil rights law prohibiting discrimination against individuals with disabilities, including the right of children with disabilities to have equal access to an appropriate education. A 504 plan documents any accommodations to be made for a student with a disability who qualifies under the law. A more detailed discussion of 504 plans and how they differ from IEPs is included in this chapter.
Specific learning disability (SLD)	Category of disability specified under IDEA, defined as a disorder of one or more basic psychological processes involved in understanding or using spoken or written language, resulting in an impaired ability to listen, think, speak, read, write, spell, or do mathematical calculations. A school district need not consider whether a child has a severe discrepancy between achievement and intellectual ability when assessing for SLD. However, school districts are encouraged to determine if the child responds to research-based intervention as part of the evaluation.

Source.   Butler 2005; Gable et al. 1998, 2000; Quinn et al. 1998; Steedman 2008; Stout and Huston 2007; Wrightslaw 2006a, 2006b; Yell et al. 2006.

Some parents may be hesitant to inform school personnel of their child's bipolar diagnosis because they are afraid the child may be stigmatized. Others may feel comfortable informing a school-based mental health professional, such as a school psychologist or social worker, but be unwilling to share information with the child's teachers. Clinicians can play a key role in combating this mind set by explaining to parents the benefits of informing all members of the child's educational support system of his or her diagnosis. Lack of information at any level of this support system can undermine parents' and clinicians' best efforts to aid a child in functioning effectively in school. Administrators and teachers, for example, should be made aware of the behavioral symptoms of bipolar disorder, both to eliminate unnecessary or inappropriate disciplinary strategies and to help them differentiate misbehavior or lack of motivation from illness presentation (National Alliance for the Mentally Ill 2004). Further, school personnel, especially teachers, can be invaluable resources in helping parents to monitor symptom progression and cycling in bipolar students.

Clinicians' responsibility to act as advocates for their pediatric patients includes helping parents approach the process of securing school-based services with a spirit of cooperativeness and rationality. Helping parents secure such services can be understandably difficult, because parents dealing with a child's new diagnosis of bipolar disorder may be frightened and confused, and have a hard time distinguishing the educational accommodations and modifications to which the child is legally entitled, if any. Too often, parents find themselves in the unenviable position of requesting services for their child with bipolar disorder, under the advisement of the child's primary mental health care provider, only to be met with resistance from the child's school district. It is at this juncture that the clinician must make a crucial decision: to allow the situation to become adversarial and lose focus on the child at hand, which can result in legal proceedings that may exact a tremendous emotional and financial toll on parents and children, or to approach the situation from a problem-solving perspective, with the sole aim of servicing the child to the extent afforded by law.

As is common in many disputes, misinformation, lack of information, and lack of communication are often at the root of the problem, and this is frequently the case when parents and schools are in disagreement as to additional services needed by a child with bipolar disorder. Perhaps, as discussed previously, the school is not adequately familiar with bipolar disorder or how it may manifest in the school environment; perhaps the school is not aware of its legal responsibilities to children with a mental illness such as bipolar disorder; or perhaps parents are expecting too much, given their child's symptom presentation and level of school functioning. The clinician conceivably is the one individual best suited to remedy this confusion and to ensure that the primary focus remains on the child and, ultimately, on how to best provide for his or her unique educational needs.

References

Abikoff H, Courtney M, Pelham WE Jr, et al: Teachers' ratings of disruptive behaviors: the influence of halo effects. J Abnorm Child Psychol 21:519–533, 1993

Axelson D, Birmaher B, Strober M, et al: Phenomenology of children and adolescents with bipolar spectrum disorders. Arch Gen Psychiatry 63:1139–1148, 2006

Bearden CE, Glahn DC, Monkul ES, et al: Patterns of memory impairment in bipolar disorder and unipolar major depression. Psychiatry Res 142:139–150, 2006

Burgeson CR, Wechsler H, Brener ND, et al: Physical education and activity: results from the School Health Policies and Programs Study 2000. J Sch Health 71: 294–304, 2001

Butler J: Individuals With Disabilities Education Improvement Act of 2004 P.L. 108-446 compared to IDEA '97. October 29, 2005. Available at: http://www.copaa.org/pdf/IDEACOMP.pdf. Accessed on July 9, 2008.

Cannon M, Jones P, Gilvarry C, et al: Premorbid social functioning in schizophrenia and bipolar disorder: similarities and differences. Am J Psychiatry 154:1544–1550, 1997

Centers for Disease Control and Prevention: Healthy Youth! Coordinated School Health Program. April 30, 2007. Available at: http://www.cdc.gov/HealthyYouth/CSHP. Accessed July 9, 2008.

Chandler J: Bipolar Affective Disorder (Manic Depressive Disorder) in Children and Adolescents. November 2006. Available at: http://jamesdauntchandler.tripod.com/bipolar/bipolarpamphlet.htm. Accessed July 9, 2008.

Child and Adolescent Bipolar Foundation: About Pediatric Bipolar Disorder. October 27, 2002. Available at: http://www.bpkids.org/site/PageServer?pagename=lrn_about. Accessed July 9, 2008.

Child and Adolescent Bipolar Foundation: Educating the Child With Bipolar Disorder. 2007. Available at: http://www.bpkids.org/site/DocServer/edbrochure.pdf?docID=166. Accessed July 9, 2008.

Clarizio HF: Assessment of depression in children and adolescents by parents, teachers, and peers, in Handbook of Depression in Children and Adolescents. Edited by Reynolds WM, Johnston HF. New York, Plenum, 1994, pp 235–248

Crick F, Mitchison G: The function of dream sleep. Nature 304:111–114, 1983

Deckersbach T, Savage CR, Dougherty DD, et al: Spontaneous and directed application of verbal learning strategies in bipolar disorder and obsessive-compulsive disorder. Bipolar Disord 7:166–175, 2005

Deglin JH, Vallerand AH: Davis's Drug Guide for Nurses, 10th Edition. Philadelphia, PA, FA Davis, 2006

Doyle AE, Wilens TE, Kwon A, et al: Neuropsychological functioning in youth with bipolar disorder. Biol Psychiatry 58:540–548, 2005

DuVal SJ: Six-year-old Thomas diagnosed with pediatric onset bipolar disorder: a case study. J Child Adolesc Psychiatr Nurs 18:38–42, 2005

Evans JR, Van Velsor P, Schumacher JE: Addressing adolescent depression: a role for school counselors. Professional School Counseling 5:211–219, 2002

Faedda GL, Baldessarini RJ, Glovinsky IP, et al: Pediatric bipolar disorder: phenomenology and course of illness. Bipolar Disord 6:305–313, 2004

Feshbach ND, Feshbach S: Affective processes and academic achievement. Child Dev 58:1335–1347, 1987

Findling RL, Gracious BL, McNamara NK, et al: Rapid, continuous cycling and psychiatric co-morbidity in pediatric bipolar I disorder. Bipolar Disord 3:202–210, 2001

Fristad MA, Goldberg-Arnold JS: Raising a Moody Child: How to Cope With Depression and Bipolar Disorder. New York, Guilford, 2004

Gable RA, Quinn MM, Rutherford RB, et al: Addressing Student Problem Behavior—Part II: Conducting a Functional Behavioral Assessment. May 12, 1998. Available at: http://cecp.air.org/fba/problembehavior2/Functional%20Analysis.PDF. Accessed July 9, 2008.

Gable RA, Quinn MM, Rutherford RB, et al: Addressing Student Problem Behavior—Part III: Creating Positive Behavioral Intervention Plans and Supports. June 2, 2000. Available at: http://cecp.air.org/fba/problembehavior3/part3.pdf. Accessed July 9, 2008.

Geller B, Luby J: Child and adolescent bipolar disorder: a review of the past 10 years. J Am Acad Child Adolesc Psychiatry 36:1168–1176, 1997

Geller B, Williams M, Zimerman B, et al: Prepubertal and early adolescent bipolarity differentiate from ADHD by manic symptoms, grandiose delusions, ultra-rapid or ultradian cycling. J Affect Disord 51:81–91, 1998

Geller B, Zimerman B, Williams M, et al: Diagnostic characteristics of 93 cases of a prepubertal and early adolescent bipolar disorder phenotype by gender, puberty and comorbid attention deficit hyperactivity disorder. J Child Adolesc Psychopharmacol 10:157–164, 2000

Geller B, Craney JL, Bolhofner K, et al: Two-year prospective follow-up of children with a prepubertal and early adolescent bipolar disorder phenotype. Am J Psychiatry 159:927–933, 2002a

Geller B, Zimerman B, Williams M, et al: DSM-IV mania symptoms in a prepubertal and early adolescent bipolar disorder phenotype compared to attention-deficit hyperactive and normal controls. J Child Adolesc Psychopharmacol 12:11–25, 2002b

Geller B, Zimerman B, Williams M, et al: Phenomenology of prepubertal and early adolescent bipolar disorder: examples of elated mood, grandiose behaviors, decreased need for sleep, racing thoughts and hypersexuality. J Child Adolesc Psychopharmacol 12:3–9, 2002c

Gilcher D, Field R, Hellander M: The IDEA Classification Debate: ED or OHI? March 8, 2004. Available at: http://www.bpkids.org/site/DocServer/field_idea_classification.pdf?docID=169. Accessed July 9, 2008.

Glahn DC, Bearden CE, Caetano S, et al: Declarative memory impairment in pediatric bipolar disorder. Bipolar Disord 7:546–554, 2005

Goldstein TR: Social skills deficits among adolescents with bipolar disorder. Doctoral dissertation, University of Colorado at Boulder, Denver, CO, 2003 [UMI Dissertation Publishing Publ No AAT 3087542]

Hammen C, Rudolph KD: Childhood mood disorders, in Child Psychopathology, 2nd Edition. Edited by Mash EJ, Barkley RA. New York, Guilford, 2002, pp 233–278

Hammen C, Rudolph K, Weisz J, et al: The context of depression in clinic-referred youth: neglected areas in treatment. J Am Acad Child Adolesc Psychiatry 38:64–71, 1999

Harris J: The increased diagnosis of "juvenile bipolar disorder": what are we treating? Psychiatr Serv 56:529–531, 2005

Karni A, Tanne D, Rubenstein BS, et al: Dependence on REM sleep of overnight improvement of a perceptual skill. Science 265:679–682, 1994

Kim EY, Miklowitz DJ: Childhood mania, attention deficit hyperactivity disorder and conduct disorder: a critical review of diagnostic dilemmas. Bipolar Disord 4:215–225, 2002

Kowatch RA, Fristad MA: Bipolar disorders, in Comprehensive Handbook of Personality and Psychopathology, Vol 3: Child Psychopathology. Edited by Ammerman RT. Hoboken, NJ, Wiley, 2006, pp 217–232

Kowatch RA, Fristad M, Birmaher B, et al; Child Psychiatric Workgroup on Bipolar Disorder: Treatment guidelines for children and adolescents with bipolar disorder. J Am Acad Child Adolesc Psychiatry 44:213–235, 2005a

Kowatch RA, Youngstrom EA, Danielyan A, et al: Review and meta-analysis of the phenomenology and clinical characteristics of mania in children and adolescents. Bipolar Disord 7:483–496, 2005b

Kumpulainen K, Räsänen E, Henttonen I, et al: Psychiatric disorders, performance level at school and special education at early elementary school age. Eur Child Adolesc Psychiatry 8 (suppl 4):48–54, 1999

Kutcher S, Robertson HA, Bird D: Premorbid functioning in adolescent onset bipolar I disorder: a preliminary report from an ongoing study. J Affect Disord 51:137–144, 1998

Lagace DC, Kutcher SP, Robertson HA: Mathematics deficits in adolescents with bipolar I disorder. Am J Psychiatry 160:100–104, 2003

Leibenluft E, Rich BA, Vinton DT, et al: Neural circuitry engaged during unsuccessful motor inhibition in pediatric bipolar disorder. Am J Psychiatry 164:52–60, 2007

Lofthouse N, Mackinaw-Koons B, Fristad MA: Bipolar spectrum disorders: early onset, in Helping Children at Home and School II: Handouts for Families and Educators. Edited by Canter AS, Paige LZ, Roth MD, et al. Bethesda, MD, National Association of School Psychologists, 2004, pp S5-13–S5-16

Malhi GS, Ivanovski B, Hadzi-Pavlovic D, et al: Neuropsychological deficits and functional impairment in bipolar depression, hypomania and euthymia. Bipolar Disord 9:114–125, 2007

McCarthy J, Arrese D, McGlashan A, et al: Sustained attention and visual processing speed in children and adolescents with bipolar disorder and other psychiatric disorders. Psychol Rep 95:39–47, 2004

McClure EB, Treland JE, Snow J, et al: Deficits in social cognition and response flexibility in pediatric bipolar disorder. Am J Psychiatry 162:1644–1651, 2005

Murnan J, Price JH, Telljohann SK, et al: Parents' perceptions of curricular issues affecting children's weight in elementary schools. J Sch Health 76:502–511, 2006

National Alliance for the Mentally Ill: Helping parents understand their rights in special education: an interview with a legal expert. NAMI Beginnings 5:3–7, 15, 2004

Packer LE: Accommodating Students With Mood Lability: Depression and Bipolar Disorder. 2002a. Available at: http://www.schoolbehavior.com/Files/tips_mood.pdf. Accessed July 12, 2008.

Packer LE: Medication Side Effects. 2002b. Available at: http://www.schoolbehavior.com/tips_sideeffects.htm. Accessed July 12, 2008.

Papolos D, Papolos J: The Bipolar Child: The Definitive and Reassuring Guide to Childhood's Most Misunderstood Disorder, 3rd Edition. New York, Broadway Books, 2006

Papolos J, Hatton MJ, Norelli S, et al: Challenging Negative Remarks That Threaten to Derail the IEP Process. 2002a. Available at: http://www.bpchildresearch.org/edu_forums/responses.html. Accessed July 12, 2008

Papolos J, Hatton MJ, Norelli S, et al: The Educational Issues of Students With Bipolar Disorder. 2002b. Available at: http://www.jbrf.org/edu_forums/issues.html. Accessed July 12, 2008

Pavuluri MN, O'Connor MM, Harral EM, et al: Impact of neurocognitive function on academic difficulties in pediatric bipolar disorder: a clinical translation. Biol Psychiatry 60:951–956, 2006a

Pavuluri MN, Schenkel LS, Aryal S, et al: Neurocognitive function in unmedicated manic and medicated euthymic pediatric bipolar patients. Am J Psychiatry 163:286–293, 2006b

Puura K, Almqvist F, Tamminen T, et al: Children with symptoms of depression: what do the adults see? J Child Psychol Psychiatry 39:577–585, 1998

Quackenbush D, Kutcher S, Robertson HA, et al: Premorbid and postmorbid school functioning in bipolar adolescents: description and suggested academic interventions. Can J Psychiatry 41:16–22, 1996

Quinn MM, Gable RA, Rutherford RB, et al: Addressing student problem behavior: an IEP team's introduction to functional behavioral assessment and behavior intervention plans. January 16, 1998. Available at: http://cecp.air.org/fba/problembehavior/funcanal.pdf. Accessed July 12, 2008.

Reynolds WM, Johnston HF: The nature and study of depression in children and adolescents, in Handbook of Depression in Children and Adolescents. Edited by Reynolds WM, Johnston HF. New York, Plenum, 1994, pp 3–17

Rich BA, Vinton DT, Roberson-Nay R, et al: Limbic hyperactivation during processing of neutral facial expressions in children with bipolar disorder. Proc Natl Acad Sci U S A 103:8900–8905, 2006

Steedman W: Independent Educational Evaluations: What? Why? How? Who Pays? 2008. Available at: http://www.wrightslaw.com/info/test.iee.steedman.htm. Accessed July 12, 2008.

Stout KS, Huston J: Special education inclusion. March 15, 2007. Available at: www.weac.org/resource/june96/speced.htm. Accessed July 12, 2008.

Warner B, Parr J, Alexander T, et al: Early Onset Bipolar Disorder in Children and Adolescents: A Brief Overview. College Park, MD, National Assembly of School-Based Health Care, University of Maryland, 2003

Waslick BD, Kandel R, Kakouros A: Depression in children and adolescents: an overview, in The Many Faces of Depression in Children and Adolescents. Edited by Shaffer D, Waslick BD (Review of Psychiatry Series, Vol 21; Oldham JM and Riba MB, series eds). Washington, DC, American Psychiatric Publishing, 2002, pp 1–36

Weckerly J: Pediatric bipolar mood disorder. J Dev Behav Pediatr 23:42–56, 2002

Weller EB, Calvert SM, Weller RA: Bipolar disorder in children and adolescents: diagnosis and treatment. Curr Opin Psychiatry 16:383–388, 2003

Wozniak J, Biederman J, Kiely K, et al: Mania-like symptoms suggestive of childhood-onset bipolar disorder in clinically referred children. J Am Acad Child Adolesc Psychiatry 34:867–876, 1995

Wrightslaw: Discrimination: Section 504 and ADA. November 27, 2006a. Available at: http://www.wrightslaw.com/info/sec504.index.htm. Accessed July 12, 2008.

Wrightslaw: No Child Left Behind—Wrightslaw. March 2, 2006b. Available at: www.wrightslaw.com/nclb/index.htm. Accessed July 12, 2008.

Yell ML, Shriner JG, Katsiyannis A: Individuals with Disabilities Education Improvement Act of 2004 and IDEA Regulations of 2006: Implications for Educators, Administrators, and Teacher Trainers. Focus on Exceptional Children. September 2006. Available at: http://www.pbis.org/files/FOEC-V39_1A-Sept.pdf. Accessed July 12, 2008.

Appendix:
Information on Bipolar Disorder for Schools

What Is Bipolar Disorder?

- *Bipolar disorder,* formerly known as *manic-depressive disorder,* is a biologically based and often genetically linked mental illness found in approximately 0.5% of children and 1% of adolescents. The distinguishing feature of bipolar disorder is a fluctuating mood that includes depression (a low mood that may appear as either sadness or irritability) and mania (a high mood that may appear as either elation or anger and irritability).

- There are several types of bipolar disorder, including bipolar I disorder, bipolar II disorder, cyclothymia, and bipolar disorder not otherwise specified. Although these various types of the disorder all share common features, they differ in the amount of time spent in depressive and manic phases and by the severity of depressive and manic symptoms.

- Although adults with bipolar disorder often have distinct periods of depression and mania that last for weeks or months, children and adolescents are much more likely to display symptoms that alternate rapidly between depression and mania, sometimes many times within a single day. In some cases, the symptoms of depression and mania may be present at the same time. Because of this complicated and often rapidly changing symptom presentation, children with bipolar disorder are often misdiagnosed as having other disorders.
- Symptoms of bipolar disorder represent a *change* from the student's usual behavior.

Manic Symptoms and Possible School Presentations

- *Elated mood:* difficulty controlling laughter, inappropriate joking or laughing at inappropriate times, inappropriate excitement over minor events.
- *Irritability:* when mild, uncooperative or oppositional behavior; when severe, aggressive or even dangerous behavior.
- *Grandiosity:* inappropriately high/unrealistic self-esteem, boasting of unrealistic abilities, harassing teachers about how best to teach class, failing subjects intentionally because of a belief the course is being taught incorrectly, telling administrators how to do their jobs.
- *Decreased need for sleep:* little or no sleep at night may affect learning, memory, and attention, although the child may appear alert and even overly energetic.
- *Fast/increased speech:* speech difficult to follow/understand.
- *Racing thoughts/flight of ideas:* difficulty processing information presented in class, talking to peers at inappropriate times, talking out of turn, jumping from topic to topic without appropriate transitions.
- *Distractibility:* difficulty concentrating.
- *Increased energy:* difficulty remaining seated/sitting still/quiet or performing fine motor tasks (e.g., writing, drawing).
- *Excessive involvement in pleasurable and risky behaviors:* inappropriate sexualized behavior, stealing, drug use, skipping school.

Depressive Symptoms and Possible School Presentations

- *Irritability:* grumpy, oppositional, or disruptive behavior.
- *Sadness:* may be easy to miss, as very sad students may be quiet and non-disruptive.
- *Loss of interest:* even students previously driven to succeed academically may find themselves unable to summon the interest or energy needed to learn.
- *Significant weight loss or gain:* this may be observable by school personnel, especially with younger students who may be more closely monitored during lunchtime.
- *Sleep disturbances:* difficulty falling or staying asleep at night, which can lead to fatigue and sleepiness, especially early in the day; wanting to sleep more than normal.
- *Restlessness:* fidgeting, trouble sitting still.
- *Sluggish behavior/fatigue:* difficulty moving or speaking at a normal rate, speaking less than normal.
- *Negative self-image:* feelings of worthlessness, inferiority, and incapability may also make it difficult for a student to be motivated.
- *Inattention:* difficulty concentrating.
- *Recurrent thoughts of death or suicidal thoughts:* students experiencing these symptoms should be closely monitored both at home and at school.

What Problems Are Associated With Bipolar Disorder?

- Students with bipolar disorder frequently have difficulties in school, ranging from an increased incidence of learning disabilities to problems in memory, attention, and behavior. These difficulties often remain even when the child's mood is stable. Approximately one-fifth to one-third of students with bipolar disorder receive special education services.
- Students with bipolar disorder usually have other co-occurring disorders, including anxiety disorders or behavioral difficulties, especially attention-deficit/hyperactivity disorder.
- Students with bipolar disorder are often socially impaired and prone to becoming bullies or victims, being very shy, misinterpreting jokes, and perceiving other students as threatening.

- Over one-half of all individuals with bipolar disorder attempt suicide at some point in their lives; over 30% of students ages 7–17 with bipolar disorder have a lifetime history of suicide attempts. Approximately 15%–20% of all individuals with bipolar disorder actually *complete* suicide.

Medication Side Effects Do Not End at Home

- Most youths with bipolar disorder require multiple medications to address their mood symptoms and co-occurring disorders. These medications, however, can produce side effects that present further school challenges. It may take quite some time for a student's physician(s) to determine the combination and dosages of medications that work best for that child. Youths undergoing medication changes may miss a lot of school or be unable to complete as much work as normal.
- Common types of medications prescribed to students with bipolar disorder include mood stabilizers, antipsychotics, antidepressants, and stimulants.
- Common side effects for these medications include drowsiness, dizziness, impaired concentration, increased thirst, increased appetite, loss of appetite, nausea, constipation, diarrhea, headache, fatigue, and tremors.

12

Special Treatment Issues

Mary A. Fristad, Ph.D., A.B.P.P.
Elisabeth A. Frazier, B.S.

Pediatric bipolar disorder can lead to considerable impairment in social, academic, and home environments. As discussed in previous chapters, the course of bipolar disorder, particularly when the disorder begins in childhood, is chronic and often severe. It frequently co-occurs with attention-deficit/hyperactivity disorder (ADHD), conduct disorder, and/or oppositional defiant disorder. Compared with adult-onset bipolar disorder, childhood-onset bipolar disorder predicts greater impairment, more frequent hospitalizations, and greater symptom severity. The multiple comorbidities seen with pediatric bipolar disorder exacerbate the course and intensity of each disorder diagnosed and complicate both diagnosis and treatment (Pavuluri et al. 2005).

Pediatric bipolar disorder leads to special concerns throughout the treatment process. Cycles of rapidly changing and mixed mood states and associated behavioral dysregulation must be addressed. To do this successfully, clinicians must build a strong alliance with the patient and his or her family and be aware of the various therapeutic issues that may arise during treatment, including medication adherence, conduct problems, hypersexuality/promiscuity, impaired peer relationships, stigma, substance abuse, and high risk of suicide. By anticipating these issues, clinicians can be prepared to deal with them as they arise over the course of the child or adolescent's illness.

Treatment and Medication Adherence

Meta-analyses suggest treatment adherence is approximately 50% for most children with chronic health conditions (Bryon 1998). This is also true in mental health care. Approximately one-third to two-thirds of children in child and adolescent psychiatry outpatient clinics do not keep scheduled appointments (Brasic et al. 2001). Among families of patients ages 12–19 with a bipolar diagnosis, only half attended all scheduled family therapy sessions, and only 54% of adolescents attended all their individual sessions (Coletti et al. 2005).

Medication adherence is similarly challenging (Coletti et al. 2005; DelBello et al. 2007; Yen et al. 2005), because even a "perfect" treatment will not benefit the patient who does not receive it, and current treatment options are not perfect. Youth with bipolar disorder often have complicated regimens that require taking multiple pills at numerous times throughout the day. This contributes to poor medication adherence, especially for patients with comorbid ADHD, because disorganization and forgetfulness are core symptoms of ADHD (Miklowitz and George 2007). Other reasons for nonadherence include unpleasant side effects and losing the highs that come with hypomania. Nonadherence can lead to serious consequences, including higher risk of relapse, more frequent hospitalizations, and longer durations of hospitalization (Miklowitz and George 2007).

When asked to estimate their children's medication adherence, parents of children with a bipolar disorder report missing an average of 2.3 doses of medication per month. However, only 34% of adolescent patients with pediatric bipolar disorder are fully adherent to their medication regimen (Coletti et al. 2005). Patients most likely to be adherent are those recently diagnosed with bipolar disorder (Coletti et al. 2005). Thus, it is critical to carefully monitor medication adherence, emphasizing its importance both at the beginning of and throughout treatment (Coletti et al. 2005).

Beliefs regarding causes, course, and consequences of mood disorders and medication are better able to predict medication adherence than other factors, such as social and demographic information (Davidson and Fristad 2006). Children and adults who have negative or distrustful beliefs about mental health, mood disorders, and medication are less likely to seek out treatment and attend sessions regularly. Those who believe a treatment's benefits outweigh its costs are more likely to adhere (Davidson and Fristad 2006). As misperceptions regarding mood disorders and their treatment can be detrimental to finding and utilizing proper care, educating patients and their families about mental illness, mood disorders, medications, and other proposed treatments may help increase adherence.

Managing medication in children and adolescents requires active involvement of both the parent and child. Treatment should be continually evaluated and altered as needed (Fristad and Goldberg-Arnold 2004). Both the youth and his or her parents may benefit from psychoeducation regarding bipolar disorder, psychotropic medications, and the importance of treatment adherence (Miklowitz et al. 2000, 2003). In addition, family therapy may be beneficial to address issues of parent-child conflict that might play out over the battles surrounding medication adherence (Jamieson and Rynn 2006).

Although adherence is an "equal-opportunity" concern, evidence suggests ethnicity plays a role in medication adherence. Patel and colleagues (2005) reported that African American patients continue being prescribed antipsychotic medication for a significantly longer time following their first psychiatric hospitalization compared with European American patients. No difference was noted in prescriptions for mood stabilizers and anticonvulsants in the two groups.

Additionally, whereas African American and European American patients both exhibit poor medication adherence, they tend to endorse different reasons for not taking all of their medication. Fleck et al. (2005) reported that over half of all adult participants with bipolar I disorder were completely or partially nonadherent in taking their medications, and over 20% denied even having bipolar disorder. When results were examined vis-à-vis ethnicity, about 40% of European Americans and 50% of African Americans attributed nonadherence to negative side effects. African American patients tended to identify patient-related factors (e.g., fear of becoming addicted to medications, taking medication is a sign of mental illness) as reasons for nonadherence more frequently than European American patients. However, there was no significant difference between patient-related and illness/medication-related factors (e.g., side effects, denial of illness) within the African American group, indicating that African Americans expressed concern for both patient-related and illness/medication-related factors. There was a significant difference between these two factors in the European American group, with significantly higher scores for illness/medication-related factors relative to patient-related factors. This indicates that European Americans are more concerned with illness/medication-related factors than patient-related factors (Fleck et al. 2005). It is important to consider these ethnic differences regarding adherence when targeting interventions to encourage improved adherence.

Although adherence is a challenge, it is considered crucial for successful treatment. An untreated or partially treated mood disorder is likely to lead to decreased school performance, participation in risky activities (e.g., multiple sexual partners), a greater likelihood of abusing drugs and alcohol, and increased suicide risk (Jamieson and Rynn 2006). Several steps can be taken to increase adherence.

First, it is essential for the youth and parents to have open communication with the prescribing physician regarding medication management. This communication should minimize the likelihood of medication discontinuation caused by frustration over manageable side effects or confusion surrounding a complex medication regimen. Second, implementing a daily ritual of taking pills at the same time and place every day makes it easier to remember to take each dose. Third, using a pillbox helps organize medications and provides a visual reminder of whether or not the day's medication has been taken (Fristad and Goldberg-Arnold 2004). Fourth, maintaining a calendar to alert the family member in charge of ordering refills prevents running out of any prescriptions (Jamieson and Rynn 2006). Finally, building insight via psychoeducation and symptom monitoring helps achieve greater adherence to treatment. Patel et al. (2005) noted that adolescents with bipolar disorder who perceive greater benefits from medication tend to display better adherence rates. Patients with bipolar disorder who show insight regarding treatment, mental health status, and psychotic experiences are more likely to have greater medication adherence rates (Yen et al. 2005).

Conduct Problems

Several conduct problems frequently overlap with the clinical presentation of pediatric bipolar disorder (Biederman et al. 2004). These may include disinhibition, lying, stealing, breaking rules, low frustration tolerance, aggression, violence, truancy, and poor academic performance. Children may fail classes, refuse to attend school, or be so disruptive in the classroom that they are suspended and/or expelled (American Psychiatric Association 2000; Kovacs and Pollock 1995; Masi et al. 2003). Comorbidity rates for youths with bipolar disorder are exceedingly high: 88%–98% met criteria for ADHD, 84%–88% met criteria for oppositional defiant disorder, and 37%–43% met criteria for conduct disorder (Biederman et al. 2004). These rates suggest that the externalizing behavior problems and delinquent actions seen in children and adolescents with bipolar disorder are complex and multidetermined. The characteristic behavioral disinhibition of bipolar disorder likely plays a role in the expression of these conduct problems and may provide a common link between bipolar disorder and conduct disorder (Biederman et al. 2003). Although pediatric bipolar disorder and conduct disorder display significant overlap, evidence suggests these are in fact two distinctive comorbid conditions with different treatment needs (Biederman et al. 2003, 2004).

Biederman et al. (2003) determined that physical restlessness, poor judgment, and vandalism were more common in children diagnosed with both bipolar disorder and conduct disorder compared with children diagnosed with bipolar disorder alone. When the clinician is attempting to differentiate between these disorders, it is important to determine whether manic-specific symptoms are present. Although these two disorders may share some behavioral manifestations, each requires unique treatment. Failure to diagnose accurately pediatric bipolar disorder because of the overshadowing of conduct problems potentially may cause a poorer outcome and delay treatment that has the potential to improve social, emotional, and educational aspects of life (Biederman et al. 2003).

Parental management and monitoring are key components to minimizing the impact of the behavioral dysregulation that can occur in youth with bipolar disorder. Similarly, maintaining clear communication with schools can lead to decreased disruption in that setting. Youths under the careful watch of their parents are less likely to steal or skip school. Creating clear, appropriate rules with direct, straightforward consequences will assist children with bipolar disorder to avoid further complications that could explode in an unstructured context.

Encouraging youths with bipolar disorder to participate in structured, supervised peer activities or to socialize with friends in their homes or the homes of friends whose parents have some awareness of the children's challenges also provides structure and containment. While in the home, parents still need to monitor the content of their child's activities. Parents should become knowledgeable about how to manage the Internet sites their child visits and, if necessary, place controls on Internet Web sites and television channels to minimize their child's ability to engage in inappropriate activities or be exposed to inappropriate content.

Hypersexuality/Promiscuity

Hypersexuality is another problematic issue for youth with bipolar disorder. In adults, hypersexuality is characterized by multiple marriages, overt sexual acts, and promiscuity. In children, the presentation of hypersexuality differs, given their developmental level. Hypersexuality in children is characterized as age- and situation-inappropriate flirtatious and sexualized behaviors. Children with bipolar disorder may excessively masturbate, attempt to engage in sexualized interactions with family members, engage in explicit sex talk (e.g., passing notes in class offering sexual favors to classmates), and appear unusually preoccupied by romantic relationships. Adolescents are more likely to have an excessive number of partners and/or rapid engagement in sexual activity while in a manic state (Geller and Tillman 2004; Kowatch et al. 2005b).

One meta-analysis by Kowatch et al. (2005b) revealed that 31%–45% of youths ages 5–18 with bipolar disorder display hypersexuality. Whenever hypersexuality is observed, it is critical to determine whether the child has been sexually abused or has been exposed to sexual material inappropriate for his or her age. However, Geller and Tillman (2004) determined that hypersexuality occurs most often in the absence of sexual abuse for youth with bipolar disorder. In a study of 93 youths with bipolar disorder, only 1% had a history of abuse, whereas 43% displayed hypersexual symptoms. Hypersexuality can help distinguish pediatric bipolar disorder from other childhood disorders and is an example of poor judgment in mania (Geller and Tillman 2004; Kowatch et al. 2005a).

Adolescents with bipolar disorder tend to have higher reported rates of hypersexuality compared with prepubertal pediatric bipolar patients (70.4% compared with 24.2%) (Geller et al. 1998). This may be an ascertainment issue, however. Clinicians tend to show discomfort in assessing hypersexuality in adults with bipolar disorder, and this discomfort seems to increase with decreasing age (Geller and Tillman 2004). The presence or absence of hypersexuality should be routinely assessed in children and adolescents (Geller and Tillman 2004). To do so, clinicians should interview parents and the child separately in addition to directly observing any sexualized behaviors or comments from the child during the interview. This may include inappropriate touching of himself or herself or the interviewer, imitating famous people who exhibit sexual behaviors, acting or speaking in a flirtatious manner, and using sexually explicit language. The clinician should also inquire about increased interest in sex, which may be reflected by the youth's increased interest in sexually explicit magazines or movies, or sex hotlines or Internet sites, and inappropriate sexual language or actions at home or at school. Special care should be taken with peripubertal children and adolescents, because they are at increased risk for unprotected sex, which may result in sexually transmitted diseases and/or unwanted pregnancies (Geller and Tillman 2004). Early intervention is important and should include preventive measures such as birth control and the human papillomavirus (HPV) vaccine.

Impaired Peer Relationships

Clinicians judge a child's functional capacity and level of impairment by exploring how he or she acts at home, in school, and with peers. When children are in preschool and kindergarten, friendship equates to playmates. As children grow, friendship is defined by mutual trust and assistance. The bond of friendship becomes increasingly important during adolescence as teenagers depend on their friends for intimacy, loyalty, and mutual understanding (Berk 2006). Therefore, impaired peer relationships become a critical area of focus for treatment in pediatric bipolar disorder. Symptoms of depression, mania, and other comorbid disorders discussed in previous chapters all contribute to impaired social interactions. The earlier the age at onset, the earlier children may veer off the normative social developmental trajectory, leading to increased difficulty with peer relations.

Many actions that may occur during a mood episode, particularly a manic episode, are considered unacceptable by societal standards. Frequent and intense mood swings, impulsive acts, and inappropriate social behaviors interrupt relationships with others. These behaviors may cause serious impairment in the life of the child with bipolar disorder as well as in the lives of other people who have significant relationships with the child (Biederman et al. 2003).

Thus, it is crucial to focus on social skills development in younger children and remediation of social skills in older children and adolescents. Symptoms of irritability and aggression can interrupt psychosocial functioning and peer relationships as early as the preschool years. Children with bipolar disorder tend to lose control over their emotions and subsequently their behavior and are in clear need of emotion-regulation skills. Only after they have the capacity to downregulate intense emotions or upregulate dysphoric mood will they be prepared to benefit maximally from training in verbal and nonverbal communication and problem-solving skills necessary for successful interpersonal relationships (Biederman et al. 2004; Fristad and Goldberg-Arnold 2004; Scheffer and Niskala Apps 2004).

Research suggests that over half of all youths with bipolar disorder have poor social skills. These children are typically teased by their peers and are unable to make or keep friends. They tend to have poor problem-solving skills and often misinterpret social cues in a negative light, further exacerbating their peer relationships (Geller et al. 2002). Youth ages 7–18 years with bipolar disorder or severe mood dysregulation make significantly more errors in judging facial emotional expressions compared with youth with other psychological disorders (e.g., anxiety, major depressive disorder, ADHD, and conduct disorder) (Guyer et al. 2007). In adolescence, it appears individuals with bipolar disorder do not differ from those not diagnosed with bipolar disorder regarding *knowledge* of appropriate social skills, but adolescents with bipolar disorder are significantly impaired in *performing* appropriate social skills compared with symptom-free youth (Goldstein et al. 2006).

Children and adolescents with bipolar disorder need the support, encouragement, and supervision of responsible adults in their lives as well as reliable peers. A strong base and support system can help to counteract the negative social effects that having bipolar disorder can produce (Copeland and Copans 2002). Structured, supervised groups such as drama clubs, music groups, athletic teams, youth groups, and volunteer organizations all can provide opportunities to interact successfully with peers who have similar interests.

Web sites such as that created by the Child and Adolescent Bipolar Foundation (www.bpkids.org) provide a safe source of support and information for teens to learn about their disorder on their own. This site has a special section for depressed teens that includes relevant articles, a gallery of artwork submitted by youth with mood disorders, a frequently asked questions section about mood disorders, and information on whom to call if a child or adolescent feels like hurting himself or herself, or knows someone else who is having suicidal thoughts. Another Web site, www.bpchildren.org, provides resources for children, teens, and adults, including games, tips from kids of all ages, and a newsletter for youth about how to deal with bipolar disorder and its challenges in everyday life.

Stigma

Stigma is real and must be addressed. *Stigma* refers to the negative attributions made about a person, in this case, a child with bipolar disorder, above and beyond the overt problems caused by the disorder. The general public often holds negative views of adults with mental illnesses, seeing a psychiatrist, and being hospitalized for mental or emotional problems. Stigma often results in a great deal of shame for both the diagnosed patient and his or her family and close friends. This shame tends to stem from feelings of being abnormal and not living up to societal expectations (Fawcett et al. 2000).

A recent national survey revealed that many people believe mental health care in childhood results in stigma toward the treated child. Nearly half (43%) of respondents believed this stigma would continue to have a negative effect on the youth into adulthood. Many survey participants were concerned with confidentiality issues, stigma directed at the entire family of a youth seeking mental health treatment, and negative side effects of medications (Pescosolido et al. 2007). Over two-thirds of respondents expressed negative attitudes toward prescribing psychiatric medication to children (Pescosolido 2007). Further, the general public considers childhood depression as more serious and perceives it as a more dangerous disorder compared with adult depression (Perry et al. 2007). Respondents endorsed formal care and treatment against the patient's will (e.g., forced hospitalization) more often for children than for adults, and they were less likely to advise discussing a child's mental health problems with friends and family compared with discussing an adult's mental disorder (Perry et al. 2007). These survey results suggest that stigma surrounding childhood mood disorders is even greater than that regarding adult mood disorders.

Whereas informing family, friends, and others about a child's mood disorder can lead to difficulties, as discussed previously, not telling anyone what is wrong can lead to another set of problems. For example, open communication with school personnel is the first necessary step to arrange for school-based services (see Chapter 11, "The Bipolar Child and the Educational System," for more details). It is also important for youth with bipolar disorder to incorporate the belief that bipolar disorder does not define who they are. It is simply another aspect of life to be mastered and lived with instead of letting the illness control their lives (Jamieson and Rynn 2006). Distinctions should be made between the youth's personality or core characteristics and the bipolar disorder symptoms he or she experiences. Negative aspects of the disorder should be identified as a separate entity from the youth's traits (Fristad et al. 1999). Stigma can be reduced by showing compassion to patients and their families; advocating for more education, research, and mental health legislation; recognizing that bipolar disorder is a real, valid illness that requires professional help; and educating others to reduce ignorance regarding bipolar disorder (Fawcett et al. 2000).

Substance Abuse

Substance abuse problems occur frequently in adolescents with bipolar disorder. Approximately 40% of adolescent-onset inpatients with bipolar disorder also have a comorbid substance use disorder (Wilens et al. 1999). Of note, adolescent-onset bipolar disorder conveys a ninefold risk of developing substance use disorder compared with childhood onset (Wilens et al. 1999). Research suggests that early-onset bipolar disorder in children is a risk factor for substance use disorder above and beyond the risk accounted for by ADHD, which is highly comorbid with pediatric bipolar disorder (Biederman et al. 2003). Adolescents with conduct disorder in addition to adolescent-onset bipolar disorder, however, were at no greater risk for developing substance use disorder compared with adolescents with only a conduct disorder diagnosis. In the absence of conduct disorder, adolescent-onset bipolar disorder confers a sixfold risk of developing substance use disorder compared with adolescents without a bipolar diagnosis. Interestingly, adolescents who had childhood-onset bipolar disorder did not differ in their rates of substance use disorder, regardless of their conduct disorder status (Wilens et al. 1999).

The presence of bipolar disorder plus conduct disorder in children each independently predicted substance use disorders in their relatives. Relatives of children with bipolar disorder or bipolar and conduct disorder tended to develop problems with alcohol abuse during adolescence, whereas relatives of children with conduct disorder but not bipolar disorder tended to develop alcohol abuse later in adulthood. Drug dependence in family members of children with conduct disorder only occurred in co-occurrence with pediatric bipolar disorder (Biederman et al. 2003).

The additional complication of substance use disorder in youth with bipolar disorder should be addressed at the beginning of treatment. Prevention, of course, is best. Monitoring medication adherence is extremely important, because it may decrease the likelihood of the youth using alcohol and drugs to self-medicate. Although alcohol and illicit drugs may produce temporary relief to the user, they actually worsen symptoms, alter the effects of prescription medications, interfere with interpersonal relationships, and may increase the likelihood of committing suicide (Copeland and Copans 2002). As substance use complicates both the assessment and treatment of bipolar disorder, these comorbid problems should be treated simultaneously (Kowatch et al. 2005a). If substance use is suspected, random drug screening may deter, or at least detect, the use of any substances in addition to prescribed medications.

Researchers have theorized that the high level of comorbidity between pediatric bipolar disorder and substance abuse is a result of patients with bipolar disorder using alcohol and drugs as a way to self-medicate their mood symptoms and comorbid anxiety (Khantzian 1997; Wilens et al. 2004). The fact that bipolar disorder predicts future substance use independently of conduct disorder suggests that careful treatment of pediatric bipolar disorder may prevent or reduce later onset of substance use disorders. It is critical for clinicians to educate both patients and their parents about the problems substance use and abuse can pose. Close communication and collaboration between patients, parents, and providers can diminish the likelihood that substance use and abuse will complicate the course of illness for youth with bipolar disorder (Wilens et al. 1999).

Suicide

The rate of suicide in all bipolar disorder patients is 30 times higher than in the general population (Ostacher and Eidelman 2006). Evidence suggests that the frequency and duration of depressive episodes in adults with bipolar disorder are associated with the high risk of suicide in this population. Time periods immediately following hospitalization and discharge are highly vulnerable periods associated with increased likelihood of suicidal behaviors (Ostacher and Eidelman 2006). Chen and Dilsaver (1996) determined that the lifetime rate of suicide attempts is higher in people with bipolar disorder (29.2%) compared with those with unipolar depression (15.9%) or other Axis I disorders (4.2%) as well as the general population (Chen and Dilsaver 1996).

Similarly, children and adolescents with bipolar disorder will attempt to end their lives through suicide at a much higher rate than their peers. Suicide risk increases with higher rates of comorbidity and greater symptom severity, both of which are common in early-onset bipolar disorder. Evidence suggests that over 25% of youth with bipolar disorder develop a suicide plan (Geller et al. 1998). Because of the increased risk for suicidal behavior in children and adolescents with bipolar disorder, clinicians need to maintain a vigilant awareness of suicidal ideation and/or suicide attempts in their patients, always keeping plans for active suicide intervention close at hand.

Evidence of psychosis is a major risk factor for attempted or completed suicide in pediatric bipolar patients. Children with bipolar disorder who also have a lifetime history of psychosis are 30.8% more likely to have thoughts of death, 51.8% more likely to experience suicidal ideation, and 49.3% more likely to make suicidal plans compared with nonpsychotic pediatric bipolar patients (Caetano et al. 2006). One-third of children ages 7–17 years with bipolar disorder have a lifetime history of suicide attempts. Those who made a suicide attempt were older and more likely to have had psychotic features, a history of mixed episodes, and bipolar I disorder compared with those who did not attempt suicide. They were also more likely to have comorbid substance use disorder or panic disorder, previous suicide attempts in their family, a history of physical or sexual abuse, previous self-harming behaviors, and/or more frequent hospitalizations compared to nonattempters (Goldstein et al. 2005).

Early onset of bipolar disorder may contribute to high rates of suicidal behaviors as a result of adverse effects that may interfere with development; longer duration of illness; and increased frequency of episodes (Chen and Dilsaver 1996). Pediatric patients who have an earlier age at onset are also at higher risk for suicide because of possible misdiagnosis with childhood behavioral disorders and large gaps between symptom onset and appropriate treatment. In addition, the more severe, rapid-cycling, chronic course of childhood-onset bipolar disorder also contributes to increased risk for suicide in younger patients. Consistent treatment and adherence to pharmacological interventions may reduce the risk of suicide in youth with bipolar disorder. Therefore, clinicians need to take extra care in the diagnosis, treatment, and maintenance of early-onset bipolar disorder patients (Ostacher and Eidelman 2006).

Risk assessment is important. Anxiety, behavioral, alcohol and substance abuse, eating, and personality disorders; severe aggression; depression; and hopelessness as well as physical ailments have all been associated with higher frequencies of suicidal behaviors in patients with bipolar disorder (Ostacher and Eidelman 2006). In addition to identifying suicide risk, preventing self-harming attempts may include coordination with family members and other individuals who have significant relationships with the bipolar patient to lock up all guns, knives, and medications in the home or temporarily hospitalize the youth at risk (Ostacher and Eidelman 2006).

Conclusion

Clinicians should have an appreciation for the complications often associated with pediatric bipolar disorder. Early diagnosis and treatment is crucial for children with pediatric bipolar disorder (Miklowitz and Cicchetti 2006). Without prompt identification and treatment, the likelihood of future, likely lifetime, problems in social, neurobiological, academic, and emotional functioning greatly increases, as does the risk of suicidal ideation and hospitalizations. Comorbidities, including disruptive behavior disorders, anxiety disorders, and alcohol and substance abuse problems, can exacerbate the already difficult to treat course of illness.

Although medication adherence is particularly important, typical rates of adherence are low. Development of a treatment team that includes a prescribing physician, a therapist, and a contact at the youth's school in addition to a supportive and knowledgeable group of family and friends will be crucial for successful treatment (Anglada 2006; Fristad and Goldberg-Arnold, 2004). This treatment team should be augmented by a social support network composed of caring adults who also will aid the patient in limiting conduct problems through monitoring at home, at school, and with friends. Careful supervision and encouragement to redirect energy into prosocial, organized activities such as athletics, music, drama, and volunteer or religious youth groups may help protect youths with bipolar disorder from engaging in maladaptive behaviors.

Participating in organized group activities may also help mend peer relations that have suffered from negative behaviors and stigma surrounding youth with bipolar disorder. The support of peers found in these groups becomes increasingly important as children with bipolar disorder grow into adolescents and turn to friends for help and comfort instead of family. As peers become increasingly important with age, it is necessary for youth with bipolar disorder to surround themselves with positive peer influences. Stigma toward youth with bipolar disorder is a very real problem that may create feelings of shame and blame for youths with bipolar disorder and their family and friends. However, by keeping essential people informed of the diagnosis and maintaining a compassionate, educated support system of people, children and adolescents with bipolar disorder can learn to take control of their illness rather than having it take control of their lives.

Problems with hypersexuality and promiscuity symptoms also increase as youths with bipolar disorder age. Again, close supervision is critical to minimizing negative consequences involving hypersexuality. Parents should be aware of what their adolescents view on the Internet and set controls to block inappropriate content. It may also be necessary to take preventive precautions such as birth control or the HPV vaccination to prevent long-term, life-changing consequences of impulsivity and promiscuity.

Youths with bipolar disorder are at an increased risk to develop substance abuse problems compared with youth in the general population. Because prevention of alcohol and drug use is a goal in treatment, parents and treatment providers may utilize random drug screenings if substance use is suspected. Because self-medication is one reason for substance use in youths with bipolar disorder, medication adherence becomes extremely important, because it may decrease the chances of youths turning to drugs and alcohol for symptom relief. Comorbid substance abuse leads to increased suicide risk in youths with bipolar disorder, so it is crucial to address these issues immediately and simultaneously. Other factors convey additional risk for suicide such as previous suicide attempts, mixed episodes, and psychotic features. Clinicians must take reports of suicidal thoughts and acts seriously and constantly assess for these features in youth with bipolar disorder. The treatment team can help reduce suicide risk by encouraging medication adherence, careful monitoring of patients, and removal of dangerous items such as guns and knives from the home. All of these special issues involved in treating youths with bipolar disorder further complicate an already complex mental illness, but by remaining educated about these issues and proactive in dealing with them, clinicians can provide appropriate care to patients and their families.

References

American Psychiatric Association: Diagnostic and Statistical Manual of Mental Disorders, 4th Edition, Text Revision. Washington, DC, American Psychiatric Association, 2000, pp 382–401

Anglada T: Intense Minds: Through the Eyes of Young People With Bipolar Disorder. Victoria, BC, Canada, Trafford Publishing, 2006

Berk LE: Child Development, 7th Edition. Boston, MA, Pearson Education, 2006

Biederman J, Mick E, Wozniak J, et al: Can a subtype of conduct disorder linked to bipolar disorder be identified? Integration of findings from the Massachusetts General Hospital Pediatric Psychopharmacology Research Program. Biol Psychiatry 53:952–960, 2003

Biederman J, Faraone SV, Wozniak J, et al: Further evidence of unique developmental phenotype correlates of pediatric bipolar disorder: findings from a large sample of clinically referred preadolescent children assessed over the last 7 years. J Affect Disord 82 (suppl 1):S45–S58, 2004

Brasic JR, Nadrich RH, Kleinrock S: Do families comply with child and adolescent psychopharmacology? Child and Adolescent Psychopharmacology News 6:6–10, 2001

Bryon M: Adherence to treatment in medical conditions, in Adherence to Treatment in Children. Edited by Myers LB, Midence K. Amsterdam, Harwood Academic Publishers, 1998, pp 163–189

Caetano SC, Olvera RL, Hunter K, et al: Association of psychosis with suicidality in pediatric bipolar I, II and bipolar NOS patients. J Affect Disord 91:33–37, 2006

Chen YW, Dilsaver SC: Lifetime rates of suicide attempts among subjects with bipolar and unipolar disorders relative to subjects with other Axis I disorders. Biol Psychiatry 39:896–899, 1996

Coletti DJ, Leigh E, Gallelli KA, et al: Patterns of adherence to treatment in adolescents with bipolar disorder. J Child Adolesc Psychopharmacol 15:913–917, 2005

Copeland ME, Copans S: Recovering From Depression: A Workbook for Teens, Revised Edition. Baltimore, MD, Paul H Brookes Publishing, 2002

Davidson KH, Fristad MA: The Treatment Beliefs Questionnaire (TBQ): an instrument to assess beliefs about children's mood disorders and concomitant treatment needs. Psychol Serv 3:1–15, 2006

DelBello MP, Hanseman D, Adler CM, et al: Twelve-month outcome of adolescents with bipolar disorder following first hospitalization for a manic or mixed episode. Am J Psychiatry 164:582–590, 2007

Fawcett J, Golden B, Rosenfeld N: New Hope for People With Bipolar Disorder. New York, Three Rivers Press, 2000

Fleck DE, Keck PE Jr, Corey KB, et al: Factors associated with medication adherence in African American and white patients with bipolar disorder. J Clin Psychiatry 66:646–652, 2005

Fristad MA, Goldberg-Arnold JS: Raising a Moody Child: How to Cope With Depression and Bipolar Disorder. New York, Guilford, 2004

Fristad MA, Gavazzi SM, Soldano KW: Naming the enemy: learning to differentiate mood disorder "symptoms" from the "self" that experiences them. J Fam Psychother 10:81–88, 1999

Geller B, Tillman R: Hypersexuality in children with mania: differential diagnosis and clinical presentation. Psychiatric Times 11:19–21, 2004

Geller B, Williams M, Zimerman B, et al: Prepubertal and early adolescent bipolarity differentiate from ADHD by manic symptoms, grandiose delusions, ultra-rapid or ultradian cycling. J Affect Disord 51:81–91, 1998

Geller B, Craney JL, Bolhofner K, et al: Two-year prospective follow-up of children with a prepubertal and early adolescent bipolar disorder phenotype. Am J Psychiatry 159:927–933, 2002

Goldstein TR, Birmaher B, Axelson D, et al: History of suicide attempts in pediatric bipolar disorder: factors associated with increased risk. Bipolar Disord 7:525–535, 2005

Goldstein TR, Miklowitz DJ, Mullen KL: Social skills knowledge and performance among adolescents with bipolar disorder. Bipolar Disord 8:350–361, 2006

Guyer AE, McClure EB, Adler AD, et al: Specificity of facial expression labeling deficits in childhood psychopathology. J Child Psychol Psychiatry 48:863–871, 2007

Jamieson PE, Rynn MA: Mind Race: A Firsthand Account of One Teenager's Experience With Bipolar Disorder. New York, Oxford University Press, 2006

Khantzian EJ: The self-medication hypothesis of substance use disorders: a reconsideration and recent applications. Harv Rev Psychiatry 4:231–244, 1997

Kovacs M, Pollock M: Bipolar disorder and comorbid conduct disorder in childhood and adolescence. J Am Acad Child Adolesc Psychiatry 34:715–723, 1995

Kowatch RA, Fristad MA, Birmaher B, et al; Child Psychiatric Workgroup on Bipolar Disorder: Treatment guidelines for children and adolescents with bipolar disorder. J Am Acad Child Adolesc Psychiatry 44:213–235, 2005a

Kowatch RA, Youngstrom EA, Danielyan A, et al: Review and meta-analysis of the phenomenology and clinical characteristics of mania in children and adolescents. Bipolar Disord 7:483–496, 2005b

Masi G, Toni C, Perugi G, et al: Externalizing disorders in consecutively referred children and adolescents with bipolar disorder. Compr Psychiatry 44:184–189, 2003

Miklowitz DJ, Cicchetti D: Toward a life span developmental psychopathology perspective on bipolar disorder. Dev Psychopathol 18:935–938, 2006

Miklowitz DJ, George EL: The Bipolar Teen: What You Can Do to Help Your Child and Your Family. New York, Guilford, 2007

Miklowitz DJ, Simoneau TL, George EL, et al: Family focused treatment of bipolar disorder: 1-year effects of a psychoeducational program in conjunction with pharmacotherapy. Biol Psychiatry 48:582–592, 2000

Miklowitz DJ, George EL, Richards JA, et al: A randomized study of family focused psychoeducation and pharmacotherapy in the outpatient management of bipolar disorder. Arch Gen Psychiatry 60:904–912, 2003

Ostacher MJ, Eidelman P: Suicide in bipolar depression, in Bipolar Depression: A Comprehensive Guide. Edited by El-Mallakh RS, Ghaemi SN. Washington, DC, American Psychiatric Publishing, 2006, pp 117–144

Patel NC, DelBello MP, Keck PE Jr, et al: Ethnic differences in maintenance antipsychotic prescription among adolescents with bipolar disorder. J Child Adolesc Psychopharmacol 15:938–946, 2005

Pavuluri MN, Naylor MW, Sweeney JA: Pediatric bipolar disorder, in Handbook of Adolescent Behavior Problems: Evidence-Based Approaches to Prevention and Treatment. Edited by Gullotta TP, Adams GR. New York, Springer, 2005, pp 185–204

Perry BL, Pescosolido BA, Martin JK, et al: Comparison of public attributions, attitudes, and stigma in regard to depression among children and adults. Psychiatr Serv 58:632–635, 2007

Pescosolido BA: Culture, children, and mental health treatment: special section on the National Stigma Study-Children. Psychiatr Serv 58:611–612, 2007

Pescosolido BA, Perry BL, Martin JK, et al: Stigmatizing attitudes and beliefs about treatment and psychiatric medications for children with mental illness. Psychiatr Serv 58:613–618, 2007

Scheffer RE, Niskala Apps JA: The diagnosis of preschool bipolar disorder presenting with mania: open label pharmacological treatment. J Affect Disord 82 (suppl 1): S25–S34, 2004

Wilens TE, Biederman J, Millstein RB, et al: Risk for substance use disorders in youths with child- and adolescent-onset bipolar disorder. J Am Acad Child Adolesc Psychiatry 38:680–685, 1999

Wilens TE, Biederman J, Kwon A, et al: Risk of substance use disorders in adolescents with bipolar disorder. J Am Acad Child Adolesc Psychiatry 43:1380–1386, 2004

Yen CF, Chen CS, Ko CH, et al: Relationships between insight and medication adherence in outpatients with schizophrenia and bipolar disorder: prospective study. Psychiatry Clin Neurosci 59:403–409, 2005

13

Resources for Clinicians, Parents, and Patients

Mary A. Fristad, Ph.D., A.B.P.P.

Empowering families through sharing resources with them, such as are found in this chapter, will aid them in becoming treatment allies. We recommend that families keep mood charts, particularly when medications are started or modified. The format families use to keep a record of their child's mood (or the child, himself or herself) matters less than the fact that the family is actively attending to and documenting relevant treatment issues—a process that should enhance their ability to recall pertinent information in an accurate manner at clinical appointments. (These issues are discussed in further detail in Chapter 10, "Working With Patients and Their Families.")

This book contains a variety of types of mood charts to share with families. Other resources reviewed here include books for children, adolescents, and parents and adults about bipolar disorder; other relevant parenting and mental health books; educational support information; national organizations and support groups for parents of and children with bipolar disorder; and information on complementary mental health interventions.

Sample Mood Charts

Mood charts can be used by parents and/or youth alone or together as a family project. Examples of mood charts are shown in Figures 10–3 and 10–4 of this manual (see Chapter 10, "Working With Patients and Their Families").

Books for Children

Brandon and the Bipolar Bear: A Story for Children With Bipolar Disorder, by Tracy Anglada, illustrated by Jennifer Taylor and Toby Ferguson, Victoria, BC, Canada, Trafford Publishing, 2004. A colorfully hand illustrated short storybook that tells the story of a young boy at the time he is initially diagnosed with bipolar disorder.

My Bipolar, Roller Coaster, Feelings Book and *My Roller Coaster Feelings Workbook,* by Bryna Hebert, illustrated by Hannah, Jessica, and Matthew Hebert. Murdock, FL, BPChildren, 2001. A short book that tells the story of a young boy diagnosed with bipolar disorder. The objective is to help elementary school–age children learn how to understand their feelings and not be alienated from the world. The workbook helps children better understand bipolar disorder in an interactive format.

The Storm in My Brain, by Child and Adolescent Bipolar Foundation, Wilmette, IL, Child and Adolescent Bipolar Foundation, 2003. An informational booklet that answers basic questions children diagnosed with bipolar disorder and depression may have. The artwork, created by children living with bipolar disorder or depression, corresponds to the given question.

Kid Power Tactics for Dealing With Depression, by Nicholas and Susan Dubuque, King of Prussia, PA, Center for Applied Psychology, 1996. Written by an 11-year-old boy who suffers from depression and his mother to aid other children in understanding what depression is and what you can do about it. The book includes 15 tactics to help control depression and live a normal life.

Matt the Moody Hermit Crab, by Caroline C. McGee, Nashville, TN, McGee & Woods, 2002. A chapter book aimed at children ages 8–12 years that uses a metaphor of a hermit crab withdrawing into his shell to portray the depressive phase of bipolar disorder. The hermit crab also goes through many episodes of aggression and paranoia to portray the manic phase. The book gives a sense of the daily struggles of those with bipolar disorder.

Anger Mountain, by Bryna Hebert, Murdock, FL, BPChildren, 2005.   A short story, illustrated by children, intended to help young children understand and deal with anger. This book was written for any child who has an unusually hard time with anger.

Children's Literature

The Phoenix Dance, by Dia Calhoun, award–winning author, New York, Farrar, Straus & Giroux, 2005.   A novel based on the Grimms' fairy tale about the 12 dancing princesses. The protagonist is diagnosed with a mythical version of bipolar disorder. The book explores what it is like to experience the diagnosis and treatment from an adolescent female's perspective.

Books for Adolescents

When Nothing Matters Anymore: A Survival Guide for Depressed Teens, by Bev Cobain, Minneapolis, MN, Free Spirit Publishing, 1998.   A survival guide divided into two parts—the first focusing on how it feels to be depressed and the second describing the benefits of treatment and staying healthy—for depressed teenagers. The book includes personal stories from teens suffering from depression, survival tips, and other resources one can go to for information, guidance, and support.

Recovering From Depression: A Workbook for Teens, by Mary Ellen Copeland and Stuart Copans, Baltimore, MD, Brookes Publishing, 2002.   An interactive workbook with an objective to help teenagers distinguish if they are depressed, learn what they can do to make themselves feel better, and learn how to make a plan to stay healthy and safe. Also included are four appendices with additional resources.

Conquering the Beast Within: How I Fought Depression and Won...and How You Can, Too, by Cait Irwin, New York, Random House, 1998.   A teenager's story, inspired by her own struggle with depression, that any age can relate to and understand. Through vivid illustrations and expressions, the author describes how depression affects not only the person but also family members and friends, and discusses the necessary steps to recovery.

Mind Race: A Firsthand Account of One Teenager's Experience With Bipolar Disorder, by Patrick E. Jamieson and Moira A. Rynn, New York, Oxford University Press, 2006.   An informative book about bipolar disorder. New information about the disorder is provided as well as a question-and-answer section for recently diagnosed adolescents.

Books for Parents

Raising a Moody Child: How to Cope With Depression and Bipolar Disorder, by Mary A. Fristad and Jill S. Goldberg Arnold, New York, Guilford Press, 2004.   A four-part book that guides parents through the difficult times of their child's bipolar diagnosis in a clear and comprehensive manner. The text provides parents with strategies to identify bipolar disorder in their child, find appropriate treatment, help their child manage and deal with his or her moods, and help the family live with a disorder.

New Hope for Children and Teens With Bipolar Disorder, by Boris Birmaher, New York, Three Rivers Press, 2000.   An informational guide to increase knowledge about bipolar disorder, specifically the genetic basis, psychosocial stress, stigmatization, treatment, and impact of the illness on loved ones.

Bipolar Kids: Helping Your Child Find Calm in the Mood Storm, by Rosalie Greenberg, Cambridge, MA, Da Capo Press, 2007.   An encouraging and compassionate book that addresses many problems families struggle with when their child is diagnosed with bipolar disorder. The author discusses family relationships and education and treatment options, and encourages parents to pay attention and listen to their children to help them through the confusion of mania and depression.

The Ups and Downs of Raising a Bipolar Child: A Survival Guide for Parents, by Judith Lederman and Candida Fink, New York, Simon & Schuster, 2003.   An informational chapter book for parents that gives suggestions and knowledge needed to cope with a child being diagnosed with bipolar disorder as well as advice about related concerns, ranging from schools and camps to legal challenges.

If Your Child Is Bipolar: The Parent-to-Parent Guide to Living With and Loving a Bipolar Child, by Cindy Singer and Sheryl Gurrentz, Los Angeles, CA, Perspective Publishing, 2004 (www.familyhelp.com). Written for parents to provide realistic ways to deal with their emotions when their child has behavioral and mood difficulties that may be a sign of a mental disorder. Personal experiences are shared to help others through the challenging process of raising a child with bipolar disorder.

The Bipolar Child, by Demitri and Janice Papolos, New York, Broadway Books, 2007. A compendium of information about childhood bipolar disorder, including diagnosis, medication, inpatient treatment, psychosocial treatment, and education. The authors explain why many are misdiagnosed and how medications given for the wrong diagnosis can actually worsen the bipolar condition.

Choosing the Right Treatment: What Families Need to Know About Evidence-Based Practices, by National Alliance on Mental Illness, Arlington, VA, National Alliance on Mental Illness, 2007. A guide to enlighten families about evidence-based practices in children's mental health. The guide provides information to make better decisions about treatment and supports.

Intense Minds, by Tracy Anglada, Victoria, BC, Canada, Trafford Publishing, 2006. Personal descriptions of symptoms shared through the words of youth with bipolar disorder and adults diagnosed with the illness in childhood. Poignant descriptions of difficulties at home, at school, and with peers are provided to improve others' understanding of childhood bipolar disorder.

Books for Adults

Out of the Darkened Room: Protecting the Children and Strengthening the Family When a Parent Is Depressed, by William R. Beardslee, Boston, MA, Little, Brown, 2002. A book that outlines symptoms and treatment programs available for depression. A preventive approach is explained to help family members become familiar with depression and reduce its possible secondary damage.

Living Without Depression and Manic Depression, by Mary Ellen Copeland, Oakland, CA, New Harbinger Publications, 1994.   A workbook that includes strategies to help people be in charge of their own lives and arrive at breakthroughs in managing their feelings so their symptoms will not have a profound impact on their lives.

Living Well With Depression and Bipolar Disorder, by John McManamy, New York, HarperCollins, 2006.   An informative book written by a writer with bipolar disorder. He distinguishes the illness from other conditions, provides treatment and coping plans, and explains the consequences of bipolar disorder on close relationships.

An Unquiet Mind, by Kay Redfield Jamison, New York, Alfred A. Knopf, 1995.   An autobiographical account of a prominent researcher of bipolar disorder. This eloquent book discusses stigma, the experience of depression and mania, the critical role of medication, and the therapeutic process.

Thoughts and Feelings: Taking Control of Your Moods and Your Life, by Matthew McKay, Patrick Fannin, and Martha Davis, Oakland, CA, New Harbinger Publications, 1998.   A handbook that uses cognitive-behavioral strategies to guide the reader through replacing negative and irrational feelings to achieve more desirable outcomes.

The Bipolar Survival Guide: What You and Your Family Need to Know, by David J. Miklowitz, New York, Guilford Press, 2002.   A guide to understanding the symptoms, diagnosis, and causes of bipolar disorder. Psychological and medical treatment options are explained as well as self-management techniques to help with mood cycles. This book is designed to improve functioning at home, with loved ones, and at work.

Winter Blues: Seasonal Affective Disorder: What It Is and How to Overcome It, by Norman E. Rosenthal, New York, Guilford Press, 1998.   A book that describes seasonal affective disorder (SAD). A self-test allows the reader to determine whether he or she might have SAD. Various treatment options are explained, including light therapy and antidepressant medication.

Loving Someone With Bipolar Disorder: Understanding and Helping Your Partner, by Julie A. Fast and John Preston, Oakland, CA, New Harbinger Publications, 2004. A book written to help the partner of a person with bipolar disorder conquer the challenges that come with the illness. The authors present supportive and useful information, methods, and real-life examples to create a warm, healthy, and close relationship with a loved one suffering from bipolar disorder.

Books for Parents on Related Topics

General Parenting

How to Talk So Kids Will Listen and Listen So Kids Will Talk, by Adele Faber and Elaine Mazlish, illustrations by Kimberly Ann Coe, New York, Avon Books, 1999. A step-by-step approach to improve relationships through communication. Cartoons, illustrations, and exercises are provided to improve parents' ability to talk and problem-solve with their children.

The Explosive Child: A New Approach for Understanding and Parenting Easily Frustrated, Chronically Inflexible Children, by Ross W. Greene, New York, Harper, 2005. An approach to helping parents lessen hostility between themselves and their child while having parents foresee and prevent situations in which the child is likely to be noncompliant.

The Optimistic Child, by Martin E. P. Seligman, with Karen Reivich, Lisa Jaycox, and Jane Gillham. New York, HarperPerennial, 1996. A book that stresses the importance of optimism in reducing the threat of depression. It outlines how to promote true self-esteem in children by teaching them to articulate their emotions better. Optimism leads to reduced depression and improved health and school performance.

Sibling Issues

Siblings Without Rivalry: How to Help Your Children Live Together So You Can Live Too, by Adele Faber and Elaine Mazlish, New York, Avon Books, 1998. A practical book illustrated with cartoons, challenging the idea that conflict between siblings is inevitable. Through the use of different stories, different ways to teach children how to get along are exemplified.

Turbo Max: A Story For Siblings of Bipolar Children, by Tracy Anglada, Murdock, FL, BPChildren, 2001.   A fictional story centered around one boy's summer diary about a sibling with bipolar disorder. The boy's journey goes from uncertainty to understanding and irritation to acceptance. The story is intended for children ages 8–12 years.

Understanding Psychiatric Disorders

It's Nobody's Fault: New Hope and Help for Difficult Children and Their Parents, by Harold S. Koplewicz, New York, Times Books, 1996.   An informational book that walks parents through the process of helping their child get the appropriate diagnosis and treatment without holding anyone responsible for the illness. Thirteen common disorders are discussed.

Understanding Psychiatric Medications

Straight Talk About Psychiatric Medications for Kids, by Timothy E. Wilens, New York, Guilford Press, 2008.   An educational guide to ensure children receive the correct diagnosis, treatment, and medications for their mental, emotional, or behavioral problems.

Miscellaneous

I Am Not Sick: I Don't Need Help, by Xavier Amador and Anna Lisa Johanson, Peconic, NY, Vida Press, 2000.   A book that guides loved ones through the steps needed to assist a family member to accept and get treatment for his or her psychiatric disorders.

The Thyroid Sourcebook, by M. Sara Rosenthal, Los Angeles, CA, Lowell House, 2000.   A book that guides the reader through conditions that can affect the thyroid and their treatments, including medication and nutrition.

Educational Resources

Information About Bipolar Disorder for Parents, Children, and Educators

www.bpchildren.org
www.schoolbehavior.com
www.bpkids.org
www.josselyn.org/Store.htm

Special Education Advocacy

www.wrightslaw.com

National Association of Therapeutic Schools and Programs

www.natsap.org

Internet Special Education Resources

www.iser.com/index.shtml

Governmental Supplemental Security Income

www.ssa.gov/notices/supplemental-security-income

National Organizations and Support Groups

National Alliance on Mental Illness

(800) 950-6264, www.nami.org

Mental Health America

(703) 684-7722, www.nmha.org

Depression and Bipolar Support Alliance

(800) 826-3632, www.dbsalliance.org

Child and Adolescent Bipolar Foundation

www.bpkids.org

Juvenile Bipolar Research Foundation

www.bpchildresearch.org

BPChildren

www.bpchildren.org

Side Effect Management

Bedwetting

General Information

(800) 214-9605, www.bedwettingstore.com

DRI Sleeper

(877) 331-2768, www.dri-sleeper.com

Weight Management

Information about children's mental and physical health via separate areas for children, adolescents, and parents, www.kidshealth.org

Complementary Treatment Information

Light Therapy

Full Spectrum Solutions

www.fullspectrumsolutions.com

The Sunbox Company

www.sunbox.com

Nutritional Intervention

EMPowerplus

(888) 878–3467, www.truehope.com

Eatwild

www.eatwild.com
Provides nutritional information about food sources.

OmegaBrite

(800) 383-2030, www.omegabrite.com

14

Conclusion and Future Directions

Robert A. Kowatch, M.D., Ph.D.

> Ask not what disease the person has, but rather what person the disease has.
>
> Attributed to William Osler

Since 2000 there have been many developments in the field of pediatric bipolar disorder. There are now two new, separate sets of treatment guidelines (Kowatch et al. 2005a; McClellan et al. 2007); data from eight large, well-controlled clinical trials; several longitudinal studies (Birmaher et al. 2006; Geller et al. 2004); neurobiological studies (Ferreira et al. 2008; Pavuluri and Passarotti 2008); and studies that document the effectiveness of family and cognitive behavioral therapy. We have moved beyond "Does bipolar disorder really exist in children and adolescents?" to "How can we best predict, diagnose, and treat this serious biologic disorder?"

Although discussion about the diagnosis of pediatric bipolar disorder has been extremely contentious in the past, a recent meta-analysis indicates emerging consensus about the clinical characteristics and phenomenology of these patients. Kowatch et al. (2005b) recently published a review and meta-analysis of the phenomenology and clinical characteristics of mania in children and adolescents. Research reports were selected that met the following criteria: a systematic method for the elicitation and reporting of symptoms and clinical characteristics of subjects; interviewing of subjects by a trained researcher or clinician; ages 5–18 years; use of a diagnostic system, use of either DSM criteria or Research Diagnostic Criteria for categorization; and a consensus method for the establishment of the diagnosis of bipolar disorder. Seven studies were found that satisfied the inclusion criteria for the meta-analysis, describing a total of 362 youths over a period spanning the last 23 years. The clinical picture that emerged was that of children or adolescents with periods of increased energy (mania or hypomania), accompanied by distractibility, pressured speech, irritability, grandiosity, racing thoughts, decreased need for sleep, and euphoria/elation. Once the effects of methodological differences are taken into account, there appears to be consistency in the description of pediatric bipolar disorder over the last 25 years in terms of symptom presentation, associated clinical features, and patterns of comorbidity. Thus, when the data are examined, there is more consensus and homogeneity about the diagnostic characteristics of pediatric bipolar disorder than the past polemics might suggest.

We have seen increasing numbers of new, very solid, and exciting young researchers enter the field of pediatric bipolar disorder. They include Dr. Melissa DelBello at the University of Cincinnati, Dr. Kiki Chang at Stanford University, Dr. David Axelson at the University of Pittsburgh, Dr. Mani Pavuluri at the University of Illinois at Chicago, Dr. Eric Youngstrom at the University of North Carolina, Dr. Rene Olvera at the University of Texas at San Antonio, and a host of other young talented researchers.

The challenges to the field include the development and testing of single medications and combinations of medications that are effective for all phases of this illness without exacerbating the manic or depressed phases of this disorder; the development of pharmacogenetic tests for the prediction of treatment response; the identification and development of genomic, proteomic, and metabolomic biological markers for diagnosis and subtyping; neuroimaging studies that are diagnostic; the development of specific cognitive and behavioral therapies that are effective for these disorders and that augment pharmacotherapy; and exploration of the basic neurobiology of this disorder to find a cure. The inherent nature of pediatric bipolar disorder is one of rapidly changing mood states affected by development, the environment, and the context in which the behaviors occur. It is also important to recognize that in many children with mood behavior problems, the phenomena of the disorder are often developing and will show themselves in time. Many children who initially do not meet the full criteria for bipolar I disorder or bipolar II disorder will develop the full illness as they mature. Birmaher and Axelson (2006; Birmaher et al. 2006) found that in a sample of 263 children and adolescents with bipolar spectrum disorder followed longitudinally for 2 years, 20% of subjects with bipolar II disorder converted to bipolar I disorder and 25% of the subjects with bipolar disorder not otherwise specified (NOS) converted to bipolar I disorder. This is the first longitudinal study of pediatric subjects with bipolar spectrum disorders and is very important because many pediatric patients first present with "bipolar spectrum" symptoms or what is referred to in DSM-IV and DSM-IV-TR as bipolar disorder NOS. It is hoped that DSM-V will take these developmental differences into consideration and offer diagnostic criteria that are developmentally sensitive. Bipolar disorder is a serious and oftentimes life-threatening disorder in children and adolescents, and we owe it to our patients and their families to accurately diagnose and effectively treat this disorder.

References

Birmaher B, Axelson D: Course and outcome of bipolar spectrum disorder in children and adolescents: a review of the existing literature. Dev Psychopathol 18:1023–1035, 2006

Birmaher B, Axelson D, Strober M, et al: Clinical course of children and adolescents with bipolar spectrum disorders. Arch Gen Psychiatry 63:175–183, 2006

Ferreira MA, O'Donovan MC, Meng YA, et al: Collaborative genome-wide association analysis supports a role for ANK3 and CACNA1C in bipolar disorder. Nat Genet Aug 17, 2008 (Epub ahead or print)

Geller B, Tillman R, Craney JL, et al: Four-year prospective outcome and natural history of mania in children with a prepubertal and early adolescent bipolar disorder phenotype. Arch Gen Psychiatry 61:459–467, 2004

Kowatch RA, Fristad MA, Birmaher B, et al: Treatment guidelines for children and adolescents with bipolar disorder. J Am Acad Child Adolesc Psychiatry 44:213–235, 2005a

Kowatch RA, Youngstrom EA, Danielyan A, et al: Review and meta-analysis of the phenomenology and clinical characteristics of mania in children and adolescents. Bipolar Disord 7:483–496, 2005b

McClellan J, Kowatch RA, Findling RL: Practice parameter for the assessment and treatment of children and adolescents with bipolar disorder. J Am Acad Child Adolesc Psychiatry 46:107–125, 2007

Pavuluri MN, Passarotti A: Neural bases of emotional processing in pediatric bipolar disorder. Expert Rev Neurother 8:1381–1387, 2008

K-SADS Mania Rating Scale

This scale was developed by David Axelson, M.D., and Boris Birmaher, M.D. at the University of Pittsburgh.

This rating scale is based on the items from the fourth revision of the K-SADS-P (Joaquim Puig-Antich, M.D., and Neal Ryan, M.D.) and some additional descriptors from the WASH-U-KSADS (Barbara Geller, M.D.). The following items are to determine the severity of manic or hypomanic symptoms during a period of time prescribed by the rater/study (usually a 1-week period). At the end of the scale, the rater should note the onset and offset of the time period being rated. If any of the items are judged present, inquire in a general way to determine how s/he was behaving at the time with such questions as, "When you were this way, what kind of things were you doing? How did you spend your time?" If there have been manic periods it is exceedingly important that they are clearly delineated.

If the subject has only described dysphoric mood, the following questions regarding the manic syndrome should be introduced with a statement such as, "I know you have been feeling (___), however, many people have other feelings mixed in or at different times too." The most difficult patients to assess are those in whom manic and depressed symptoms simultaneously coexist, superimposed on each other during the same times (Mixed States). The rater should keep this possibility in mind as s/he goes through this section.

This is a semistructured scale, so the rater is to use his or her judgment about how many of the suggested questions will be asked for each symptom. The rater should also make additional inquiries or clarifications as indicated.

The ratings are based on all available information about the time period rated (parent and child interview, records or other reports if available). The rater is to use his or her best clinical judgment and take into account the available information about the frequency, intensity, duration, and impairment of each symptom in order to formulate a summary rating for each item.

K-SADS Mania Rating Scale

1. Elation, expansive mood

Elevated mood and/or optimistic attitude toward the future which lasted at least 4 hours and was out of proportion to the circumstances. Differentiate from normal mood in chronically depressed subjects. Do not rate positive if mild elation is reported in situations like Christmas gifts, birthdays, amusement parks, which normally overstimulate and make children very excited.

Have (there been times when) you felt very good or too cheerful or high or terrific or great, or just not your normal self?

If unclear:

When you felt on top of the world or as if there was nothing you couldn't do? ...That this is the best of all possible worlds? Have you felt that everything would work out just the way you wanted? If people saw you, would they think you were just in a good mood or something more than that? Did you get as if you were drunk? Did you laugh a lot, get silly? Did you feel super happy? When did this happen?
(example)

0 No Information

1 Not at all, normal, or depressed

2 Slight: Good spirits, more cheerful than most people in his/her circumstances, but of only possible clinical significance.

3 Mild: Definitely elevated mood and optimistic outlook that is somewhat out of proportion to his/her circumstances.

4 Moderate: Mood and outlook are clearly out of proportion to circumstances. Noticeable to others.

5 Severe: Quality of euphoric mood way out of proportion to circumstances.

6 Extreme: Clearly elated, almost constantly exalted expression, overexpansive.

K-SADS Mania Rating Scale (continued)

2. Irritability and anger

Subjective feeling of irritability, anger, crankiness, bad temper, short tempered, resentment, or annoyance, externally directed, whether expressed overtly or not. Rate the intensity and duration of such feelings. Do not rate here if irritability is due to depression or disruptive disorders.

Do you get annoyed and irritated or cranky at little things? What kinds of things?

Have you been feeling mad or angry also (even if you don't show it)? How angry? More than before?

What kinds of things make you feel angry?

Do you sometimes feel angry and/or irritable, and/or cranky and don't know why? Does this happen often?

Do you lose your temper?

With your family? Your friends? Who else? At school? What do you do? Has anybody said anything about it?

How much of the time do you feel angry, irritable, and/or cranky: All of the time? Lots of the time? Just now and then? None of the time?

When you get mad, what do you think about?

Do you think about killing others? Or about hurting them or torturing them?

Whom: Do you have a plan? How?

0　No Information

1　Not at all, clearly of no clinical significance

2　Slight and doubtful clinical significance.

3　Mild: Often (at least 3X3 hrs. ea. week) feels definitely more angry, irritable than called for by the situation. relatively frequent but never very intense. Or often argumentative. quick to express annoyance. No homicidal thoughts.

4　Moderate: Most days irritable/angry or over 50% of awake time. Often shouts, loses temper. Occasional homicidal thoughts.

5　Severe: At least most of the time child is aware of feeling very irritable or quite angry or has frequent homicidal thoughts (no plan) or thoughts of hurting others. Or throws and breaks things around the house.

6　Extreme: Most of the time feels extremely angry or irritable, to the point s/he "can't stand it." Or frequent uncontrollable tantrums.

K-SADS Mania Rating Scale (continued)

3. Decreased need for sleep

Less need for sleep than usual in order to feel rested (average for several days when needed less sleep). (Refer to norms on insomnia)

Have you needed less sleep than usual to feel rested?
How much sleep do you ordinarily need?
How much do you sleep when you are feeling so good?
When you wake up do you feel good and rested?

When you cannot fall asleep or when you get up through the night, what types of things do you do?
Watch TV? Read? or do you do active things? (e.g., rearrange furniture? clean house? exercise?)

Do you have a lot of thoughts go through your mind when awake? What kinds of thoughts?

Do you worry? About what types of things?
How long are you awake? How often during the night? During the week?

0   No information
1   No change or more sleep needed
2   Up to 1 hour less than usual
3   Up to 2 hours less than usual
4   Up to 3 hours less than usual
5   Up to 4 hours less than usual
6   4 or more hours less than usual

K-SADS Mania Rating Scale (continued)

4. Unusually energetic

More active than his/her usual level without expected fatigue.

Have you had more energy than usual to do things?
Did people tell you that you were (are) non-stop?
Did it seem like too much energy? Do you know why? Were you doing too many things? Did you feel tired?
When did this happen? (example)

0   No information
1   No difference than usual or less energetic
2   Slightly more energetic but of questionable significance
3   Little change in activity level but less fatigued than usual
4   Somewhat more active than usual with little or no fatigue
5   Much more active than usual with little or no fatigue
6   Unusually active all day long with little or no fatigue

5a. Increase in goal-directed activity

As compared with usual level. Consider changes in scholastic, social, sexual, or leisure involvement or activity level associated with work, family, friends, new projects, interests, or activities (e.g., telephone calls, letter writing)

Is there any time when you were more active or involved in things compared to the way you usually are? What about in school, at your club, scouts, church, at home, friends, hobbies, new projects or interests?
Were you doing a lot of things?
How much of your day has been spent in this?
Were you trying to do so many different things that you couldn't keep up?
When did this happen? (example)

0   No information
1   No change or decrease
2   Slightly more interest or activity but of questionable significance
3   Mild but definite increase in general activity level involving several areas
4   Moderate generalized increase in activity level involving several areas
5   Marked increase and almost constantly involved in numerous activities in many areas
6   Extreme, e.g., constantly active in a variety of activities from awakening until going to sleep

K-SADS Mania Rating Scale (continued)

5b. Motor hyperactivity

Visible manifestations of generalized motor hyperactivity which occurred during a period of abnormally elevated, expansive, or irritable mood. Make certain that the hyperactivity actually occurred and was not merely a subjective feeling of restlessness. Make sure it is not chronic but episodic hyperactivity.

When you were (___), were there times when you were (high, feeling so good, so angry) that you were always moving, could not stay put, were unable to sit still or you always had to be moving, pacing up and down? Or are you always like that?

0 No information

1 Not at all or retarded

2 Slight increases which is of doubtful clinical significance

3 Mild: Unable to sit quietly in a chair

4 Moderate: Paces about a great deal

5 Marked: Almost constantly moving and pacing about

6 Extreme: so hyperactive that s/he would exhaust her/himself if not restrained

6. Grandiosity

Increased self-esteem and appraisal of his/her worth, power, or knowledge (up to grandiose delusions) as compared with usual level. Persecutory delusions should not be considered evidence of grandiosity unless that subject feels the persecution is due to some special attributes of his/her (e.g., power, knowledge).

Have you felt more self-confident than usual? Have you felt much better than others? ...smarter? ...stronger? Why?

Have you felt that you are a particularly important person or that you had special talents or abilities?

What about special plans?

When did this happen? (example)

0 No information

1 Not at all or decreased self esteem

2 Slight: somewhat more confident about himself but of doubtful clinical significance

3 Mild: Definitely overestimates or exaggerates at least two of his talents, prospects or plans

4 Moderate: Disproportionately inflated self-esteem involving several areas of functioning

5 Severe: Marked, global, overevaluation of her/himself and her/his abilities, but falls short of true delusions

6 Extreme: Clear grandiose delusions

K-SADS Mania Rating Scale (continued)

7. Accelerated, pressured, or increased amount of speech

When you were (___), were there times that you talked very rapidly or talked on and on and couldn't be stopped? Did people say you were talking too much? Could people understand you?

0   No information

1   Not at all of retarded speech

2   Slight increase which is doubtful clinical significance

3   Mild: Noticeably more verbose than normal but conversation is not strained

4   Moderate: So verbose that conversation is strained

5   Marked: So rapid that conversation is difficult to maintain

6   Extreme: Talks rapidly or continuously and cannot be interrupted. Conversation extremely difficult or impossible

8a. Racing thoughts

Subjective experience that thinking was markedly accelerated.

When you were (___), were there times when your thoughts raced through your mind? Did you have more ideas than usual or more than you could handle?

0   No information

1   Not at all

2   Doubtful

3   Mild: Occasional racing thoughts at least 3 times per week

4   Moderate: Racing thoughts at least 50% of awake time

5   Severe: Racing thoughts most of the time

6   Extreme: Almost constant racing thoughts

K-SADS Mania Rating Scale (continued)

8b. Flight of ideas (observed or reported by informant)

Accelerated speech with abrupt changes from topic to topic, usually based on understandable associations, distracting stimuli or play on words. In rating severity consider speed of associations, inability to complete ideas and sustain attention in a goal-directed manner. When severe, complete or partial sentences may be galloping on each other so fast that apparent sentence to sentence derailment and/or sentence incoherence may also be present. An extreme example of this symptom is "You have to be quiet to be sad. Everything having to do with 's' is quiet-on the q.t., -sit, sob, sigh, sin, sorrow, surcease, sought, sand, sweet mother's love and salvation."

Have there been times when people could not understand you? When they said you did not make sense? Could you give me an example?

0   No information

1   Not at all or some other form of

2   Slight: Occasional instances, which are of doubtful clinical significance

3   Mild: Occasional instances of abrupt change in topics with some impairment in understandability. >5% of sentence to sentence transitions are abrupt

4   Moderate: Frequent instances with moderate impairment in understandability. >10%

5   Severe: Very frequent instances with definite impairment in understandability. >25%

6   Extreme: Most of speech consists of such rapid changes of topic that is impossible to follow. >50%

K-SADS Mania Rating Scale (continued)

9. Poor judgment

Excessive involvement in dangerous activities without recognizing the high potential for painful consequences.

When you were (___), did you do anything that caused trouble for you or your family...or friends? What about anything that could have? Did you do things you normally wouldn't do (like giving away a whole lot of things or taking a whole lot of chances)? Did you think of what would happen before you did it? Was there anything that you did that you now think you should not have done?

0   No information

1   Not at all

2   Slight: Of doubtful clinical significance

3   Mild: e.g., Calls friends at odd hours

4   Moderate: e.g., Purchases many things she/he doesn't need and can't afford or gives money away

5   Severe: e.g., On impulse, goes to places without plans or money and takes too many chances

6   Very Severe: Attempts activities with potentially very dangerous consequences

10. Distractibility (observed or reported by informant)

Child presents evidence of difficulty focusing his/her attention on the questions of the interviewer, jumps from one thing to another, cannot keep track of his/her answers, and is drawn by irrelevant stimuli he cannot shut off. Not to be confused with avoidance of uncomfortable themes.

Have you ever been told that you have trouble sticking to what you are supposed to do? did you? Can you give me an example? Has a teacher told you that you "always" get distracted?

0   No information

1   Not at all

2   Slight: Of doubtful clinical significance

3   Mild: Present but responds to structuring and repetition

4   Moderate: Difficult to complete interview because of child's inattentiveness which doesn't respond to structure

5   Severe: Impossible to complete interview because of child's inattentiveness

K-SADS Mania Rating Scale (*continued*)

11. Hallucinations

Sometimes children, when they are alone, hear voices or see things, or smell things and they don't quite know where they come from.

Has this happened to you?
Do you ever hear voices when you are alone?
Have you ever seen things that were not there?
When did you?
What did you see?
What did you hear?
Has there been anything unusual about the way things sounded?
How often have you heard these voices (noises)? (smell, feeling, visions) Is it some of the time, only now and then, most of the time, or all of the time?
What do you think it is?
Do you think it is your imagination or real?
Did you think it was real when you (heard, saw, etc.) it?
Do you think it's real or your imagination now?
What did you do when you (heard, saw, etc.) it?

0   No information or N/A

1   Not at all—Absent

2   Suspected/Possible

3   Mild: Definitely present but subject is generally aware it is his imagination and usually able to ignore it. Occurs no more than once per week.

4   Moderate: Generally believes in the reality of the hallucinations, but it has little influence on his behavior. (Or) Occurs at least once per week.

5   Severe: Convinced his hallucination is real and significantly effects his actions. i.e.: locks door to keep pursuers away. (or) Occurs frequently.

6   Extreme: Actions based on hallucinations have major impact on him or others: Unable to do school work because of constant "conversations." (or) Occurs most of the time.

K-SADS Mania Rating Scale (continued)

12. Delusions

Do you know what imagination is? Tell me.

Sometimes does your imagination play tricks on you? What kind of tricks? Tell me more about them.

Do you have any ideas about things that you don't tell anyone because they might not understand? What are they?

Do you have any secret thoughts? Tell me about them.

Do you believe in other things that other people don't believe in? Like what? Is anybody out to hurt you?

Does anybody control your mind or body (like a robot)?

Is anything happening to your body?

Do you ever feel the world is coming to an end?

Do you ever think you are an important or great person? Who?

Are you sure that this (....?) is this way?

Could there be any other reason for it?

Who do you know that it happens as you say?

Any other possible explanation?

Do you enjoy making up stories like this?

Or is it different from making up stories?

(you might suggest other possible explanations and see how the subject reacts to them)

Did you ever think that this was your imagination?

Do you think it could be your imagination?

What did you do about . . . ?

0   No information

1   Definitely not delusional

2   Suspected

3   Mild: Delusion definitely present but at times subject questions his false belief.

4   Moderate: Generally has conviction in his false belief.

5   Severe: Delusion has a significant effect on his actions, e.g., often asks family to forgive his sins, preoccupied with belief that he is a new Messiah.

6   Extreme: Actions based on delusions have major impact on him or others, e.g., stops eating because believes food is poisoned

K-SADS Mania Rating Scale (continued)

13. Mood lability

Changability of mood; rapid mood variation with several mood states (angry, elated, depressed, anxious, relaxed) within a brief period of time; appears internally driven without regard to circumstances or not related to anything external to the patient. Could be an exaggerated mood change in regard to minor slights, frustrations or positive events.

Number of days during rating period with 4 hours of manic symptoms: _____

Percentage of rated time period that subject had manic symptoms: _____ %

0 No information

1 Not at all

2 Slight: Some moodiness or mood variation possibly out of proportion to circumstances, but of doubtful significance

3 Mild: Definite mood changes, internally driven or somewhat out of proportion to circumstances, occurring several times per day. Noticeable by others, but does not cause significant impairment in functioning or relationships

4 Moderate: Many mood changes throughout the day, can vary from elevated mood to anger to sadness within a couple of hours; changes in mood clearly out of proportion to circumstances and causes impairment in functioning

5 Severe: Rapid mood swings nearly all of the time, with mood intensity way out of proportion to circumstances

6 Extreme: Constant, explosive variability in mood, several mood changes occurring within minutes, difficult to identify a particular mood; changes in mood radically out of proportion to circumstances.

Scoring:

Take maximum of 5a and 5b
to determine score of Item 5

Take maximum of 8a and 8b
to determine score of Item 8

Add scores of the 13 items

Subtract 13 from total to zero the scale

Total score is 0–64

General Guidelines for Correlation of MRS scores to CGI-BP Mania Severity Scores:

No or minimal – MRS ≤ 11

Mild: MRS ~ 12–17

Moderate: MRS ~ 18–25

Marked or Worse: MRS ≥ 26

Index

*Page numbers printed in **boldface** type refer to tables or figures.*